Gerontological Social Work in Action

Gerontological Social Work in Action introduces "anti-oppression gerontology" (AOG), a critical approach to social work with older adults, their families, and communities. AOG principles are applied to direct and indirect practice and a range of topics of relevance to social work practice in the context of a rapidly aging and increasingly diverse world.

Weaving together stories from diverse older adults, theories, research, and practical tools, this unique textbook prompts social workers to think differently and push back against oppressive forces. It pays attention to issues, realities, and contexts that are largely absent in social work education and gerontological practice, including important developments in our understanding of age/ism; theories of aging and social work; sites and sectors of health and social care; managing risk and frailty; moral, ethical and legal questions about aging including medical assistance in dying; caregiving; dementia and citizenship; trauma; and much more.

This textbook should be considered essential reading for social work students new to or seeking to specialize in aging, as well as those interested in the application of anti-oppressive principles to working with older adults and researching later life.

Wendy Hulko is an associate professor in the School of Social Work and Human Service at Thompson Rivers University. She conducts interdisciplinary research on aging and health with equity-seeking groups, including Secwepemc Elders, racialized older adults, and rural residents. Wendy is co-editor of *Indigenous Peoples and Dementia: New Understandings of Memory Loss and Memory Care*, published by UBC Press in 2019.

Shari Brotman is an associate professor at the McGill School of Social Work. Her research explores issues of access and equity in the design and delivery of health and social care services to older adults, their families, and communities (racialized, immigrant, and LGBTQ communities). Shari is a member of the Centre for Research and Expertise in Social Gerontology (CREGES).

Louise Stern is the Chair of Social Work at Vancouver Island University. She was a practicing social worker for over 20 years in the field of gerontological social work. Her current research and teaching interests are focussed on trauma and aging, food security issues and older adults, and gerontological curriculum development.

Ilyan Ferrer is an assistant professor in the University of Calgary's Faculty of Social Work. His research focusses on aging, immigration/migration, and caring labour of racialized communities in Canada. Ilyan also works with qualitative and oral history methodologies and anti-oppressive social work theory and practice.

Gerontological Social Work in Action

Anti-Oppressive Practice with Older Adults, their Families, and Communities

Wendy Hulko, Shari Brotman, Louise Stern, and Ilyan Ferrer

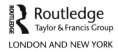
Routledge
Taylor & Francis Group

LONDON AND NEW YORK

First published 2020
by Routledge
2 Park Square, Milton Park, Abingdon, Oxon OX14 4RN

and by Routledge
52 Vanderbilt Avenue, New York, NY 10017

Routledge is an imprint of the Taylor & Francis Group, an informa business

© 2020 Wendy Hulko, Shari Brotman, Louise Stern, and Ilyan Ferrer

British Library Cataloguing-in-Publication Data
A catalogue record for this book is available from the British Library

Library of Congress Cataloging-in-Publication Data
A catalog record has been requested for this book

ISBN: 978-1-138-63330-8 (hbk)
ISBN: 978-1-138-63331-5 (pbk)
ISBN: 978-1-315-20773-5 (ebk)

Typeset in Bembo
by Integra Software Services Pvt. Ltd.

We dedicate this book to all of our parents who have inspired and supported us throughout our lives:

Sandy and Alan Hulko
Lila and Nathan Brotman
Dennis Stern
Annette Stern
Chito Javier and Avelino Ferrer

Contents

Tables and figures

Tables

Figures

Preface

This book represents a journey of several decades. Although together as a team we only started putting pen to paper (or fingers to keyboard) a few years ago, individually and collectively it has been a dream of ours to write anti-oppressive perspectives into social gerontology for many, many years. For example, the eight principles for anti-oppression gerontology (AOG) that underpin this book began life as five principles created by Wendy and Shari for a presentation on *The integration of anti-oppressive perspectives in gerontological social work* at the 2002 Canadian Association for Social Work Education (CASWE) conference. Ilyan, who started collaborating with Shari in 2009 on immigration and aging, joined our AOG team in 2016 to co-author a chapter on ageism and older adults for Baines (2017) in which we published a revised version of these five principles. With the addition of Louise, with whom Wendy began collaborating in 2008 on critical dementia studies, we updated our AOG principles, including adding three, and this 2.0 version appears in the introduction and the concluding thoughts.

This book has been a collective endeavour from start to finish; although there was a lead author for each of the 15 chapters, each of us contributed to every chapter, and we are all immensely pleased with the result. It is through this recent collaboration and exchange that we have found the synergy and opportunity to write together about the things that have sustained and challenged us, both personally and professionally, in our encounters with older people, their families, and communities. We speak from our unique positions as individuals, members of families, members of communities, and, most importantly, social work service providers and scholars. As you read the book, we hope that you will enter into a dialogue with us, the writers, and with others with whom you come into contact, including colleagues, students, organizations, institutions, and your own families. The book is premised on sharing stories, stories that reflect both current contexts and a re-visioning of possibilities in doing social work with older people across various sites and sectors, regions, and contexts that represent the diverse and dynamic realities present across Canada. When you read these stories, you will get to know us as a team, and our intent is to situate a form of praxis [reflection and action] that can facilitate your process of storytelling, engagement, and critique with our work and your own. No doubt, you will find the answers to some of your questions and concerns in these pages, but you will also identify gaps and challenges that leave your questions and concerns unanswered. This is the nature of any journey, but particularly one embedded in critical reflection. We hope that this book begins a dialogue that foregrounds critical concepts such as voice, power, recognition, discourse, equity, and social justice and facilitates the process of questioning taken-for-granted assumptions in the design and delivery of health and social care services for older adults as they are currently articulated. To this end, the book provides the reader with questions for consideration at the start of each chapter and exercises at the end through which you can flex your anti-oppressive practice muscles in the context of social gerontology.

Although we are now all scholars working in university contexts across Canada, we have not forgotten our professional social work roots in putting this book together. In fact, this book is predominantly about practice, how it is shaped, configured, constrained, and prioritized. While we met each other in university contexts (as students and/or professors), we found immediate connection through our links to practice and our penultimate interest in infusing anti-oppressive principles into a field in which there is little recognition of the way oppression shapes service delivery models and the power (or lack thereof) afforded to older people – and often the social workers working with them. We come at this critical reflection from different vantage points and social locations (positions of oppression and privilege), which is reflected in our varying perspectives and has resulted in some interesting and challenging discussions at times about the nature of social problems and potential resolutions. To best keep room for agreement and dissent in the current book, we have relied significantly on case studies and counter-stories as a means of enacting diversity and difference and reflecting the unique configurations of individual identity, both for ourselves and in the context of institutional and historical oppression. While we do not identify who wrote which story or chapter, except for a few personal ones, we hope that you will read our identities into the book as a whole. We agree, and what inspires us without any doubt, that social gerontology and gerontological social work practice to date have done little to incorporate anti-oppressive perspectives or to provide a working framework for social workers to consider within their own practice. In our view, this is unacceptable. We hope that this book begins a journey of dialogue, reflection, and collaboration, not only amongst ourselves, but with you the reader and with the fields of anti-oppressive practice, social gerontology, and social work practice and scholarship more generally.

Acknowledgements

First, we would like to thank our funders who supported the research featured in this book and/or the completion of the book itself, including Thompson Rivers University, Michael Smith Foundation for Health Research, Interior Health, the Social Sciences and Humanities Research Council of Canada, the Canadian Institutes for Health Research, the Centre for Research and Expertise on Social Gerontology (CREGÉS), and the Equipe VIES (Viellissements, exclusion sociales et solidarités).

We would also like to thank our respective universities (Thompson Rivers University, McGill University, Vancouver Island University, and University of Calgary), our colleagues (past and present), and our families (near and far) for their support of this passion project of ours, particularly during the final/most intense phase. Thank you to Donna Baines for kick-starting this process by including us as contributors to the third edition of her AOP social work textbook and to Routledge Press for turning our dream of writing a book on AOG social work into a reality.

Several social work students and alumni assisted with the book completion as research assistants, including Zoe Silverberg and Nauveen Dubash (McGill) who worked on the references for the book (Zoe) and chapters in Part 2 (Nauveen); Rob Long (TRU) who prepared the tables in Chapter 5 and the index for the book; Caitlin Orteza (TRU) who searched for and summarized the literature in Part 1; Katrina Kusari (U of C) who did a literature and policy scan for Chapter 12; and Kristiana Cruz (U of C) who made the graphic designs of all the figures in this book. We extend our appreciation to all the collaborators and accomplices with whom we have had dynamic, inspiring, and at times challenging discussions about anti-oppression gerontology (AOG) and/or anti-oppressive practice (AOP) in social work. A special thank you goes to Amanda Grenier and Sharon Koehn for previous collaborations that contributed to the development of the intersectional life course as theory and method featured in this book.

Our gratitude goes to Danielle Wilson for reviewing most of the Indigenous stories and content for accuracy and cultural appropriateness; other colleagues who reviewed particular chapters, including Pam Orzeck; and all those who shared their reflections on particular stories (John Kinloch, Wanda Gabriel, Genny Gray). We especially thank Danielle Wilson and Paulo Roberto Fumaneri for sharing their inspiring reflections on the important role of social workers (Danielle) and doing anti-oppressive practice (Paulo), which appear in our concluding thoughts.

We are grateful to Georgia Priestley and the other editorial staff at Routledge Press, who were responsive and enthusiastic throughout this process. Any errors or omissions are our own, however.

Finally, and most importantly, we extend a heartfelt thank you to all of the older adults with whom we have worked over the past 15 to 30 years for sharing their everyday lives and realities with us, teaching us about resilience and resistance as a means of both surviving and pushing back against oppression, and helping us revision gerontological social work.

Introduction

Social work as a profession has evolved from one focussed on either individual treatment or social reform (Carniol, 1984; Haynes, 1998) to one that attends to both personal troubles and public issues (Mills, 1959) in a collective pursuit of social justice (Kennedy-Kish (Bell), Sinclair, Carniol, & Baines, 2017). Anti-oppressive practice (AOP) is part of this critical tradition and seeks to eliminate oppression at the structural level and oppressive practices in our daily interactions as social workers while promoting equity, diversity, and inclusion[1] (Baines, 2017; Dumbrill & Yee, 2019; Mullaly & West, 2018; Whebi & Parada, 2017). One of the core skills of an AOP social worker is critical self-awareness or reflexivity. We cannot begin to address the oppression faced by the service users and service providers with whom we work without being aware of our own fluid, contextual, and temporal relationships to the dynamics of privilege and oppression (i.e., our social location - see textbox 0.1 below) (Hulko, 2009).

Textbox 0.1

Social location refers to our position in society based on the social groups to which we belong and the extent to which these groups are subject to oppression and/or afforded privilege – historically and contemporaneously. Various tools can be used to depict one's relationship to the margin (oppression) and the centre (privilege) (i.e., one's social location). This requires critical self-reflection on our multiple (intersecting) identities, specifically those associated with categories of difference like race, class, gender, and age, and the corresponding (interlocking) systems of oppression (e.g., racism, classism, sexism, and ageism).

In addition to appreciating the impact of social location, AOP social work involves (critical) consciousness-raising with individuals and groups about ageism and other forms of oppression, as well as advocacy for systemic changes like the application of *gender-based analysis plus* (GBA+) and/or an *equity, diversity, and inclusion* (EDI) lens in policy work. Multiple forms of oppression have been accounted for in the broader research and writing situated within an AOP framework, including sexism, racism, classism, homophobia/heterosexism, transphobia/cissexism, able-ism, and their intersections.

> **Textbox 0.2**
>
> **Ageism** is discrimination directed towards older adults on the basis of their chronological age or the perception that they are "elderly" and therefore frail and/or incompetent.

Unfortunately, ageism as a form of oppression and as defined in textbox 0.2, has been largely neglected by AOP social work scholars and practitioners, and gerontological social work has failed to incorporate AOP perspectives (Hulko, Brotman, & Ferrer, 2017). For example, aging is addressed just once – in the context of ableism devaluing all human life (p. 54) – and the descriptor "elderly" is used in relation to older adults in Dumbrill and Yee's (2019) otherwise welcome addition to the AOP social work literature. Laura Funk's (2016) critical gerontology text addresses ageism in depth, has substantial content on inequalities in later life, and is a great resource for social work students interested in aging; however, it does not incorporate key AOP terms like oppression and privilege (see textbox 0.3) or provide guidance for practice as it is aimed at sociology students. Thus, there is a gap to be filled, and that is what we have attempted to do with this book. We provide practical guidance for social work students interested in working with older adults and their families and communities, as well as those in aging studies seeking AOP content.

> **Textbox 0.3**
>
> **Oppression and privilege** are concepts that are often paired together to reference the workings of power. **Oppression** evokes a state of being pressed down upon (without power), while **privilege** indicates freedom from societal constraints (with excess power), including the ability to impose penalties on oppressed groups.

The Canadian Association of Social Work (CASW) (2017) estimates there were 50,000 social workers practicing in Canada in 2016; however, the number of people actually doing social work is likely double this figure if social service workers, child and youth care workers, and others are counted (Dumbrill & Yee, 2019, p. 344). These others could include gerontological social workers with titles like care coordinator, case manager, discharge planner, or project coordinator, for example. The Canadian Institutes for Health Information (CIHI) (2017) names social work in the 30 health professions for which it collects data and determined there to be slightly more social workers (52,000) across Canada than the CASW estimate. More importantly, the CIHI data indicate there is great variability in the rate of social work across the country, with Newfoundland and Labrador having the most social workers per capita (288: 100,000) and BC having the fewest (89: 100,000). Further, our profession remains highly gender imbalanced with women making up the majority, very much like nursing and very unlike medicine; in 2017, 86.6% of the 51,859 social workers in Canada were women, compared with 91.5% of nurses in the same year and 38.2% of physicians in 2013.[2] Nursing and medicine are just two of the professions with which gerontological social workers regularly interact and/or collaborate in the care of older adults. The continued growth in the health and aging sectors makes gerontological social work a sustainable field of practice as well as a rewarding one (Service Canada, 2015). This applies to social work not only in Canada, but also in many other countries in the Global North and Global South (see textbox 0.4), as population aging has become a global phenomenon and social work an international profession.

Textbox 0.4

Global North and Global South refers to a division between geographic locations and represents a shift away from the colloquial terms "developed" and "developing" worlds. The terms Global North and Global South underscore not only the social, political, and economic inequality between the two regions, which is tied to settler colonialism, globalization, and neoliberalism, but also the increasingly fluid movement of capital, people, and goods between North and South nations around the world. **Eurocentrism** is a worldview based on the inherent superiority of Western (Global North) nations. It implicitly assumes a stance that is biased in favour of European colonialism and other forms of imperialism.

The aging of Global North and South societies requires that social workers meet the multiple and complex needs of older adults (Cummings et al., 2005). At the same time, there has been a shortage of social workers competent to work with older adult populations (Cox & Burdick, 2001), especially in long-term care facilities (Allen et al., 2007). Despite progress in promoting the importance of gerontology among social work faculty and students, lack of student interest in gerontology as a field of practice remains an issue with only a small percentage of social work students choosing to specialize in gerontology (Wang & Chonody, 2013; Tompkins, 2007). Dominant narratives in health and social care that portray older adults as in decline or as challenging to work with (Clark, 2015; de Medeiros, 2016) undoubtedly impact social work students. The opinion among students that child welfare practice is more interesting than gerontological social work may relate to the belief that interventions with older adults are futile and have limited benefits (Olson, 2011). For these reasons, it is extremely important that we infuse aging content across the curriculum, develop strategies to eliminate ageist assumptions among students, and enhance capacity and connection with social gerontology as a dynamic career path.

It is well recognized that Canada, along with the rest of the world, is rapidly becoming an aging society with adults over the age of 65 already comprising a larger percentage of the population than children and youth under the age of 15 (Statistics Canada, 2015).[3] The median age of the Canadian population has risen from 26.2 years in 1971 to 40.5 years in 2015, largely due to the baby boom cohort (those born after the second world war), and it is predicted that the median age could reach 44 years by 2040 (Statistics Canada, 2019). At the same time, the Canadian population is becoming increasingly diverse, largely due to immigration;[4] this trend is reflected in the older adult population and will continue into the future (Statistics Canada, 2016). Importantly, Statistics Canada (2016) reports that the aging of the Canadian population will continue beyond 2031 when the last of the baby boomers reach age 65, due to not only lower mortality rates but also immigration. Thus, the need to adapt to an aging society, including preparing gerontological social workers, will not end in 2031, and our profession has a responsibility to reshape itself accordingly.

These twin phenomena – the aging and diversification of the Canadian population – have implications for the provision of health and social care and the need for social work students and practitioners to have a strong foundation in gerontological social work, including skills, knowledge, and values. Social work in health and social care and aging services are the two practice areas of greatest growth for social work careers according to both provincial and federal labour market projections. For example, in Quebec, 56.6 % of the jobs in health care and social assistance involve working with older people (ambulatory healthcare, hospitals, and residential care) (Service Canada, 2015). This growth does not necessarily mean that we should decrease the emphasis placed on child welfare within the social work profession, but rather we need to increase the attention paid to social work with older adults, as well as adopt a life course perspective that allows for linkages to be made between the early and the later years of life.

Social workers have been known to move between child welfare practice and gerontological social work practice and to work across generations, with both children *and* older adults. Since children, youth, adults, and older adults are all part of families and communities, social workers are required to work with people of all ages. Thus, all social workers need to understand that age – as a category of difference – is the basis upon which children (and youth) *and* older adults are subject to discrimination, as well as learn the importance of and possibilities for intergenerational work. This is especially important for social workers that, like us, are committed to AOP and therefore support a shift from dependence to interdependence and actively counter the crisis discourse associated with population aging.

This book addresses social work with older adults, their families, and communities through the lens of AOP, what we have termed anti-oppression gerontology (AOG) (Hulko et al., 2017). In doing so, we foreground the development of a contextualized, nuanced approach to understanding older adults (i.e., as situated personally, historically, and structurally). We call into question some of the beliefs and practices prominent in social work with older people, seeking to move beyond notions of frailty and dependence, and to situate older adults as actors in their own lives. Further, we position social workers not only as service providers, but also as agents of social change in their work with older people, their families, and communities – across diverse social conditions and structures.

This textbook is unique in that it (1) employs a critical gerontology lens; (2) showcases the diversity of older adults' experiences through counter-storytelling and case studies; (3) provides guidance for social work practice that is both direct or micro (interventions primarily with individuals, families, and groups) and indirect or meso/macro (mainly community and/or policy interventions and research); and (4) includes content situated in large urban areas, small cities, and rural and remote communities across Canada. Further, foundational values of social work including social justice, anti-discrimination, and resistance to oppression (CASW, 2005) are woven throughout the text. Building on our earlier collaborative work (Brotman & Ferrer, 2015; Brotman, Ferrer, Sussman, Ryan, & Richard, 2015; Ferrer, Grenier, Brotman, & Koehn, 2017; Hulko et al., 2017; Hulko & Stern, 2009; Stern & Hulko, 2016), we define and explore in this book other key concepts for social work in the field of aging, including social location, bio-medicalization of aging, intersectionality and interlocking oppressions, decolonization, globalization and neoliberalism, cultural safety, familism, hetero/cis-normativity, chosen family, and transmigration (see text-boxes and index). These key concepts do not stand alone; rather, they form part of a comprehensive view on aging that links the personal, the historical, and the structural (Ferrer et al., 2017).

Anti-oppression gerontology (AOG) and counter-storytelling

As AOG scholars, we propose a re-visioning of gerontological social work in Canada that troubles normative understandings and dominant narratives of aging and shows how social workers can support agency, equity, resilience, and resistance to oppression in their daily work with older adults, their families, and communities. This includes groups or communities that have been and continue to be subject to oppression due to their gender identity, gender expression, Indigenous ancestry, sexual orientation, racialization, ethno-cultural identity, and dis/ability, for example. As part of our individual and collective efforts to infuse an appreciation for aging and ageism into anti-oppressive social work practice, we introduce in this book eight principles for AOG which are outlined in Table 0.1 (adapted from Hulko et al., 2017, p. 205) and apply them to the 13 main chapters that follow. We do not do so in a prescriptive way, however, as we believe that "once critical thinking relies on a formula, it is no longer critical" (Dumbrill & Yee, 2019, p. 52); checklists or formulas do not serve social workers well when faced with the complexities and constraints of practice. Critical thinking skills and an AOG lens do, however.

This text uses a critical lens with an emphasis on highlighting the voices and experiences of older adults from equity seeking groups[5] and their families and communities.

Table 0.1 Anti-oppression gerontology (AOG) principles version 2.0

1.	Be critically **self-reflexive** and **humble**, understanding that you are part of the process and have your own biases and triggers;
2.	Focus on the complex notion of **identity**, including questioning taken-for-granted **privilege** and the rationale for **dominance** in society, using age and ageism as the starting point;
3.	Explicitly name the issue of social **difference** as an issue of **power** and **equity** rather than a matter of cultural and ethnic variation;
4.	Go beyond individual actions, prejudices, and ideas to examine the ways that individual and **everyday oppressive acts** are entrenched in and (un)consciously supported by **institutional structures**;
5.	View **social justice** and **cultural safety** as both process and goal, which entails affirming **difference** and sharing **power** in interactions with patients, clients, and/or service users;
6.	Value individuals as **self-determining and interdependent** actors who have a sense of their own **agency** and **social responsibility** and appreciate that **resilience and resistance** are important strategies of **agency** enacted by individuals and communities in response to oppressive forces.
7.	Centre **voice** and **access** as foundational rights in the design and delivery of policy and services and make use of **GBA+** (gender-based analysis plus) in policy and planning to foreground **intersectionality** and related concepts like **equity, diversity** and **inclusion** (EDI).
8.	Live your **values** and **ethics** by working towards a more **socially just** and **equitable** world.

In an AOG practice context, this includes Indigenous Elders, LGBTTsIQ[6] older adults, racialized and ethno-cultural minority older adults, and older women. Stories and suggestions for practice are situated not only in large urban centres, but also in small cities and rural and remote communities across Canada. While we situate our work in Canada, we do so with an understanding and critique of a global context that is increasingly marked by an unwavering commitment to globalization and neoliberalism, which has had profound effects on sites and sectors of health and social care and social work as a profession. As Funk (2016) notes,

> Western societies in particular have seen an expansion of individualistic thinking tied to neoliberal political and economic discourse that accompanies globalization and shifts within postmodern society. This perspective emphasizes individual responsibility for risk management (and, for example, successful aging) … [and thus] it becomes difficult to view an individual's actions and decisions as rooted in forces beyond one's personal control.
>
> (p. 3)

Grande (2018) challenges critical gerontology's linking of austerity measures and "precarity" in particular (see textbox 0.5) to neoliberal policy and governance, suggesting instead that it is part and parcel of the normative order introduced and sustained by settler-colonialism: "precarity-as-instigated-by-settler colonialism is best understood as a condition premised upon the dispossession of Indigenous peoples from land and Black peoples from labor and within these communities, the most vulnerable: the sick, young, and elderly" (p. 169). She stresses the need to pursue a "decolonial option" and offers a glimpse of what this "Indigenous elsewheres" might look like, which we share with readers as a counter-story in **Theorizing later life and social work praxis**.

Textbox 0.5

Austerity measures are the cutbacks and restrictions placed on sites and sectors of health and social care due to neoliberal political-economic systems and settler-colonialism. **Precarity** refers to the vulnerable state in which workers and citizens are placed under globalized capitalism.

As authors we represent senior (Hulko and Brotman), mid-career (Stern), and emerging (Ferrer) gerontological social work scholars based at four different schools/faculties of social work across Canada. We have extensive experience in British Columbia, Alberta, Ontario, and Quebec in direct and indirect practice, including hospital and long-term care, home and community care, community development, and policy and planning, as well as educating social work students at the undergraduate and graduate level. Our social locations are varied: While all of us are cisgender, middle-class, Canadian-born adults, one of us is a bisexual woman with a recently acquired disability, two of us are Jewish women, one of whom has a lifelong disability, and one of us is a racialized younger man. This book reflects our collective experience and knowledge, derived from practice, research, teaching, and service with and on behalf of older adults, their families, and communities. It integrates current and emerging theoretical developments and research findings in critical aging studies and gerontological social work.

Counter-storytelling is a key feature of this book, building on our chapter in the third edition of Donna Baines' *Doing anti-oppressive practice* (Hulko et al., 2017). Developed by critical race theorists (Delgado, 1989, 1995), counter-storytelling is "the process of creating and sharing stories that challenge dominant or normative understandings of the social worlds in which we live and work" (Hulko et al., 2017, p. 198). As we assert in that chapter, counter-storytelling is not only an effective way to introduce the voices of diverse older adults, but also stands as an important example of an AOP strategy that social workers can adopt in practice. Solorzano and Yosso (2002) define counter-storytelling as "a method of telling the stories of those people whose experiences are not often told" (p. 26), including older adults (de Medeiros, 2016). Counter-stories of older adults and their encounters with health and social care services and social workers are present throughout this book.[7] Sometimes these counter-stories are as told to us by a specific older adult, and other times they are composites of stories we have heard from older adults with whom we have worked in practice, research, and teaching over the past 30 years or more. We have included as well our personal experiences as social workers and researchers, presented in the form of case studies or counter-stories (see textbox 0.6). We encourage you to consider – or "re-vision" (vision anew) – stories you have heard from older adults or experiences you have had in professional and/or personal contexts. While the book includes a diversity of older adults, we draw mostly from our own experiences working within Indigenous, Jewish, immigrant, LGBTTsIQ and rural communities.

Textbox 0.6

Counter–stories are stories told by (and in solidarity with) marginalized peoples about their experiences and worldviews in order to disrupt or destabilize dominant discourse(s) and challenge systems of oppression. **Case studies** are detailed descriptions of social work clients and practice encounters that may or may not explicate AOP/AOG principles.

While we focus on the identities of older adults throughout this book, this is not to suggest that social workers and other service providers are "identity neutral". In some instances, we situate the social worker as "the reader" so you should read imagining yourself as part of the story. We also ask you at times to imagine how an intervention might shift (e.g., direct to indirect forms of practice and/or in consideration of relational, professional, and institutional/structural change) if the social worker were themselves a member of a marginalized community, such as racialized or queer, for example. In some of the cases drawn from our own practice histories, we identify categories of differences that had particular relevance in terms of oppression and/or privilege. The social work literature has been critiqued for placing identity on clients while assuming mainstream (white) identity of providers (Lee & Ferrer, 2014; Yee & Dumbrill, 2003). The same can be said about other dominant social positions such as cisgender, heterosexual, and/or able-bodied. A related critique is that when social work engages with whiteness it does so by drawing attention to the concept of *white privilege* and fails to name and address *white supremacy* as the root/source (Beck, 2019). These errors and omissions render invisible the experiences of social workers who must navigate power relations very differently than their mainstream colleagues, yet are provided with little guidance on how to do so, including how to manage discrimination by others when faced with it. Although this is not the focus of our book, as we are primarily addressing oppression faced by older adults, we have tried to open this conversation by including stories that address this specifically, along with strategic questions in other chapter exercises.

Structure and content of the book

This book is composed of 15 chapters, including an introduction and concluding thoughts. We have divided the 13 substantive chapters into three parts that move from the more theoretical/conceptual and macro to the more practical and micro/meso and then outwards again, paralleling a gerontological social work course.

Part 1: Shifting our lens on gerontological social work

The first chapter – **Age/ism: age as a category of difference** – sets the context of AOP with older adults in Canada through critically analyzing current demographic trends, including the aging and diversification of the population. The experiences of a new social worker – Maria – are interwoven with our theoretical discussion of age as a category of difference. We address how older adults are positioned as a homogenous group with similar experiences and needs and how this contributes to ageism in the lives of older adults; ageism is interrelated with other forms of oppression like heterosexism and racism that older adults may have experienced throughout their life course. This chapter reviews key terminology in aging studies including ageism, cohort, and generation and introduces the intersectional life course perspective.

We then move to **Theorizing later life and social work praxis**, building on the core concept of ageism and the intersectional life course perspective introduced in **Age/ism: age as a category of difference**. This second chapter begins with a discussion of theory (what it is and why it is useful) and a review of social work practice theories commonly used with older adults. We follow this with an exploration of theories of aging, including early functional theories like disengagement, activity, exchange, and age stratification, before turning to the political economy of aging and other theories associated with critical gerontology, including feminist, queer, and post-structural, and end with Indigenous conceptualizations of aging. The latter theories are more aligned with AOP as they take into account both the lived experience of older adults and the structural realities in which they live and seek to reduce or eliminate oppression and promote EDI. Praxis (linking reflection and action) is woven throughout this chapter through the use of exercises and stories, and it concludes with an exercise on visually depicting the relationship of the theories discussed to the three levels of social work practice (micro/personal, meso/socio-cultural and relational, macro/structural), along with our own attempt to draw these connections.

The third chapter details the different **Sites and sectors of health and social care** older adults must navigate as they age and where social work practitioners most often work. We introduce a continuum model that situates the spaces and contexts in which older people and their families and communities come into contact with health and social care service delivery systems. This chapter not only explains the linkages between the different sectors, but it also illuminates the discourses shaping their mandates, philosophies, and practices, whether explicitly or implicitly, and calls attention to the relative power or voice that older people and their families and communities have in shaping priorities and claiming ownership over services. Through counter-storytelling, this chapter illuminates challenges in the construction of older adults as passive and dependent recipients of care and addresses the important role that social workers can play within these sites and sectors of care (e.g., as discharge planners) to counteract hegemonic (dominant/master) narratives and contextualize the lives of older adults. As with other chapters, the significance of place is addressed and jurisdictional differences noted.

Part 2: Doing AOP social work with older adults

Deconstructing risk and frailty is the focus of the fourth chapter which begins this part on doing AOP social work with older adults. It shows how the concepts of risk and frailty are used to label and categorize older people at individual and structural levels, arising from the bio-medicalization of aging and the dominance of the medical model. Frailty and risk are strongly linked to the idea that as people age they become more dependent, overlooking interdependency. This chapter describes and critically analyzes assessment tools and processes used to measure and understand frailty and risk and identifies how these processes are constructed through risk management and aversion in sites and sectors of health and social care. Counter-storytelling is used to explore the experiences of social work practitioners in the field and give voice to older adults as they strive to enact agency in the context of aging-related changes.

Chapter 5 focusses on **Moral, legal, and ethical issues** in gerontological social work practice and provides a framework for the chapters that follow. It starts with a case study of an older woman and her neuro-diverse adult son whose story is taken forward into the overview of social work ethical guidelines and regulatory mechanisms and the description and analysis of legislation on health care consent and substitute decision-making across Canada. This chapter also addresses medical assistance in dying (MAiD) as an example of a new legal, ethical, and moral issue that gerontological social workers are facing in practice and that requires an AOP lens as well as comfort/skills in talking about death and dying. As one of several emerging debates in social work practice that raise moral, legal, and ethical issues, MAiD is illustrative of the complexity of gerontological social work practice. Our review of guidance from professional and regulatory bodies and the role of social workers across Canada with respect to consent, capacity, and decision-making is paired with stories and exercises to make the links between legislation/guidelines and practice visible/understandable, including the role an AOP social worker can play in policy and planning to promote EDI.

Caregiving and aging are seen as intertwined in gerontological social work and we know that both are highly gendered activities, thus we pose the question "**Who cares about caregiving?**" in this next chapter. We challenge the invisibility of caregivers in health and social care settings, contest the dominant discourse and assumptions of who counts as a caregiver, and address caregiving as a human rights issue. Social service providers tend to identify and define caregivers as members of biological and nuclear families. Moreover, these assumptions often frame older adults as recipients of care, downplaying their caring contributions and the reciprocal nature of caring exchanges. Counter-storytelling in this chapter centres on the impact of transnational migration on care practices within families, highlighting the lack of culturally safe responses available in most sites and sectors of health and social care. The chapter ends by re-visioning what is possible if we apply an AOG lens in our work as social workers, at both individual and organizational levels of intervention.

Chapter 7 focuses on **Dementia, personhood and citizenship as practice**, with the goal of having students understand dementia as a bio-psycho-social phenomenon and integrate approaches to care more consistent with AOG. The chapter follows Harpreet, a newly hired social worker in a care home as she learns about the residents and starts to appreciate the need/potential for an AOP approach in this setting. We start by deconstructing current paradigms of dementia and dementia care that inform sites and sectors of health and social care and often marginalize and exclude people with dementia by privileging the voices and experiences of caregivers and service providers. After discussing risk factors, symptoms, prevalence, and types of dementia and their connections to the social determinants of health, we discuss social work contributions to dementia care/practice, focussing on validation therapy, personhood, cultural safety, and citizenship as practice in particular. This chapter introduces ways to facilitate the voices and inclusion of persons living with dementia and demonstrates AOG through moving beyond person-centred care and towards cultural safety and citizenship as practice.

Mapping trauma across the life course, the next chapter in this part, attends to the impact of trauma over the life course and its interaction with the aging process. Trauma and its effects have been largely ignored in the aging field, and social work practitioners (and the settings in which they work) are often unprepared to recognize, assess, and respond to it. This chapter explores the relationship of aging to both individual and collective traumas. Individually experienced traumas include childhood abuse, domestic or intimate partner violence, sexual assault, combat experience, and exposure to violence from childhood to old age. Collectively experienced traumas are those that occur (and endure) over a prolonged period of time, target specific groups of people, and tend to leave wounds that impact the individuals within it, the group as a whole, and the generations that come after it. These include residential school survivors, refugees, Holocaust survivors, and survivors of genocide. The chapter draws on a trauma-informed practice framework that social workers (and the organizations they work within) can use that is strengths-based, relationship-centred, and culturally safe.

Social work with older adults seeking assistance with **Mental health, mental wellness, and substance mis/use** is the focus of the next chapter in this part of the book, including an exploration of the process of aging with a pre-existing mental health condition as well as the later onset of mental illness and the connection of mental illness to substance mis/use throughout the life course. We look specifically at how bio-medical notions of mental illness can be both the consequence and cause of inequalities and exclusion in older adults' lives. This chapter critically reviews the ways in which sanism and ageism intersect in the treatment and care of older adults diagnosed with mental illness, thereby creating forms of oppression that stigmatize them in unique ways. AOP approaches, including harm reduction and the recovery model of care, are introduced and applied to practice scenarios.

Addressing mistreatment and violence, the final chapter of Part 2, links the direct practice themes presented in this part to the life course and structural issues that impact the everyday experiences of older adults addressed in Part 3 which follows. What makes this chapter unique is that it builds connections between interpersonal forms of violence and mistreatment commonly referred to in the elder abuse literature (e.g., intimate and domestic partner violence, family violence, neglect) with structural forms of violence enacted upon marginalized communities such as homophobia and colonial violence.

Linking direct and indirect practice, the chapter addresses the ambiguous and ethically challenging context of social work practice in this area through the integration of harm reduction, least intrusive, and client-centred approaches.

Part 3: Re-visioning gerontological social work

Building inclusive communities begins the final part of the book, and focusses on working with communities to facilitate social inclusion, civic participation, and belonging among older adults. Central to this is an overview and discussion of how an inclusive community is defined and how the concept of community is not only time and context specific, but also fluid and contested. We elaborate on three types of communities: (1) communities that are defined by local geographic boundaries, (2) communities that emerge through shared interests or concerns and lead to advocacy or collective action, and (3) communities that develop as a result of shared identities. This chapter explores what it means to build communities inclusive of diverse older adults, their families, and networks and how social workers can encourage agency (both resilience and resistance) in order to build community and advocacy initiatives.

Chapter 12 addresses **Policy and planning for an aging society** and focusses on not only describing and analyzing current social policies that impact older adults in the context of globalization and neoliberalism, but also the role social workers play in shaping inclusive policies. Along with EDI, we see human rights and citizenship as integral social work values that should underpin aging policies, rather than a narrow focus on meeting needs. We introduce GBA+ (gender-based analysis plus), a framework for analyzing policies that foregrounds intersectionality and operationalizes the language of EDI (equity, diversity and inclusion) currently favoured by policymakers and planners. Topics include specific policies on work and retirement, health and social care, im/migration, and pensions. We address how these policies might be re-visioned, and the role of both social workers and older adults in the policy planning process is explored to make clear this form of AOG.

The final substantive chapter highlights the **Everyday lives and realities** of older adults through the use of their own voices and narratives (stories). This chapter emphasizes counter-storytelling by a wide range of older adults to draw attention to the unique challenges and strengths that have a direct impact on their everyday lives. Examples of how older adults engage with precarious housing, mental health, trauma, belonging, identity, sexuality, and recognition by health and social service providers are ways in which we reveal both the taken-for-granted and invisible experiences that older adults grapple with in their everyday lives. This chapter applies the intersectional life course perspective presented in Chapter 1. We ask students to attempt their own re-visioning of gerontological social work in relation to the four older adults they meet in this chapter, using the step-wise narrative exercise we present. This will increase appreciation for each older adult and their distinct life history, including varied experiences with sites and sectors of health and social care.

In **Concluding thoughts**, we provide a brief summary of the main ideas discussed throughout this book and offer our final reflections. The conclusion gives an opportunity for the authors and readers to engage in a kind of virtual dialogue through our talking about our experience of writing the book and challenging readers to think about all the issues raised in the stories we shared. We invite you to dialogue with those issues and stories by making use of your subjectivity, positionality, and critical reflexivity. Finally, we return to the eight principles for AOG that we introduced in the introduction as these emphasize how gerontological social work practice can be re-visioned through an anti-oppressive lens, and we encourage students and practitioners to join with us and older adults to put AOG into practice.

Notes

1 While we prefer the term "interaction" developed by critical disabilities scholar Mary Bunch (2017) over "inclusion", we retain "inclusion" in this book as it is a core concept in AOP social work and social gerontology. The problem with "inclusion" is that it is rarely accompanied by the question "inclusion into what?" and therefore can be perceived to be assimilationist. A goal of "inclusion" (in neoliberal policies and programs) is different than "interaction" with said policies and programs in order to change them.
2 2017 data were not available for Medicine.
3 This trend is not consistent across all population groups. For example, both Black and Indigenous populations have higher proportions of children and youth and lower rates of older adults 65+ than the Canadian average as a whole (for example over 43% of people who identified as Black (Visible Minority Status) in the 2016 Canadian Census, were under the age of 25, and only 7.3% were 65+); nevertheless these communities will witness a substantial increase in the proportion of older adults 65+ over the next 20 years.
4 This does not mean that all ethnocultural diversity is due to immigration. Not all racialized people in Canada are immigrants. Black communities are an important example of a group with long-standing and important historical roots dating back centuries, particularly in Nova Scotia which served as the main terminus of the underground railroad. While only 12% of the older (65+) Black population in Nova Scotia are first generation (immigrants), the vast majority of Canadian older Black persons today identified themselves as such in the 2016 Census (92%). Overall, 96% of older visible minority people identify as first generation (immigrants) (Statistics Canada, 2016). The Japanese population 65+ has the lowest rate of first generation immigrants (40%).
5 Equity-seeking groups refers to those groups that have been subject to oppression historically and/or contemporaneously and therefore require special attention to ensure equality of outcome. This includes not only the four federally designated groups (Indigenous people, persons with disabilities, women, and visible minorities), but also LGBTTsIQ people, ethno-cultural minorities, and poor people. EDI policy initiatives focus on these groups of people in particular.
6 The acronym LGBTTsIQ is meant to be inclusive of lesbian, gay, bisexual, transgender, transsexual, two-spirit, intersex, queer and questioning individuals and groups. We recognize this is not an exhaustive list of sexual and gender minorities and note that it is one attempt to balance visibility, inclusion, and accessibility. Other possibilities include LGBTQ+ or LGBTQ★, both of which might be read as leaving out two-spirit and intersex people.
7 While counter-storytelling was developed within Critical Race Theory (see endnote 4 in **Theorizing later life and social work praxis**) as a strategy of resistance enabling marginalized people to claim space and tell their own stories, we have adapted it in this book to provide a mechanism for both re-telling stories from our research and practice with older adults and re-visioning social work, *in solidarity with marginalized people* and in line with the critical pedagogy principles of counter-storytelling. As such, all of our "counter-stories" are re-created or co-constructed by us as authors for the purpose of demonstrating solidarity, challenging oppressive structures and expanding our knowledge-base to include the perspectives and experiences of older adults from equity-seeking groups. This includes older adults who may need assistance to story their lives and experiences due to cognitive and/or physical impairment(s).

References

Allen, P., Nelson, W., & Netting, F. E. (2007). Current practice and policy realities revisited. *Social Work in Health Care*, *45*(4), 1–22. doi:10.1300/J010v45n04_01

Baines, D. (Ed.). (2017). *Doing anti-oppressive practice: Social justice social work* (3rd ed.). Halifax, NS: Fernwood Publishing.

Beck, E. (2019). Naming white supremacy in the social work curriculum. *Affilia: Journal of Women and Social Work*, 1–6. doi:10.1177/0886109919837918

Brotman, S., & Ferrer, I. (2015). Diversity within family caregiving: Extending definitions of 'who counts' to include marginalized communities. *Healthcare Papers*, *15*(1), 47–53. Retrieved from www.ncbi.nlm.nih.gov/pubmed/26626117

Brotman, S., Ferrer, I., Sussman, T., Ryan, B., & Richard, B. (2015). Access and equity in the design and delivery of health and social care to LGBTQ older adults: A Canadian perspective. In N. Orel & C. A. Fruhauf (Eds.), *The lives of LGBT older adults: Understanding challenges and resilience* (pp. 111–140). Washington, DC: American Psychological Association.

Bunch, M. (2017). Julia Kristeva, disability and the singularity of vulnerability. *Journal of Literary & Cultural Disability Studies*, *11*(2), 133–150. doi:10.3828/jlcds.2017.11

Canadian Association of Social Workers. (2005). *Code of Ethics*. Ottawa, ON. Retrieved from www.casw-acts.ca/en/what-social-work/casw-code-ethics.

Canadian Association of Social Workers. (2017). *What is social work?* Retrieved from www.casw-acts.ca/en/what-social-work

Canadian Institute of Health Information. (2017). *Canada's health care providers: Provincial profiles, 2008 to 2017 – Data tables*. Retrieved from www.cihi.ca/en/social-workers.

Carniol, B. (1984). Clash of ideologies in social work education. *Canadian Social Work Review*, *2*(84), 184–199. Retrieved from www.jstor.org/stable/41669968

Clark, P. (2015). Emerging themes in using narrative in geriatric care: Implications for patient-centred practice and interprofessional teamwork. *Journal of Aging Studies*, *34*, 177–182.

Cox, L. E., & Burdick, D. C. (2001). Integrating research projects into field work experience: Enhanced training for undergraduate geriatric social work students. *Educational Gerontology*, *27*(7), 597–608. doi:10.1080/036012701753122929

Cummings, S. M., Adler, G., & DeCoster, V. A. (2005). Factors influencing graduate-social-work students' interest in working with elders. *Educational Gerontology*, *31*(8), 643–655. doi: 10.1080/03601270591003382

de Medeiros, K. (2016). Narrative gerontology: Countering the master narratives of aging (Invited). *Narrative Works*, *6*(1), 63–81. Retrieved from https://journals.lib.unb.ca/index.php/NW/article/view/25446

Delgado, R. (1989). Storytelling for oppositionists and others: A plea for narrative. *Michigan Law Review*, *87*(8), 2411–2441.

Delgado, R. (Ed.). (1995). *Critical race theory: The cutting edge*. Philadelphia, PA: Temple University Press.

Dumbrill, G. C., & Yee, J. Y. (2019). *Anti-oppressive social work: Ways of knowing, talking, and doing*. Don Mills, ON: Oxford University Press.

Ferrer, I., Grenier, A., Brotman, S., & Koehn, S. (2017). Understanding the experiences of racialized older people through an intersectional life course perspective. *Journal of Aging Studies*, *41*, 10–17. doi:10.1016/j.jaging.2017.02.001

Funk, L. (2016). *Sociological perspectives on aging*. Don Mills, ON: Oxford University Press.

Grande, S. (2018). Aging, precarity, and the struggle for Indigenous elsewheres. *International Journal of Qualitative Studies in Education*, *31*(3), 168–176. doi:10.1080/09518398.2017.1401145

Haynes, K. (1998). The one hundred-year debate: Social reform versus individual treatment. *Social Work*, *43*(6), 501–509. Retrieved from www.jstor.org/stable/23717766

Hulko, W. (2009). The time and context contingent nature of intersectionality and interlocking oppressions. *Affilia: Journal of Women and Social Work*, *24*(1), 44–55. doi:10.1177/0886109908326814

Hulko, W., Brotman, S., & Ferrer, I. (2017). Counter-storytelling: Anti-oppressive social work with older adults. In D. Baines (Ed.), *Doing anti-oppressive practice: Social justice social work* (3rd ed., pp. 193–211). Halifax, NS: Fernwood Publishing.

Hulko, W., & Stern, L. (2009). Cultural safety, decision-making and dementia: Troubling notions of autonomy and personhood. In D. O'Connor & B. Purves (Eds.), *Decision-making, personhood and dementia: Exploring the interface* (pp. 70–87). London: Jessica Kingsley Press.

Kennedy-Kish (Bell), B., Sinclair, R., Carniol, B., & Baines, D. (2017). *Case critical: Social services and social justice in Canada*. Toronto, ON: Between the Lines.

Lee, E., & Ferrer, I. (2014). Examining social work as a Canadian settler colonial project: Continual continuities of circles of reform, civilization, and in/visibility. *Journal of Critical Anti-Oppressive Social Inquiry, 1*(1), 1–20.

Mills, C. W. (1959). *The sociological imagination*. New York: Oxford University Press.

Mullaly, B., & West, J. (2018). *Challenging oppression and confronting privilege: A critical approach to anti-oppressive and anti-privilege theory and practice* (3rd ed.). Toronto, ON: Oxford University Press.

Olson, C. A. (2011). Blending continuity and change. *Journal of Continuing Education in the Health Professions, 31*(1), 1–2. doi:10.1002/chp.20094.

Service Canada. (2015, October 30). *Social workers*. Retrieved from www.servicecanada.gc.ca/eng/qc/job_futures/statistics/4152.shtml

Solorzano, D. G., & Yosso, T. J. (2002). Critical race methodology: Counter-story telling as an analytical framework for education. *Qualitative Inquiry, 8*(1), 23–44. doi:10.1177/107780040200800103

Statistics Canada. (2015, September 29). *Canada's population estimates: Age and sex, July 1, 2015*. Retrieved from https://www150.statcan.gc.ca/n1/en/daily-quotidien/150929/dq150929b-eng.pdf?st=r0LMDKu3

Statistics Canada. (2016, March 9). *The contribution of immigration to the size and ethno cultural diversity of future cohorts of seniors*. Statistics Canada. Retrieved from www.statcan.gc.ca/daily-quotidien/160309/dq160309a-eng.htm

Statistics Canada. (2019, July 1). *Age and sex structure: Canada, provinces and territories, Statistics Canada*. Retrieved from https://www150.statcan.gc.ca/n1/en/daily-quotidien/190930/dq190930a-eng.pdf?st=LSRBxTFj

Statistics Canada. (2019, Oct 20). *Data tables, 2016 Census. Visible Minority (15), Generation Status (4), Age (12) and Sex (3) for the Population in Private Households*. Retrieved from https://www12.statcan.gc.ca/census-recensement/2016/dp-pd/index-eng.cfm

Stern, L. & Hulko, W. (2016). Historical trauma, PTSD and dementia: Implications for trauma-informed social work. *The Gerontologist, 56*(Supplement 3), 311.

Tompkins, C. J. (2007). Are we really teaching our students an aging perspective when we use the term intergenerational? Are we encouraging the stigmas associated with aging if we use a "backdoor approach" in recruiting students to become interested in working with older adults? *Journal of Intergenerational Relationships, 4*(4), 109–112. doi:10.1300/J194v04n04_11

Wang, D., & Chonody, J. (2013). Social workers' attitudes toward older adults: A review of the literature. *Journal of Social Work Education, 49*(1), 150–172. doi:10.1080/10437797.2013.755104

Whebi, S., & Parada, H. (Eds.). (2017). *Reimagining anti-oppression social work practice*. Toronto, ON: Canadian Scholars' Press.

Yee, J., & Dumbrill, G. (2003). White-out: Looking for race in Canadian social work practice. In A. Al-Krenawi & J. Graham (Eds.), *Multicultural social work in Canada: Working with diverse ethno-cultural communities* (pp. 98–121). Don Mills, ON: Oxford University Press.

Part I

Shifting our lens on gerontological social work

Chapter 1

Age/ism

Age as a category of difference

Questions to consider as you read this chapter

- Given the diversity of experiences of aging, how do we know when someone is considered "old"?
- What perceptions do we have of someone who is older?
- How do identity categories such as age, race, and gender distinguish people?
- What is ageism and age discrimination?
- How do we – as social workers – challenge dominant perceptions of aging and ageism?
- What role can older people's counter-stories play in this process?

Maria is an undergraduate social work student who has been placed in an agency that provides services to older adults. Having spent most of her volunteer time and her first practicum experience working with children, Maria is upset about having to work with older adults. Maria does not know much about older people beyond what she sees in the news. She agrees with politicians who speak about a rapidly aging population and express concerns over current social and health care services not being able to care for the number of older community members. She associates aging with physical and cognitive decline and thinks all older people are frail and grumpy. Maria expects there to be less diversity amongst the older adult population than the children with whom she has worked and the work to be uninteresting. After several weeks at her practicum, Maria is surprised at just how different her clients are in terms of age, gender, class, sexual orientation, ability, interests, and experiences. For instance, she notices that there are older people who are in their 80s who do not require as much homecare assistance as their younger counterparts.

There is no question that the world is encountering a global aging demographic. Known as *population aging*, the median age of the global population is rising due to declining fertility rates and rising life expectancy (United Nations, 2017). A recent report by the United Nations' Population Division of the Department of Economic and Social Affairs (2017) noted several trends within Global North and Global South societies (see textbox 0.4 in introduction):

- The global population of people aged 60+ years numbered 962 million in 2017. This is more than double the size recorded in 1980. The number of older people 60+ years is projected to double to nearly 2.1 billion by 2050.
- In many Global North and Global South societies, older persons are expected to outnumber children under age ten (1.41 billion versus 1.35 billion) by 2030. The

number of persons 80+ years is projected to rise from 137 million to 425 million by 2050.

• Two thirds of the world's older persons live in the Global South, and their numbers and growth are outpacing the number of older people in Global North societies. The United Nations projects eight out of ten of the world's older people will be living in the Global South by 2050.

• The United Nations (2017) noted significant differences in the rates of intergenerational family cohabitation between Global North and Global South societies. For example, more than half of persons aged 60+ co-resided with a child in Asia, Africa, and Latin America and the Caribbean. However, only about 20% of older people lived with their children in Europe and North America. In general, older women are more likely than older men to live alone.

The fact that we are experiencing an aging society has implications for social workers in Canada and across the globe. When you read the statistics above, what was your initial reaction? Was it closer to excitement or closer to concern? The aging of the Canadian and global population should be taken as a success, yet it is often portrayed as problematic. Scholars have noted how society tends to view the aging population as an impending disaster that will negatively affect social and health care programs (Gee, 2002; Longin, 1995). This perspective is known as *apocalyptic demography*[1] (Robertson, 1991) and presupposes that an aging population will undoubtedly create challenges and burdens to society due, in large part, to significant and negative long-term effects on our economy (see textbox 1.1).

Textbox 1.1

Apocalyptic Demography uses demographic data and economic indicators to forecast that an aging population will create challenges for societal functioning. People living longer is seen to place a burden on society as an increase in the number of older people relative to younger people, especially those aged 19 to 64 years old, is believed to have significant and negative long-term effects on our economy. Economists and critical gerontologists have countered these assertions.

Apocalyptic demography is based on a figure called the "dependency ratio", which is a calculation of the number of people under the age of 19 and over the age of 65 ("the dependents") in relation to all those aged 19–64 years old (the working age population). Obviously, there are assumptions built into this (e.g., that all those aged 19–64 are (fully) employed and that all those under 19 and over 65 are not working at all). Yet, how many teenagers and older adults have you encountered in restaurants and stores (the service industry)? The labour force participation (and exploitation) of both younger and older people has grown in recent years since the introduction of training wages for the former and the elimination of mandatory retirement for the latter. Further, the "dependency ratio" does not reflect the volunteering and caregiving work performed by either group as this is not recognized as having economic value (see **Who cares about caregiving?**).

Within popular media, there are references to a *silver tsunami*, which present the aging population as an incoming tidal wave that will not only overburden sites and sectors of health and social care but also destroy our welfare state. Most concerns about an aging population position older people as chronically ill, using up health care resources like hospital beds with the pejorative term "bed blockers" being applied to the latter stereotype. Take for instance, the following excerpts from well-known news-papers and note how their focus is on the costs of taking care of our aging population.

- **Media Snapshot 1:** "The older they get, the more they cost" (*The Economist* as cited in Martin, Williams, & O'Neill, 2004).
- **Media Snapshot 2:** "Given that they all agree that a demographic 'pension time-bomb' is ticking, Europe's policy makers have done remarkably little to diffuse it" (*The Economist* as cited in Martin et al., 2004)
- **Media Snapshot 3:** "Far too many people, including health professionals and policy-makers, believe that older people are hopeless and burdensome, so they make little effort" (*Globe and Mail* as cited in Fraser, Kenyon, Lagace, Wittich, & Southall, 2016).
- **Media Snapshot 4:** "There is much angst these days about the impact of the aging population on health care utilization and spending" (*Globe and Mail* as cited in Fraser et al., 2016).

Apocalyptic demography and the silver tsunami are predominant interpretations of what it means to have an aging society and how we as a society should respond to this contemporary phenomenon. The problem with these kinds of perceptions is that they essentialize, overgeneralize, and treat older people as a burden to society. In addition, perceptions that frame "aging as a burden" categorize older people as passive members of society who hold little to no agency and who contribute very little to society. Reflecting on these media portrayals, do you think these assumptions about our aging population are accurate? Social gerontologists have criticized apocalyptic demography arguments by suggesting that perceptions of "aging as a burden" are incorrectly predi-cated on highly speculative as well as biased economic predictions and inaccurate and damaging portrayals of older people (see endnote 1 and Barusch, 2013).

Before we proceed further, ask yourself: What do I know about aging? And more importantly, how do we know when people are older? These questions and others will be addressed in this opening chapter that critically examines current demographic trends in and across Global North and Global South societies, including the aging and diversification of the Canadian population. This chapter also examines and problem-atizes age as a form of social division, or what we call a category of difference, where older adults are seen as a homogenous group with similar experiences and needs (see textbox 1.2). These perceptions are oftentimes reinforced by societal and personal beliefs regarding aging and working with older people.

Textbox 1.2

A category of difference refers to characteristics, identities, and traits that can be used to distinguish and categorize a person, people, or community. Examples include race, gender, age, sexual orientation, class, and dis/ability.

This chapter outlines some of the ways in which these assumptions and understandings contribute to age as a category of difference and underpin ageism. We then situate the field of social work within historical and contemporary forms of aging and ageism and the ways in which older people are discriminated against as they reach and live through their later lives. Age being a category of difference has also contributed to ageism in the lives of older adults, which when combined with other identity positions (or categories of difference such as race, gender, sexual orientation, gender identity, and class) contributes to multiple and interlocking oppressions of older adults. We conclude this chapter with a discussion of the life course perspective, including the original formulation by Elder (1974) and a recent update by social work scholars that integrates intersectionality, diversity, and subjective interpretations to ensure our understandings of aging reflect the heterogeneity and complexity of older adults as a cohort and the socio–cultural and geo–political contexts in which they live.

The objectives of this chapter are to

- Understand shifts within the aging population in Canada and across the globe;
- Acknowledge and discuss how age is a category of difference and ageism is a form of oppression;
- Understand the life course and intersectionality and their interrelationship; and
- Consider the ideologies that shape and structure expectations of aging.

Age as a category of difference and distinguishing older people as "old"

We begin this chapter by exploring the ways in which older people have been defined in research and practice. While there are distinctions between younger and older people, have you ever wondered how we determine when someone can be classified as "older"? Is there a magic threshold after which one becomes "old"? Do we recognize people according to physical markers such as greying hair and wrinkled skin? Does old age depend on when people require care? Or does the federal and provincial government have a say in how we distinguish older people from the rest of society? Society tends to see people as old in a myriad of ways, which include societal expectations, professional approaches common to the field of aging (such as social work, nursing, and medical professions), and personal and cultural values/experiences of growing old. Within Global North societies, there are a number of ways to categorize and perceive someone as older. An early conceptualization was that of Bytheway (1997) who suggested six common ways of thinking about aging and questions that are or could be asked.

1. **Chronology:** How old are you in years?
2. **Description:** What words describe how old you are?
3. **Relations**: How do other people affect your experience of aging?
4. **Body:** How are changes in your body affecting your sense of aging?
5. **Pressures:** How do social expectations and institutional regulations regarding age affect your experience of aging?
6. **Biography:** How do you view your past and your future?

The most common of these are likely chronology, body, and biography, which align with the three categories in the model proposed by Grenier and Ferrer (2010): (1) chronological age, (2) functional age, and (3) life stage. The sections that follow are based on the model developed by these two social work scholars though we have integrated the work of other critical gerontologists on ways to think about or conceptualize aging, as well as our own thoughts and examples.

Chronological, functional age and life stages

When we think about the study of aging, the fields of **geriatrics** and **gerontology** come to mind.

Geriatrics focusses on the health, biological, or physical aspects of aging (e.g., longevity, morbidity). On the other hand, gerontology examines the social, cultural, and psychological aspects of aging. While the foci of geriatrics and gerontology are different, both fields tend to classify age according to chronological age, as well as capacity and functional ability, and the roles and life stages of older adults.

Chronological age

The most well-known and understood way of knowing someone is older is through their chronological age. Chronological age is determined by a person's numerical age in relation to their date of birth. This type of classification is based on a linear chronology and is typically used by institutions to develop programs and/or entitlements based on someone's age of eligibility (Bytheway & Johnson, 1990). However, there is no one specific age at which someone becomes "old" – researchers, practitioners, and society at large have differing criteria for deciding that someone has reached old age or later life. The most widely assumed definition for when one turns old is generally when one starts to access or is eligible to receive services, and this is often connected to retirement from the labour market. It should be noted, however, that the age of retirement – and the commencement of a state pension – was set at 65 at a time when life expectancy was much lower (Funk, 2016). In fact, in the 1920s it was only 59 years of age for men and 61 years of age for women; these figures both rose steadily from the 1970s until 2017 when life expectancy for men dropped to 79.9 years of age (from 82 years in 2013) while remaining at 84 years of age for women (Auger, Tedford-Litle, & Wallace-Allen, 2018; Statistics Canada, 2019).

Old Age Security in Canada is a universal provision offered to Canadians who are 65 years of age and over and eligible to receive state pensions (see **Policy and planning for an aging society**). With the aging of the population, there have been proposals to raise this age to 70 years. In Britain, older men aged 67+ and older women aged 65+ are eligible for the State Pension, while in Cuba men receive a pension at 65 and women at 60 (Social Security Office of Retirement and Disability Policy, 2017). In these instances, the age at which people are considered to be "old" varies according to the specific policy or service and their gender. Moreover, the age at which people access programs for older people is widely used as a marker of being considered older. Note that the idea of a retirement age was first introduced in 1889 by German Chancellor Otto von Bismarck who initially selected 70 years based on life expectancy that was below 60 years at that time (Von Herbay, 2014). The World

Health Organization (WHO) uses 50+ as their age marker, due to variability in life expectancies around the world. While 50+ undoubtedly makes more sense as a marker of age in the Global South, it is also relevant to specific populations in Canada for whom rates of morbidity and mortality have been negatively impacted by long-standing experiences of stigma and discrimination across the life course, such as is the reality among Indigenous peoples. Although life expectancy is now trending upwards within Indigenous and other marginalized communities in Canada, the impact of colonialism and other forms of oppression continue to play an important role in shaping negative health outcomes and lowered life expectancy.

As a society, we tend to categorize people according to their chronological ages. Chronological classifications of age are also sometimes further broken down according to age-based groupings in order to better link age with other factors that have an impact upon aging such as life stage or variations in health status. Such groupings include the "*3rd age*" or "*young-old*" (people who are between 65 and 74 years old), "*middle-old*" (people who are between 75 and 84 years old) and the "*4th age*" or "*oldest-old*" (people who are 85+ years old) (see for example Forman, Berman, McCabe, Baim & Wei, 1992; Grenier, 2012; Grenier and Ferrer, 2010; Higgs and Gilleard, 2015 for the ways these terms are used in theory and research on aging). In her work on later life transitions, Grenier (2012) noted that these demarcations not only represent chronological age but also align with expectations of physical and cognitive status, most notably that of decline. It is for this reason that policy-makers and planners are particularly concerned about the "*oldest-old*" as the rate of disability and illness among this group of older people is markedly greater, as are their health care needs, when compared with those aged 65–84 years.

As Maria familiarizes herself in her placement, she notices that there are people of different ages and capabilities. There are some folks who she assumes to be older but are actually younger and others who are older but who Maria would assume were younger based on their physical appearance or activity level. Maria jokes with a few of the older residents and asks, "My gosh, you don't look your age! What's your secret to looking so young?"

Have you noticed that some people age differently than others? As we see in Maria's story above, we sometimes meet and work with people who might be younger than they physically appear to be or a lot older than we initially think. Part of these dynamics can be attributed to the experiences and processes that make aging so varied. This is an idea that we will explore in more detail throughout this book.

Functional age

Another way in which older people are identified as being "old" is in relation to physical markers. Greying hair, wrinkles, use of assistive mobile devices such as canes or wheelchairs, and vision and hearing difficulties are all examples of how we commonly understand older people to be "old" (Grenier and Ferrer, 2010). These signs of aging vary by gender, however. For example, in Global North societies women letting their hair "go natural" is considered a signifier of aging, but men whose hair turns grey, white, or silver are considered distinguished, not "old". While some older men are labelled "silver foxes", there is no corollary for older women that links their aging to virility rather than frailty (see Clarke, 2012). These are simple markers of aging, but they are built upon stereotypes that centre and normalize old age as a time of decline and, by extension, youth as a time of vitality (Grenier & Ferrer, 2010). Global North societies, in particular, emphasize and valorize youth. If youth is the centre, then the aging body is neglected and/or placed into the margins of society (Featherstone & Hepworth, 1990; Gilleard & Higgs, 2005). Yet, while older people often resist these stereotypical functional markers (for example by asserting that "age is simply a number and has no meaning"), they may also, at times, conceal their age in order to minimize experiences of exclusion, marginalization, and stigma (Woodward, 1999).

Life stages or roles

Grenier and Ferrer (2010) note that life stages, as conceptualized by psychologists such as Erik Erikson, is another common way in which older people come to be known as older. Life stages are understood in relation to events and/or social roles throughout the life course. For example, childhood and adolescence are life stages marked by physical and mental changes and development. Children and teenagers learn new responsibilities as they transition into adulthood. As adults reach their 20s and 30s, they enter a life stage where jobs and family represent the dominant norms. Life stage theories have for the most part paid more attention to early stages of human development than later life stages. Only one of the eight stages of human development in Erikson's (1958, 1963) model pertains to older adults while five pertain to children and youth, for example. Common life stages and/or roles associated with later life tend to be associated with retirement, being a grandparent, and/or preparing for death. However, gerontologists have spent their careers questioning how older people experience the later stages of their lives. Grenier (2012) in particular has focussed on the ways in which older people experience transitions and life stages. While classification based on chronological age, functional age, and life stages are the most well-known approaches to distinguishing "older" people and form the basis of eligibility criteria in policy contexts, they tend to essentialize people solely by age while ignoring the considerable diversity that exists among older people as well as the various historical, structured, and lived experiences that shape their experiences of aging (Grenier & Ferrer, 2010).

> At Maria's placement, she meets older adults who are different ages from 62 to 108 years. She meets older people who survived the Great Depression and/or served in World War II, and then she meets others who speak about more recent events like the Stonewall Riots in 1969 and the fall of the Berlin Wall in 1989. She is surprised to learn that not everyone has the same ideas or even the same experiences about world events despite all being "older adults". Maria had thought that all older people could be lumped together with similar pasts and identical presents. Some of the family caregivers – daughters and daughters-in-law mostly – who were visiting were also retired and "older". This got Maria thinking about generations and how different people can live through several generations and belong to more than one cohort.

Cohort versus generation

Social gerontologists have used the terms *cohort* and *generation* to account for aging experiences across time and other historical events. These terms were created to take into account the differences that can exist between older people across different socio-historical periods. According to the *Oxford English Dictionary*, cohort is "a group of persons having a common statistical characteristic, especially that of being born in the same year" (2019). Generation on the other hand, is "all of the people born and living at about the same time, regarded collectively" (Oxford English Dictionary, 2019). This could be the difference between children in grade one or grade five (cohort) versus all children in primary and elementary school (generation), for example. See textboxes 1.3 and 1.4 below for definitions of cohort and generation.

Textbox 1.3

Cohort is defined as group of persons having a common statistical characteristic (for instance, being born in the same year).

Textbox 1.4

Generation refers to all of the people born and living at about the same time who share cultural and social attitudes.

The definition of generation also implies shared cultural and social attitudes. One generation that receives significant media attention is known as the Baby Boomer Generation. This is the generation of people born following World War II. The population grew exponentially during that period and has aged alongside advances in health and technology. Relevant generations include:

- **The Greatest Generation**: People born between 1910 and 1924.
- **The Silent Generation**: People born from 1925 to 1945.
- **Baby Boomers**: People born in the years following World War II (until 1966).
- **Generation X**: Following the baby boomer generation, Gen Xers are people born in the early to mid-1960s to the early 1980s.
- **Generation Y/Millennial Generation** is the demographic cohort proceeding Generation X, generally understood to represent people born in the early 1980s to the early 2000s.

Thus, in the 20th century, there were at least five different generations, the most recent being the Baby Boomer generation, Generation X, and Generation Y/Millennial Generation. What generation are you part of? Do you know the main traits and characteristics of your generation? Do you identify with them? What about your parents', grandparents', or colleagues' generations?

While the connection between cohort and generation is being born within the same time period, an important question we must ask is: Do people born in the same cohort or generation have similar aging experiences? How would people from previous generations experience aging if they lived their later lives today? It's also important to note the complexity and considerable diversity that exists within a generation. For instance, while the Baby Boomer generation is commonly characterized by postwar productivity and prosperity that led to greater rights and welfare of many older people, it continues to be marked by multiple forms of social and institutional discrimination among historically marginalized communities. This means that not all baby boomers have the same experience of prosperity simply because they were born within the same time period. For example, baby boomer members of LGBTTsIQ communities and Black communities have experienced significant oppression across the life course (Brotman, Ryan, Collins & Chamerland, 2007; Gee, Walsemann & Brondolo, 2012). Despite the fact that older people in Canada have witnessed significant changes in the past 50 years, which has led to increased recognition of their social and political rights, older members of Black and LGBTTsIQ communities to this day continue to experience subcultural status within society generally and within various institutions (Benjamin, Este et al., 2010; Fredriksen-Goldsen & Muraco, 2010). This is particularly problematic for older racialized LGBTTsIQ people who are exposed to intersectional forms of discrimination (Mullings, 2016; Pino, 2017). Within homecare settings that are sites of hetero-/ cis- normative and white privilege, for instance, some community members might be exposed to both homo/bi/transphobia and racism. For older LGBTTsIQ people, hiding their identity is still a commonly adopted survival strategy. Much research has documented that today's cohort may neither self-identify as LGBTTsIQ nor feel a sense of community belonging because of these experiences and the limited opportunities afforded them earlier in their life course to find and build solidarity with others through community networks. These networks and organizations remained underground in order to avoid exposure to political, legal, and social repercussions, including arrest and various forms of violence. Among racialized older LGBTTsIQ people, finding and building solidarity within spaces in which they are accepted as both LGBTTsIQ and racialized can be particularly challenging and may make them hesitate to engage with health, social, and community care systems and be more vulnerable to invisibility and marginalization within them.

Introduction to ageism

The classification of older people as a separate group can result in ageism and often does. Ageism is defined as discrimination on the basis of age and relates to the lowered social value afforded older people due to their chronological age (Butler, 1969). Ageism expresses itself in the form of negative stereotypes, inequitable treatment, and discriminatory practices against older people. According to Comfort (1979) ageism is the perception that "people cease to be the same by virtue of their age" (p. 35). As Figure 1.1, "Expectations of aging", shows, there are both negative and positive expectations of aging, the former including dying, death, and decline and the latter retirement, benefits, and living a long and healthy life. While society expects aging to be either positive or negative, there are experiences in between these binary views that tend to be forgotten. Within Global North (capitalist) societies where productivity is a core value and therefore prioritized, issues of ageism place older people in predominately subordinated or marginalized positions. Hendricks and Hendricks (1977) suggest that older people's physical appearance and capacities become the basis for viewing and treating people differently. Through personal essays on being rendered invisible

Expectations of Aging

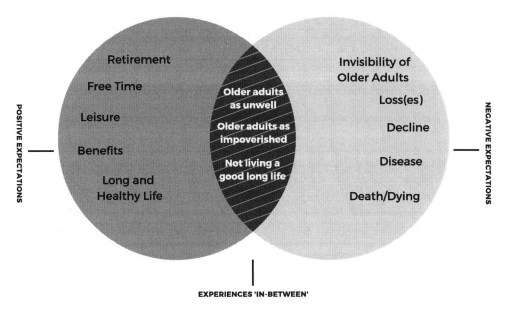

Figure 1.1 Expectations of aging

through the aging process, Macdonald and Rich (1983) identified this focus on physical appearance as not only ageist but also sexist and issued a call for older women to be seen by society and to be "looked in the eye" by individuals. Bytheway (1997) discusses how ageism is manifested through chronological age and the ways in which policies and programs are structured. This important text showcases how ageism is more than a by-product of social values, a mechanism by which government and other institutions have the power to provide and deny opportunities to older people (Bytheway, 1997). After reviewing Figure 1.1, consider the questions in Table 1.1. Do you think that policies which give benefits to people at a certain age should also be considered ageist?

Table 1.1 Is this ageist?

These are some benefits offered to older adults. Do you think that these policies are ageist? Why or why not?

At the Vancouver Island ferry, BC residents over the age of 65 receive free rides from Monday to Thursday from 9:00 AM to 4:00 PM.
Older adults receive a "seniors discount" on specific days of the week for restaurant and retail chains such as Denny's and Bulk Barn.
Parks Canada: Older adults can receive a discount for a Discovery Pass (unlimited admission for 12 months to over 80 Parks Canada spaces). Ages 65+ are eligible.

Inequalities in later life

Policymakers and program planners often use population-based data to make decisions about services. Statistical information can be used to predict patterns of aging, service use, and vulnerability to particular forms of inequalities. The outcome variables used most often to provide evidence of inequalities in later life are rates of poverty, physical and mental health conditions, and discrimination in health, community support, and housing services. This information can be used to help older people by allocating much-needed resources or it can harm them by restricting their access to entitlements. Older people, their families, and communities also can use these data to make claims and gain access to programs and services. Data can help educate the broader society regarding the realities, issues, and inequalities older people confront in order to advance social recognition of aging.

Inequalities in later life are often explained by the use of *cumulative advantage/disadvantage theory,* which posits that both the disadvantages and the advantages held by various social groups compound with age, as in the adage "the rich become richer and the poor become poorer" (Crystal & Shea, 1990; Dannefer, 2003). The *feminization of poverty theory* (Pierce, 1978, as cited in Gonyea, 1994) is associated with cumulative disadvantage in that it argues that women endure higher levels of poverty throughout the life course. In terms of gender, aging, and health, the later lives of [cisgender] women are more marked by sickness and disability, while [cisgender] men more often have acute illnesses. As a result, policymakers are advised to

> pay as much attention to living as to dying – to mom's grimace [due to arthritis] as she opens a car door and Dad's empty chair [due to death].
>
> (Verbrugge, 1989, p. 70)

Dressel (1991) expanded on critiques of the feminization of poverty and the way it overlooks the racial dimensions of poverty by highlighting the limitations of the concepts of *double* and *triple jeopardy* so popular in the gerontological literature since the 1960s. Double jeopardy is defined as "falling into two or more social categories, which increase the risk of having some poor outcome" (Hammond, 1995, pp. 5–6), and triple (or multiple) jeopardy added age to race and sex to explain the compound effect of discrimination (Havens & Chappell, 1983). The multiple jeopardy models that include minority ethnic and racialized women are termed "add and stir" approaches as "racial-ethnic women's experiences are forced into the model rather than being utilised to refine or critique the model itself" (Dressel, 1991, p. 247). Indeed, it has been argued that "the feminization of poverty" as well as "the advantaged elder" further relegate sub-groups of older people to the margins of society and that the way forward rests in taking a life span approach with an integrated analysis of race, class, gender, and age (Gonyea, 1994; see also Browne, 1995; Hooyman, Browne, Ray, & Richardson, 2002). The intersectional life course (Ferrer, Grenier, Brotman, & Koehn, 2017), which we elaborate on later in this chapter, extends this focus on inequalities in later life and proposes an integrated analytical framework.

Introducing the life course theory and approach

Midway through her practicum, Maria is assigned caseloads with older people. She begins to see how older adults are categorized according to age and physical functioning. In one of her cases, Maria works with Kamali, an older immigrant from Ethiopia. Kamali is 59 years old but requires extensive physical care and would like to be placed in a long-term care home as he has no family to help him with his daily activities. Working with Kamali has opened Maria's eyes to some of the complexities of aging. In particular, Maria learns that Kamali came to Canada in search of employment. He was an engineer in Ethiopia but couldn't find work in Canada because of racist assumptions regarding his educational and professional accreditations, skills, and capabilities, which were not recognized by potential employers. As such, he worked as a manual labourer where he was subject to daily experiences of isolation and rejection by his coworkers. He often sat alone during lunch and found that some of his coworkers would refuse to work with him because they said he was "unqualified" to do his job, a statement he knew was only subtly concealing their prejudice against him. One day, he was forced to work overtime without compensation and was so tired, he did not step properly and experienced a workplace accident. Now with a physical disability, Kamali is looking for a place that will provide assistance within an environment free of discrimination in order to improve his quality of life. Maria has come to appreciate Kamali's identity as a provider to his family in Ethiopia even though he is separated by thousands of kilometres. Maria is intrigued by Kamali's story and realizes that his experiences of racism get lost in his assessments (focussing mainly on his extensive physical care and functioning).

In response to the criticisms of ageism and age as a category of difference, some social gerontologists have incorporated a life course perspective in order to better account for the ways in which historical and social dimensions experienced earlier in the life course impact people as they age (Grenier, 2012; McMullin, 2010). This approach has generally been used to understand how transitions and trajectories impact one's life (see Clausen, 1986; Grenier, 2012; Hareven, 1994). While there are different interpretations of the life course (Dannefer & Settersten, 2010), the best-known iteration in North America is that proposed by Glen Elder (1974, 1994). Elder outlines how structured pathways (i.e., social institutions and organizations) and individual trajectories (i.e., roles, status, and development) shift over time and shape individual identities and behaviors. Elder's (1974, 1994) life course perspective is based on four major concepts. First, *human lives and historical times*, suggests lives are intertwined and defined by significant events that have long-lasting effects. Second, *the timing of lives* highlights how events occurring at specific points in one's lifetime could have different consequences for people. The third key concept, *linked lives*, identifies the interrelatedness and interdependence of human relationships across the life span. Finally, the life course takes into account the key concept of *human agency* and the ways in which people make choices, adopt strategies, and articulate experiences of resilience when encountering structural constraints (Ferrer et al., 2017; also see Dannefer & Settersten, 2010; Settersten, 2003).

The life course perspective has been widely used in social gerontology, including to analyze processes of racialization and ethno-cultural minority status in the United States. Studies examining health disparities are the most representative type of life course research, with predictive models being used to situate identity categories such as class, race, and gender (Brown, Richardson, Hargrove, & Thomas, 2016; Warner & Brown, 2011). Research in this area has focused on individual trajectories and key life events such as health outcomes in later life, and the links between multiple identities and interlocking oppressions in everyday experiences of structural inequality have not been well theorized (Dannefer & Settersten, 2010).

Taking into account life course and intersectionality

In order to move towards an integrated theory of class, age, gender, and ethnicity/race,[2] McMullin (2000) argues that class, age, gender, and ethnicity/race need to be seen as categories of social relations and as interlocking sets of power relations. This is in line with the *intersectionality approach to aging* articulated by feminist gerontologists (Calasanti & Slevin, 2001; Dressel, Minkler & Yen, 1997). Calasanti (1996) expanded the critique of additive approaches to oppression by engaging with privilege and oppression, noting that privilege on one axis does not cancel out oppression on another and that social life is relational. This analysis was echoed and extended in recent work by Krekula and colleagues on gendered ageism: "intersectionality stresses the need to understand the powerful alongside the powerless and opens a discourse of mutual shaping while recognizing the flexibility and the unfinished projects of creating differences" (Krekula, Nikander & Wilińska, 2018, p. 36). Krekula et al. (2018) put forth the argument that "gendered ageism can be understood as a dynamic social positioning practice" (p. 42). That is, age is doing and is also a power relation.

Textbox 1.5

Intersectionality and interlocking oppressions is a theoretical framework that explicates the way in which (1) social identities interact to produce unique experiences of oppression and privilege for individuals and (2) systems of domination reinforce and sustain one another (Hulko et al., 2017). The power to oppress those with stigmatized social identities and to guard unearned privilege is embedded within and distributed through oppressive systems.

As authors, we argue that an intersectional life course perspective can provide a key roadmap for understanding "multiple pathways" of care, linking lived experience to macro structures and policy that shape everyday life as people age. The intersectionality perspective focusses on the examination of the multiple and interlocking systems of domination that shape and structure people's lives (Collins, 2000) through the interplay between categories of difference (such as age, race, class, sexual orientation) with wider systems of domination (see textbox 1.5). Hulko (2009) notes that "intersectionality is used in conjunction with identities and categories, while interlocking oppressions applies more to processes and systems" (p. 47), this being the micro and macro distinction that Collins (2000) intended. Further,

> intersectionality can be seen to operate at more of a theoretical level and to refer to the way in which identity categories interact, whereas social location [see textbox 0.1] indicates the result of this interaction in terms of privileges and disadvantages and functions at more of a practical or everyday level and is thus of critical importance to AOP social work practice.
>
> (Hulko, 2009, p. 45)

Accounting for the intersecting identities and interlocking oppressions that impact experiences of aging requires that we understand the role of categories of difference within society as well as the role of subjective interpretations of age (e.g., how people come to experience their social location) (Grenier & Ferrer, 2010). Critical gerontologists such as Calasanti (1996) have noted that understanding diversity allows us to examine "groups in relation to interlocking structural positions within a society" (p. 148). We can then focus on the situation, special problems, and/or experiences of specific groups and inquire about ways in which power operates in relationships between dominant groups and subordinate groups within society, including diverse categories of difference among older people in society; in that way, we can gain a deeper understanding of processes of differentiation and oppression (McMullin, 2000).

Using an intersectional life course perspective would enable a nuanced examination of aging in Global North and South societies, linking lived experiences to state and institutional policies and practices in health and social care, labour, retirement, and immigration sectors. An intersectional life course perspective can also be used to connect the impact of state and institutional policies with the everyday choices and experiences of older adults, their families, and communities. This includes a focus on how "individual choices" are shaped and constrained by social, political, and economic forces which older adults may not be able to see or control. Perhaps most importantly, an intersectional life course perspective makes space for exploring **resilience** as strength in coping with exclusion and oppression and **resistance** as pushing back against forces of exclusion and oppression. As such, examining the diversity of aging through an intersectional life course perspective opens up possibilities to link state and institutional policies and practices with the unique and varied lived experiences of older adults who face historical and current marginalization and oppression.

Considering social and cultural constructions of older adults

At this point, it is worth asking about the popular conceptions and social constructions of older people in Global North and Global South societies. Social constructions are our socially constructed understandings of the world and realities in which we live. Thus far, we have presented ways in which research and policy conceptualize the category "older". People and communities also use different markers to recognize older people. There are many examples of Indigenous nations and communities where age is conceptualized through a lens of respect and honour. For example, the teachings within the Elders of the Blackfoot Confederacy assert that Elders should be respected and honoured for their teachings and knowledge as the safe keepers of cultural protocol and history and give Elders a central role in educating and counselling community members (Livingstone Regional School Division No 68, 2016). While the history of many nations and communities includes valuing older people for their wisdom and leadership, settler colonialism and associated processes of industrialization, globalization, and neoliberalism have undermined the place of Elders as teachers, leaders, and counsellors. Thus, a key part of decolonization and resurgence efforts is returning Elders to a place of respect and honour.

As social workers, we must understand aging as socially constructed and that there are tensions between personal, cultural, social, and structural definitions of aging. While most people would individually abide by the "respect your elders" doctrine and have learned to do so in their families, with their grandparents, the way one lives in a personal way doesn't always translate to the way in which society is governed. As social workers, we live every day the tension between our own values, our professional values, and the values of society generally; at times these values may connect seamlessly, sometimes they may be in conversation with one another, and at times they may be in conflict. We can see this as a clash of ideologies or belief systems (see

Theorizing later life and social work praxis). We need to constantly reflect on and make visible these tensions and distinctions to better serve the needs of our clients. In other words, we need to examine our own value systems as well as those of our profession and the sites and sectors of health and social care in which we work. Further, we need to understand and make visible values across cultures and be willing to learn from others and be open to differing points of view. This includes differing cultural constructions of age and how these dynamics play out in people's lives at the micro, meso, and macro levels. We conclude this chapter by returning to Maria's story, highlighting how Maria's journey of critical self-reflection has enabled her to identify the limitations of her previous assumptions regarding older adults and the ways in which her placement afforded her a unique opportunity to expand her perspective on the diversity and lived experiences of older adults. In particular, Maria is excited about how interesting and dynamic a career path in social gerontology could be.

> *After months at her placement, Maria has learned that there is considerable diversity in later life and that the assessments she makes with her clients are often based on eligibility and restrictions, almost ignoring the differences in social constructions of age between actors and systems. Maria begins to reflect on what she has learned about aging in her BSW program. She realizes that her faculty does not have a dedicated, required course on aging and that discussions on later life are framed by physical and cognitive decline or what she has come to know as positive or successful aging. Maria speaks to some of her colleagues who have shared similar concerns. With the help of a faculty member, she starts a reading group to spark discussions about dominant perceptions of aging among emerging social workers. Through her reading group, Maria realizes that she can integrate different ways of knowing to inform her practice and understanding of aging.*

Exercises

- Consider Maria's journey in gerontological social work practice. How do your experiences and perceptions of aging compare and contrast to hers?
- In thinking about your social work program and the undergraduate/graduate courses you've taken to date, how is content related to age and aging taught or presented?
- Create a case example of one of your older clients. How would you incorporate an intersectional life course perspective in your write up?

Takeaways

- We are currently experiencing a global aging trend.
- Like race and gender, age is a category of difference used to distinguish a group of people. However, age as a category of difference positions older adults as a homogenous group with similar needs.
- Experiences of ageism are interrelated with other forms of oppression such as heterosexism, cissexism and racism.
- An intersectional life course perspective links lived experiences to macro structures that shape everyday lived experience as people age.
- Gerontological social workers must consider their own views on aging and how these perspectives impact their work with older adults.

Notes

1 Apocalyptic demography is also known as voodoo demography (Gee & Gutman, 2000) and alarmist demography (Katz, 1992).
2 While we do not recommend conflating race and ethnicity as these are distinct concepts, we retain the framing used in earlier critical gerontological scholarship when appropriate. Ethnicity, culture and race are distinct but related terms that often mistakenly get used interchangeably. Ethnicity refers broadly to a connection to ancestry, region (and at times may also be linked to religious affiliation and/or language); culture to a shared set of values, beliefs and practices within groups (ethnocultural refers to the combination of both ethnicity and culture). Race is a term which refers to the social construction of assigned group membership based upon 'visible' markers of difference/distinguishing physical characteristics (such as skin/eye colour or facial features). 'Racialization' calls attention to the socio-political process of assigning subordinate status to individuals and communities based upon their imposed/assumed membership within 'specific' racial groups in order to deny rights, entitlements, resources etc. Those with the power to 'racialize others' are, as a consequence, implicitly assigned superordinate status and granted rights, entitlements, resources, etc.

References

Auger, J., Tedford-Litle, D., & Wallace-Allen, B. (2018). *From the inside looking out: Competing ideas about growing old* (2nd ed.). Halifax, NS: Fernwood Publishing.

Barusch, A. (2013). The aging tsunami: Time for a new metaphor? *Journal of Gerontological Social Work, 56*(3), 181–184. doi:10.1080/01634372.2013.787348

Benjamin, A., Este, D., James, C., Lloyd, B., Thomas Bernard, W., & Turner, T. (2010). *Race and wellbeing: The lives, hopes and activism of African Canadians.* Halifax: Fernwood Publishing.

Brotman, S., Ryan, B., Collins, S., & Chamberland, L. (2007). Coming out to care: Caregivers of gay and lesbian seniors in Canada. *The Gerontologist, 47*(4), 490–503. doi:10.1093/geront/47.4.490

Brown, T., Richardson, L., Hargrove, T., & Thomas, C. (2016). Using multiple-hierarchy stratification and life course approaches to understand health inequalities: The intersecting consequences of race, gender, SES, and age. *Journal of Health and Social Behavior, 57*(2), 200–222. doi:10.1177/0022146516645165

Browne, C. (1995). Empowerment in social work practice with older women. *Social Work, 40*(3), 358–364. doi:10.1093/sw/40.3.358

Butler, R. N. (1969). Age-ism: Another form of bigotry. *The Gerontologist, 9*(4), 243–246. doi:10.1093/geront/9.4_Part1.243

Bytheway, B. (1997). Talking about age: The theoretical basis of social gerontology. In A. Jamieson, S. Harper, & C. Victor (Eds.), *Critical approaches to ageing and later life* (pp. 7–15). Milton Keynes: Open University Press.

Bytheway, B., & Johnson, J. (1990). *Welfare and the ageing experience: A multidisciplinary analysis.* Aldershot: Avebury.

Calasanti, T. (1996). Incorporating diversity: Meaning, levels of research, and implications for theory. *Gerontologist, 36*(2), 147–156. doi:10.1093/geront/36.2.147

Calasanti, T., & Slevin, K. (2001). *Gender, social inequalities, and aging.* Lanham, MD: AltaMira Press.

Clarke, L. H. (2012). Researching the body and embodiment in later life. In M. Leontowitsch (Ed.), *Researching later life and ageing* (pp. 24–40). Basingstoke: Palgrave Macmillan.

Clausen, J. A. (1986). *The life course: A sociological perspective.* Englewood Cliffs, NJ: Prentice Hall.

Collins, P. H. (2000). *Black feminist thought: Knowledge, consciousness, and the politics of empowerment.* New York: Routledge.

Comfort, A. (1979). Clinical aspects of aging. *The Western Journal of Medicine, 130*(5), 491. Retrieved from www.ncbi.nlm.nih.gov/pmc/articles/PMC1238695/

Cronin, A., Ward, R., Pugh, S., King, A., & Price, E. (2011). Categories and their consequences: Understanding and supporting the caring relationships of older lesbian, gay and bisexual people. *International Social Work, 54*(3), 421–435. doi:10.1177/0020872810396261

Crystal, S., & Shea, D. (1990). Cumulative advantage, cumulative disadvantage, and inequality among elderly people. *The Gerontologist, 30*(4), 437–443. doi:10.1093/geront/30.4.437

Dannefer, D. (2003). Cumulative advantage/disadvantage and the life course: Cross-fertilizing age and social science theory. *The Journals of Gerontology. Series B, Psychological Sciences and Social Sciences, 58*(6), S327–S337. doi:10.1093/geronb/58.6.s327

Dannefer, D., & Settersten, R. A. (2010). The study of the life course: Implications for social gerontology. In D. Dannefer & C. Phillipson (Eds.), *The SAGE handbook of social gerontology* (pp. 3–19). Los Angeles, CA: SAGE Publications.

Dressel, P. L. (1991). Gender, race, and class: Beyond the feminization of poverty in later life. In M. Minkler & C. L. Estes (Eds.), *Critical perspectives on aging: The political and moral economy of growing old* (pp. 245–252). Amityville, NY: Baywood.

Dressel, P., Minkler, M., & Yen, I. (1997). Gender, race, class, and aging: Advances and opportunities. *International Journal of Health Services, 27*(4), 579–600. doi:10.2190/7XAY-PYBN-AA5L-3DRC

Elder, G. H. (1974). *Children of the great depression: Social change in life experience*. Chicago, IL: University of Chicago Press.

Elder, G. H. (1994). Time, human agency, and social change: Perspectives of the life course. *Social Psychology Quarterly, 57*(1), 4–15. doi:10.2307/2786971

Erikson, E. H. (1958). *Young man Luther*. New York: W. W. Norton & Company.

Erikson, E. H. (1963). *Childhood and society*. New York: W. W. Norton & Company.

Featherstone, M., & Hepworth, M. (1990). Ageing and old age: Reflections on the postmodern lifecourse. In B. Bytheway, T. Kiel, P. Allat, & A. Bryman (Eds.), *Becoming and being old* (pp. 143–157). London: Sage.

Ferrer, I., Grenier, A., Brotman, S., & Koehn, S. (2017). Understanding the experiences of racialized older people through an intersectional life course perspective. *Journal of Aging Studies, 41*, 10–17. doi:10.1016/j.jaging.2017.02.001

Fraser, S. A., Kenyon, V., Lagace, M., Wittich, W., & Southall, K. E. (2016). Stereotypes associated with age-related conditions and assistive device use in Canadian media. *The Gerontologist, 56*(6), 1023–1032. doi:10.1093/geront/gnv094

Fredriksen-Goldsen, K., & Muraco, A. (2010). Aging and sexual orientation: A 25-year review of the literature. *Research on Aging, 32*(3), 372–413. doi:10.1177/0164027509360355

Funk, L. (2016). *Sociological perspectives on aging*. Don Mills, ON: Oxford University Press.

Forman, D. E., Berman, A. D., McCabe, C. H., Baim, D. S., & Wei, J. Y. (1992). PTCA in the elderly: The "young-old" versus the "old-old". *Journal of the American Geriatrics Society, 40*(1), 19–22. doi:10.1111/j.1532-5415.1992.tb01823.x. PMID 1727842

Gee, E. M. (2002). Misconceptions and misapprehensions about population ageing. *International Journal of Epidemiology, 31*, 750–753. doi:10.1093/ije/31.4.750

Gee, E. M., & Gutman, G. M. (2000). *The overselling of population aging: Apocalyptic demography, intergenerational challenges and social policy*. Don Mills, ON: Oxford University Press.

Gee, G., Walsemann, K., & Brondolo, E. (2012). A life course perspective on how racism may be related to health inequities. *American Jouurnal of Public Health, 102*(5), 967–974.

Gilleard, C., & Higgs, P. (2005). *Contexts of ageing: Class, cohort, and community*. Cambridge: Polity.

Gonyea, J. G. (1994). The paradox of the advantaged elder and the feminization of poverty. *Social Work, 39*(1), 35–41. doi:10.1093/sw/39.1.35

Grenier, A. (2012). *Transitions and the lifecourse: Challenging the constructions of "growing old"*. Bristol: Policy Press.

Grenier, A., & Ferrer, I. (2010). Age, ageing and growing old: Contested definitions of age. In N. Guberman, M. Charpentier, & A. Grenier (Eds.), *Gerontologies sociale: Problemes sociaux et interventions sociales* (pp. 35–54). Quebec, QC: Presses de l'Universite du Quebec.

Hammond, D. (1995). Perspectives from the bouldering files. *Systems Research, 12*(4), 281–290. Retrieved from http://web.a.ebscohost.com.proxy3.library.mcgill.ca/ehost/pdfviewer/pdfviewer?vid=1&sid=21d6abba-a63e-41f1-8d3a-bfd68faee617%40sdc-v-sessmgr01

Hareven, T. K. (1994). Aging and generational relations: A historical and life course perspective. *Annual Review of Sociology, 20*(1), 437–461. doi:10.1146/annurev.so.20.080194.002253

Havens, B., & Chappell, N. L. (1983). Triple jeopardy: Age, sex and ethnicity. *Canadian Ethnic Studies = Etudes Ethniques Au Canada, 15*(3), 119. Retrieved from https://proxy.library.mcgill.ca/login?url=https://search.proquest.com/docview/1293146670?accountid=12339

Hendricks, J., & Hendricks, C. D. (1977). *Aging in mass society: Myths and realities.* Cambridge, MA: Winthrop Publishers.

Higgs, P. & Gilleard, C. (2015). *Rethinking old age: Theorizing the fourth age.* London: Palgrave Macmillan.

Hooyman, N., Browne, C. V., Ray, R., & Richardson, V. (2002). Feminist gerontology and the life course. *Gerontology & Geriatrics Education, 22*(4), 3–26. doi:10.1300/J021v22n04_02

Hulko, W., Brotman, S., & Ferrer, I. (2017). Counter-storytelling: Anti-oppressive social work with older adults. In D. Baines (Ed.), *Doing anti-oppressive practice: Social justice social work* (3rd ed., pp. 193–211). Halifax, NS: Fernwood Publishing.

Hulko, W. (2009). The time- and context-contingent nature of intersectionality and interlocking oppressions. *Affilia, 24*(1), 44–55. doi:10.1177/0886109908326814

Katz, S. (1992). Alarmist demography: Power knowledge, and the elderly population. *Journal of Aging Studies, 6*(3), 203–225. doi:10.1016/0890-4065(92)90001-M

Krekula, C., Nikander, P., & Wilińska, M. (2018). Multiple marginalizations based on age: Gendered ageism and beyond. In L. Ayalon & C. Tesch-Römer (Eds.), *Contemporary perspectives on ageism* (pp. 33–50). New York, NY: Springer International Publishing. doi:10.1007/978–3–319–73820–8_24

Livingstone Range School Division No 68. (2016). *First Nation elders/resource directory.* Retrieved from www.lrsd.ca/documents/general/2015-01-28%20Elders%20Directory%201%20revision.pdf

Longin, C. F. (1995). *Retirement migration in America.* Houston, TX: Vacation.

Macdonald, B., & Rich, C. (1983). *Look me in the eye: Old women, aging and ageism.* San Francisco, CA: Spinster's Ink.

Martin, R., Williams, C., & O'Neill, D. (2004). Retrospective analysis of attitudes to ageing in the economist: Apocalyptic demography for opinion formers? *British Medical Journal, 339*(7735), 1435–1437. doi:10.1136/bmj.b4914

McMullin, J. (2000). Diversity and the state of sociological aging theory. *The Gerontologist, 40*(5), 517–530. doi:10.1093/geront/40.5.517

McMullin, J. (2010). *Understanding social inequality: Intersections of class, age, gender, ethnicity, and race in Canada.* Don Mills, ON: Oxford University Press.

Mullings, D. V. (2016). Caring for older black LGBTQ people: A new challenge for the social work profession. In S. Hillock & N. Mule (Eds.), *Queering social work education* (pp. 205–226). Vancouver, BC: UBC Press.

Oxford English Dictionary. (2019). *Cohort.* Retrieved from www-oed-com. ezproxy.lib.ucalgary.ca/view/Entry/35953?rskey=Gne6uL&result=1#eid

Pino, F. L. (2017). Older Filipino gay men in Canada: Bridging queer theory and gerontology in Filipino-Canadian studies. In R. Diaz, M. Largo, & F. Pino (Eds.), *Diasporic intimacies: Queer Filipinos and Canadian imaginaries* (pp. 163–181). Evanston, IL: Northwestern University Press.

Robertson, A. (1991). The politics of Alzheimer's disease: A case study in apocalyptic demography. In M. Minkler & C. Estes (Eds.), *Critical perspectives on aging: The political and moral economy of growing old* (pp. 135–152). Amityville, NY: Baywood.

Ryan, B., & Canadian AIDS Society. (2003). *A new look at homophobia and heterosexism in Canada.* Ottawa, ON: Canadian AIDS Society.

Settersten, R. A. (2003). Age structuring and the rhythm of the life course. In J. T. Mortimer & M. J. Shanahan (Eds.), *Handbook of the life course* (pp. 82–102). New York: Kluwer.

Social Security Office of Retirement and Disability Policy. (2017). Social security programs throughout the world: The Americas. Retrieved from www.ssa.gov/policy/docs/progdesc/ ssptw/2016-2017/americas/cuba.html

Statistics Canada. (2019, September 26). Table 13-10-0134-01 life expectancy at various ages, by population group and sex, Canada. doi: 10.25318/1310013401-eng

United Nations. (2017). *World population ageing 2017 – Highlights.* Retrieved from www.un.org/ en/development/desa/population/theme/ageing/WPA2017.asp

Verbrugge, L. (1989). The Twain meet: Empirical explanations of sex differences in health and mortality. *Journal of Health and Social Behavior, 30*(3), 282–304. doi: 10.2307/2136961

Von Herbay, A. (2014). Otto Von Bismarck is not the origin of old age at 65. *The Gerontologist, 54*(*1*), 5. Retrieved from https://doi-org.ezproxy.lib.ucalgary.ca/10.1093/geront/gnt111

Warner, D. F., & Brown, T. H. (2011). Understanding how race/ethnicity and gender define age-trajectories of disability: An intersectionality approach. *Social Science & Medicine, 72*(8), 1236–1248. doi:10.1016/j.socscimed.2011.02.034

Woodward, K. (1999). *Figuring age: Women, bodies, generations.* Bloomington, IN: Indiana University Press.

Chapter 2

Theorizing later life and social work praxis

Questions to consider as you read this chapter

- What is theory, and how are theories related to and useful for social work practice?
- How do you explain the process of aging? What ideologies underpin your theory/ies of aging?
- How do we connect theories of aging, subjective or lived experiences of aging, and practice wisdom in AOP with older adults? Whose knowledge do we prioritize in personal and professional settings?
- Which theories of aging are most closely associated with AOG & AOP? How does/should theory inform our practice with older adults, their families, and communities?

My (Wendy's) Dad's best friend who is 84 years old has a theory that "street rodding" (restoring and modifying vintage cars to drive and show at events) prevents dementia. He first presented this idea to me several years ago and reminded me of it in June 2018 when I brought my 1957 Nash Metropolitan to a car show with them in Osoyoos, BC. This theory comes from his observation that within his circle of older, white, higher-income male street rodders who live in or near Victoria, BC – The Over the Hill Gang – no one has been diagnosed with dementia or shown symptoms of cognitive impairment to date. As a critical gerontologist well versed in the social determinants of health,[1] I think his theory is worth exploring for the same reason that I don't discount another dementia prevention strategy suggested to me by Secwepemc (First Nation in BC) Elders: Bring back bingo. The latter activity entailed walking to a community centre, sharing a meal prepared by community members, exercising one's mind by playing bingo, socializing/talking with other Elders, and receiving prizes such as a sack of potatoes. What both theories have in common is that they place emphasis on the socio-cultural and geo-political context in shaping experiences of aging and health and attribute agency to the older adult, without placing blame. The first theory has more of a chance of being taken up than the second one, as the theorist is an older, white, higher-income man, and that is generally who has theorized our social world. However, the second theory created by Secwepemc Elders (who are lower income and predominantly women) is more likely to be empirically valid than the one suggested by the Over the Hill Gang as the latter's higher-income, non-Indigenous status, and male gender reduce their risks of dementia.

We make and use theories on a daily basis, whether to explain why our partner left dirty dishes in the sink (e.g., they think it's our job to wash dishes, they ran out of time as their boss or one of our children called, a clean house is not as important as a happy household) or to understand why more women than men are caregivers (e.g., women are naturally more caring than men, women are socialized to care for family members, women's inequality in the workplace forces them to give up or reduce paid work to provide care, men's caring labour is less visible). Theories can be used to make decisions as basic as how to dress for the weather or to understand more complex matters like the state of the economy. Ask yourself if it makes a difference to you that the evidence for the former decision was a meteorologist giving a weather report on TV, while the latter opinion was informed by friends at the coffee shop. In other words, does the source affect the legitimacy of the theory? We don't usually think of our attempts to explain the social world that surrounds us and/or events in our daily lives as theorizing, yet it is. This does not make us theorists, however. Were we to test our theories through empirical research and then subject them to peer review, then perhaps we would be recognized as theorists.

Most dominant social theories have been developed by white, upper/middle-class, straight, able-bodied cisgender men, and the knowledge of those who deviate from this "mythical norm" (Lorde, 2001) is not seen to be as legitimate or get as much cir-culation and application. The everyday theorizing of older adults – the way they make sense of their social worlds – is usually dismissed or discounted as theory despite the results being similar to the explanations and insights of professionals and academics (Auger, Tedford-Litle, & Wallace-Allen, 2018; Gubrium & Wallace, 1990). *Active aging* is one example of this and indicates the power of neoliberal ideology and health promotion discourse, which instruct people to take responsibility for doing all that they can – by being physically active and eating healthily for example – to maintain their health and avoid life-limiting illnesses and disabilities.

Bruce is a retired insurance agent and a high-performance athlete who lives in a small city in BC's Interior. Bruce started running marathons when he retired at age 66 and took up triathlons a few years later; he continues to average four triathlons per year. I (Wendy) met Bruce over 14 years ago when we ran a relay race together, during which he took the hardest section (middle leg up a long steep hill) and I had the easiest (flat stretch to the finish line). After getting to know one another through this experience, I invited Bruce to co-teach a class on the aging process with me – first at a Philosopher's café to which I had been invited to speak and then in the aging class I had recently developed. We did this for several years, and each time Bruce would share with social work students his story of coming to competitive sports and distance running later in life and then present them with his formula for success-ful aging: thinking (positive outlook) and doing (physical activity). I would then share with them the physiology of aging (i.e., the decline narrative, according to geriatrics, as well as critical gerontological views on life extension) (Olshansky, Carnes, & Butler, 2015; see also Funk, 2016). While Bruce's formula aligns with active aging theory, much of his experience of aging counters the dominant narrative on aging as decline, as he is thriving rather than failing.

This chapter builds on the discussion of ageism and the intersectional life course per-spective introduced in the previous chapter. It starts with an overview of what theory and ideology are and how they relate to social work practice and a review of key social work theories relevant to gerontological social work, including the strengths perspective, solution-focussed practice, client/person-centred practice, and structural social work. After building on what students and practitioners might already know about theory and ideology from social work education and practice, we introduce key theories of the aging process and later life. This includes early theories (e.g., activity, disengagement, age stratification, exchange) and theories like political economy that are associated with critical gerontology along with those centred in particular standpoints (i.e., feminist, queer, post-structural, Indigenous). The latter theories are more aligned with AOG as they take into account lived experiences of older adults *and* the structural realities in which they live. Throughout this chapter, we focus on *praxis* – the integration of theory and practice – through the use of exercises and counter-stories.

The objectives for this chapter are to

- Make clear the relationship between social work theories and aging theories and their connections to ideology;
- Critically analyze theories from an AOG perspective;
- Illustrate the relevance and application of theories to practice; and
- Provide guidance on the use of theory in social work with older adults, their families, and communities.

The use of theory and ideology in social work

Theory guides social work practice, whether we are consciously aware of this or not. For example, students and practitioners may use genograms and ecomaps[2] routinely in their work yet be unaware that these tools are associated with systems theory and ecological perspectives (see Payne, 2014). Further, our ideological positioning affects which theories we draw upon in our practice. For example, those who position themselves as Marxists or Social Democrats are more likely to be drawn to structural and anti-oppressive theories than problem-solving or solution-focused theories, which are more closely aligned with Liberalism and Conservativism since these latter theories focus on helping the individual fit into the system rather than changing the system to better meet clients' needs. That said, we should always choose the theory that best fits the practice scenario (i.e., population, issue, setting), and social workers can make solution-focussed or problem-solving approaches more critical or transformative by applying a feminist or AOP perspective, for example.

Ideologies are worldviews or "systems of beliefs that guide our choices and behaviors and, indeed, justify our thoughts and actions" (Bailey & Gayle, 2008, p. 2). Unlike theories, which we consciously apply to the people or problems with which we interact in practice, we are often unconscious of our ideological positioning and/or the ideological framework that has led us to select a particular theory, model, framework, or perspective. Table 2.1 is an exercise that tests your knowledge of various ways to categorize social work theories. The response key is listed at the bottom of the Table.

Ideologies may be political as represented by the left to right spectrum of Marxism, Social Democracy, (Neo-)Liberalism, (Neo-)Conservatism, and Fascism (Freeden, 2003; McCullough, 2017). Ideologies may also be connected to the "isms" associated with social movements such as environmentalism and feminism (Bailey & Gayle,

Table 2.1 Exercise on types of social work theories

Which description best fits each of these different types of social work theories?
A. Explanatory theory   B. Models   C. Perspectives   D. Frameworks

1.	Extract patterns of activity from practice and structure how you approach a situation to ensure consistency.
2.	Express ways of thinking of the world based on principles that help you see situations from different points of view.
3.	Accounts for why an action results in or causes consequences and tells you what works and why.
4.	Organize bodies of knowledge in a systematic way so can select and use them in practice.

Answer key: 1-B, 2-C, 3-A, 4 -D

Based on Payne (2014, p. 93).

2008). One of the first tasks students face in becoming social workers is to identify their values and beliefs and gain an appreciation for how their personal ideologies have affected their lives to date. It is a process of becoming aware of "what we carry in our minds" (Dumbrill & Yee, 2019) before opening our minds to new/alternative under-standings of the social world in which we and others (including clients and colleagues) live, work, and play. While the definition of explanatory theory (why A causes B or what works and why) may be the one we think of when we think of theory, social work uses "theory" more broadly than other disciplines such as sociology and psychology. Healy (2014) refers to social work theories as "formal theories that are intended to guide and explain social work practices" (p. 111), while Payne (2014) defines social work theories as "generalized sets of ideas that describe and explain our knowledge of the world in an organized way" (p. 3). The latter more expansive definition allows for models, perspectives, and frameworks to fall under the umbrella of theory, alongside explanatory theories. We note that Indigenous theories are often framed as perspectives or worldviews, rather than theory. Basically, there are three types of theories that inform social work practice: theories of what social work is, theories of how to do social work, and theories of the client's world (Payne, 2014). The second group are usually called models, frameworks, and approaches.

Table 2.2 charts common social work theories in the field of aging and brief descriptions. All of these can be recognized as theories though they may not typically be termed as such (e.g., task-centred approach, narrative therapy, systems theory, structural social work). Some of the theories commonly used in social work such as attachment, psychodynamic, cognitive-behavioural, and crisis are not applied very often in Gerontological Social Work. This may be because we don't see older adults as capable of changing (e.g., "you can't teach an old dog new tricks") and/or dominant theories like disengagement run counter to attachment. You may have been exposed in social work to these theories that have applications to the process of aging and social work with older adults. In addition to the emphasis or key concepts associated with each practice theory, in the right column, we direct you to counter-stories and case studies in this book that relate most closely to each of these theories. Also, consider how each theory applies to your experiences to date with older adults.

Table 2.2 Praxis worksheet: 13 theories used in gerontological social work

	Theory	Emphasis/key points	Example in this book
1	Human development	Posits that individuals progress from birth to death through 8 stages, including trust vs. mistrust (birth to 12 months), identity vs. role confusion (12–18 years), and integrity vs. despair (mid-60s to end of life/death)	Bruce – Chapter 2 (theory) Charlene – Chapter 4 (risk) BB – Chapter 8 (trauma) Estella – Chapter 9 (mental health)
2	Task-centred/ goal-oriented/ problem solving	Practitioner identifies and/or isolates a problem, task, or goal and instructs the client/s on a step-wise approach to solving it	Louise – Chapter 4 (risk) Charlene – Chapter 4 (risk) Sachika – Chapter 6 (caregiving) James, Fannie, Peter, and Jeannie – Chapter 13 (everyday lives)
3	Client-centred (person-centred)	Positions the client as the expert and tailors intervention to them through use of congruence, unconditional positive regard, and empathy	Eleanor – Chapter 4 (risk) Robin – Chapter 5 (moral, legal, and ethical) Olive, Jimmy, Clara, Michael – Chapter 7 (dementia)
4	Solution-focussed	Practitioner assists client/s to envision a future with a desired solution and determines steps to arrive there via a specific line of questioning that includes 'the miracle question'	Louise – Chapter 4 (risk) Estella – Chapter 9 (mental health) South Cariboo (age friendly) – Chapter 11 (communities)
5	Systems	Seeks balance between different systems affecting individuals or families	Shari – Chapter 3 (sites and sectors) Mrs. P and Miles – Chapter 5 (moral, legal, and ethical)
6	Strengths	Sees individuals, families, and communities as resilient and capable with challenges to overcome	Les – Chapter 3 (sites and sectors) Charlene – Chapter 4 (risk) Sachika – Chapter 6 (caregiving) Olive - Chapter 7 (dementia) BB – Chapter 8 (trauma) Amina – Chapter 8 (trauma)
7	Feminist	Values the experiences and knowledge of women and strives for gender justice; considers the intersection of gender with other categories of differences	Olive – Chapter 7 (dementia) Penny – Chapter 10 (violence)
8	Narrative	A postmodern approach that assists client/s to re-story their lives by recognizing problems as external to them and rewriting difficult or challenging stories	Les – Chapter 3 (sites and sectors) Eleanor – Chapter 4 (risk) Sachika – Chapter 6 (caregiving) BB – Chapter 8 (trauma) Amina – Chapter 8 (trauma)
9	Structural	Recognizes the interplay between individual experiences and societal structures and works at all levels (micro, meso, macro)	Maria– Chapter 1 (age/ism) Shari – Chapter 3 (sites and sectors) Les – Chapter 3 (sites and sectors)

(Continued)

Table 2.2 (Cont).

	Theory	Emphasis/key points	Example in this book
		through covert and overt strategies	Wendy – Chapter 5 (moral, legal, and ethical) Michael – Chapter 7 (dementia) Ahnjong – Chapter 11 (communities) Alejandra – Chapter 11 (communities) Romero – Chapter 11 (communities) Ilyan – Chapter 12 (policy)
10	Queer	Disrupts binaries (e.g., man/woman, gay/straight) & challenges heteronormativity and cissexism	Les – Chapter 3 (sites and sectors) Olive – Chapter 7 (dementia) Josephine – Chapter 11 (communities)
11	Culturally safe	Sees need to move beyond being aware, sensitive, or competent to shifting power in order to create safety (as defined by the client/service user)	Les – Chapter 3 (sites & sectors) Sachika – Chapter 6 (caregiving) Michael – Chapter 7 (dementia) Amina – Chapter 8 (trauma) Francesko and Chantele – Chapter 11 (communities) Mr. Nguyen – Chapter 12 (policy)
12	Critical Race	Focusses on experiences of racialized people and uses counter-storytelling to disrupt master/dominant narratives	Kamali – Chapter 1 (age/ism) Sachika – Chapter 6 (caregiving) Amina – Chapter 8 (trauma) Romero – Chapter 11 (communities)
13	Indigenous	Emphasizes (physical, spiritual, emotional, mental) holism, balance, respect, and interconnectedness	Ona – Chapter 2 (theory) Secwepemc Elders – Chapter 2 (theory) Michael – Chapter 7 (dementia)

Theories of aging: expanding outward from the individual

Theorizing aging began with early individualistic theories based on order views of society and grew to include more structurally focussed theories located within a conflict perspective[3] (Bengston, Burgess, & Parrott, 1997). This theoretical shift outward from the individual to the wider society and then coming to rest on the individual within society that occurred in aging studies is similar to the history of social work theory. Theorizing about older people and the aging process has largely been the work of "the aging enterprise" (Estes, 1979, 1993), not of older people themselves (Gubrium & Wallace, 1990); older people's attempts at making meaning of their experiences of getting older and "being old" are not usually acknowledged as theories by "the aging enterprise" (see textbox 2.1). It has been argued successfully, however, that there are remarkable parallels between the intellectual products of "the aging enterprise" and those of older people themselves (Auger & Tedford-Litle, 2002; Gubrium & Wallace, 1990). For example, older adults particularly like activity and continuity theory (Auger, Tedford-Litle & Wallace-Allen, 2018). We also saw this alignment of views on aging earlier in the story of Bruce, the marathoner and triathlete.

Textbox 2.1

A conceptual term created by critical gerontologist Carroll Estes in 1979, **the aging enterprise** refers to all those who work within the gerontology and geriatrics sector and thus are invested in sustaining an industry created to respond to, and more importantly, profit from, population aging.

Early (micro) theories of aging

The first- and second-generation theories of aging included disengagement, activity, exchange, modernization, socio-environmentalism, age stratification, sub-culture, and continuity (Bengston et al., 1997). We describe most of these theories to expose their ideological differences and show how the focus has expanded outward from the individual to their social environment and societal structures (Katz, 1996), the latter being of more interest/relevance to AOP social workers. In the brief overview that follows, we note connections to social work theories and/or when these theories of aging have been adopted/promoted by gerontological social workers as well as newer theoretical developments associated with these more micro theories. As a visual guide to this chapter and the relationship between theory and practice (praxis), we include our diagram of **theorizing later life and social work praxis** in Figure 2.1 that shows how the social work theories in Table 2.2 are associated with the theories of aging that follow and how these theories link to levels of social work practice.

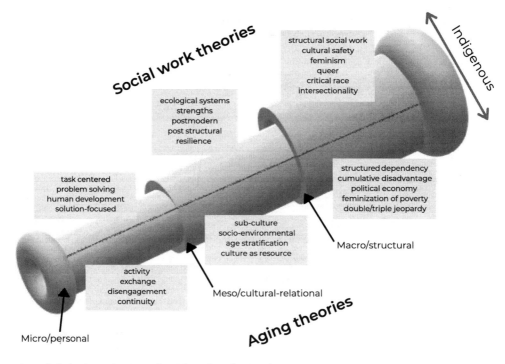

Figure 2.1 A telescopic view of social work and aging theories

Disengagement theory (Cumming & Henry, 1961) argued that older people all go through a process of gradual disengagement from society in preparation for death. Older people choose to exclude themselves and are expected to do so, as this contributes to the functioning of society. A criticism of this "functional" theory of aging is that it "condones a policy of indifference" (Bond, Briggs, & Coleman, 1993, p. 32) and ignores structural influences on the lives of older people. *Exchange theory* (Dowd, 1975) also portrayed older adults as non-contributory (i.e., having fewer resources to exchange, and this was identified as the reason for their disengagement). The key difference between this and disengagement theory is that the latter sees withdrawal (e.g., from the labour market or the housing market) as being beneficial to older adults (and functional to society), while exchange theory suggests that older adults are forced to disengage due to unequal exchange relationships (i.e., they have less to offer than younger/working-age people). Exchange theory has been critiqued for its marketization of familial/intergenerational relationships (Funk, 2016).

Associated with *disengagement theory* and *exchange theory*, as it too focussed on the individual actor, is *activity theory*. Activity theory proposed that successful aging can be achieved by denying or rejecting the "onset of old age" through the maintenance of and/or replacement of lost relationships, networks, and activities (Havighurst, 1961). Activity theory has been critiqued for being idealistic and enforcing a normative view of aging (Katz, 2000), yet it appears to resonate with older adults themselves (Auger et al., 2018). Further, this theory has been promoted by gerontological social workers who see it as aligned with social work values and ethics as it challenges ageism, focusses on autonomy and choice, and considers the person in their socio–cultural and political-economic environment (Chonody & Teater, 2017), the latter being limited in our opinion. The concept of active aging has been criticized for being oppressive to marginalized and disadvantaged older adults (Katz, 2000; Ranzijn, 2010). This includes Indigenous Elders in Australia for whom alternative conceptualizations like "aging well" or "authentic aging" are more culturally appropriate and better able to promote social inclusion (Ranzijn, 2010).

There is a close association between activity theory and the discourse of *successful aging* (Rowe & Kahn, 1987) and *healthy, positive, and productive aging,* as all of these terms are connected to neoliberal ideology and governmentality (Katz, 2000; Rudman, 2015; Sandberg & Marshall, 2017). Some critical gerontologists have attempted revisions of *successful aging* to bring it more in line with Indigenous views on later life (Lewis, 2010; Pace & Grenier, 2017) while others have rejected this discourse (Chonody & Teater, 2017), seeing it as incompatible with social work values and ethics due to its individualism (p. 174). The *theory of model aging* builds on this conceptual coherence and proposes that "the discourses of active and successful aging model the social representations of later life, as well as the practices and narratives of older people" (Timonen, 2016, as cited in São José, Timonen, Amado, & Santos, 2017, p. 50). In other words, these discourses tell older adults how they should be, act, and talk. While AOP social workers are unlikely to find much use for activity theory and associated discourses of active and successful aging, another micro theory called the *capabilities approach* (Robeyns, 2005) is promising as it focusses on what older adults are able "to do and to be", thus resonating with the strengths perspective in social work (Saleebey, 1996). This approach has been recommended for older adults with disabilities in particular due to its incorporation of "care, dependence, and dignity" and has been used "to claim injustice in unmet needs and the oppression of those who provide care" (Berridge, 2012, p. 18), thereby allowing for a focus on both care recipients and care providers.

Socio-environmentalism (Gubrium, 1972, 1973) was one of the first theories of aging to describe meaning as derived through social interaction and behavior as learned through interactions between individuals and other members of their social worlds (i.e., society), in the tradition of symbolic interactionism (see Manis & Meltzer, 1967). Older people's responses to the aging process were thought to be shaped through their socio-cultural environment and social life to arise from society itself (i.e., the social actors), not from external structures (e.g. government, economy) per se. Another theory that takes into consideration the socio-cultural context surrounding the individual is *age stratification theory* (Riley, 1971), which put forward the idea that society is structured on the basis of age strata (young, middle, old age) with key activities associated with each strata (education, work, leisure). This theory has been critiqued for its normative approach to roles and activities, much like systems theory.

Critical gerontology

Power is a central focus of *critical gerontology,* which arises from three strands of intellectual thought: (1) political economy perspectives, (2) the humanities with its focus on the moral economy, and (3) biographical and narrative approaches (Phillipson, 1998, p. 13). Critical gerontology has its roots in critical social theory, which is concerned with seeking not only to understand the world, but also to transform it (as Marx advised) and can be seen as a reaction to traditional gerontological theorizing about aging and older people (Bengston et al., 1997; Estes, 1993; Estes, Biggs, & Phillipson, 2003; Holstein & Minkler, 2003; Minkler & Estes, 1991). Katz (1996, p. 4) summarized the work of critical gerontology as

- admonishing gerontology for its narrow scientificity;
- advocating closer ties to the humanities;
- endorsing reflexive methodologies;
- historicizing ideological attributes of old age;
- promoting radical political engagement; and
- signifying the aging process as heterogeneous and indeterminate.

Underpinning the critical gerontology tradition is the recognition that old age is socially constructed and that structural inequalities differentially shape experiences of later life (Phillipson, 1998). Social exclusion has been recommended by critical gerontologists in social work as a promising framework for explicating "the various intersecting ways in which elderly people are excluded from public services, participation in public life and community, and are increasingly relegated to the home" (Grenier & Guberman, 2009, p. 122). For example, poor public transportation can exclude older adults from both social events and diagnostic medicine.

The *political economy of aging perspective* (Walker, 1981) and *structured dependency theory* (Townsend, 1981; Wilson, 1997) are examples of work that falls within the critical gerontology tradition. The political economy of aging perspective is concerned with the interrelationships between the economy, society, and polity (politics) and how they impact resource distribution and the lives of older people. Political economy of aging has been critiqued for its class emphasis, yet is thought to be flexible enough to incorporate gender, race, and ethnicity. Feminist critical gerontologists expanded political economy to include the moral economy as well (Holstein & Minkler, 2003; Minkler & Estes, 1991). Structured dependency refers to the dependent position in which older people, or more accurately "pensioners", are placed in order to meet the needs of a capitalist society. Thus, retirement is an important institution for moving people out of the labour market so that others can move in and is responsible for the creation of a dependent class of people – pensioners or retirees.

Feminist theory

A feminist perspective on aging furthers the feminist goal of achieving gender justice and destabilizing the sex/gender system by focussing on the disadvantages experienced by older women, thereby adding an analysis of aging and ageism to gender and (hetero & cis) sexism (Ginn & Arber, 1995; Krekula, 2007). Such disadvantages could be part of a lifelong pattern (e.g., cumulative) or newly experienced later in life. Poverty is a good example of this, with divorce and widowhood resulting in a sharp decrease in income for older women compared to older men (Davis, Grant, & Rowland, 1990) and older ethno-cultural minority and racialized women having significantly lower incomes than white women and men (Brotman, 1998). Feminist perspectives on aging have illuminated the gendered dimensions of the aging process not only in terms of how the physiological changes associated with aging are experienced differently by men and women – and more recently transgender people – but also how the visible signs of aging are responded to differently.

Hooyman, Browne, Ray, and Richardson (2002) proposed nine elements to consider in analyzing policies from a feminist gerontological perspective:

1. Inequality and oppression;
2. Diversity and aging;
3. Production and reproduction;
4. Separate spheres and familism;
5. Political and structural change;
6. Power and empowerment;
7. Holistic and ecological view;
8. Solidarity; and
9. Alternative methodology (as cited in Netting, 2011, p. 241).

Many of these concepts are foregrounded in this book, including inequality, oppression, diversity, familism, and power, and are foundational to an AOP approach. Social work has been a leader in feminist gerontology, though our profession has mostly applied feminist theory to social work practice with older adults with theoretical developments happening more recently. The latter includes the "provisioning" work of older women (Neysmith & Reitsma-Street, 2009), the temporal and contextual nature of intersectionality and interlocking oppressions (Hulko, 2009), transitions and ruptures in later life (Grenier, 2012), the intersectional life course perspective (Ferrer, Brotman, Grenier, & Koehn, 2017), and anti-oppression gerontology (Hulko, Brotman, & Ferrer, 2017). Much earlier than this, feminist gerontological social work scholars were promoting AOP perspectives, person-centred practice, and the life course, with Chambers (2004) stressing the need to "introduce future social workers to knowledge, theories and practice which enable them to engage in sensitive, creative, anti-oppressive practice with those older women who are in receipt of personal social services" (p. 375). Further, applying critical social gerontological theories and taking a narrative approach can allow us to appreciate how

> older women have an acute awareness of both 'age' and 'gender' as integral to their multiple narratives. 'Age' in terms of both belonging to a particular gener- ation and also 'personal' ageing, and 'gender' as a social construction over the life course, combining with personal aging in recent years.
>
> (Chambers, 2004, p. 756)

This too aligns nicely with the AOG approach detailed in this book.

Intersectionality, aging, and the social model of disabilities

In **Age/ism: age as a category of difference**, we addressed how *intersectionality and inter- locking oppressions* (see textbox 1.5) is an important theoretical framework arising from critical race theory[4] and feminist theory and brought into aging studies by critical feminist gerontolo- gists. Those adopting this theoretical framework reject additive (e.g., *double jeopardy*) and reductionist approaches in favour of an integrative analysis that sees inequalities as intersecting and as structuring life course opportunities and people as cohesive units, not divided into strands of identity (Calasanti, 1996; Dressel, Minkler, & Yen, 1997; Vincent, 1995). This includes disability scholars looking at aging with a disability and referring to the additive approach as "serving to atomise, distort and marginalize" experiences (Zarb & Oliver, 1993, p. 16).

Regarding the connection between aging theories and disability models, Putnam (2002) advocates not only for the incorporation of intersectionality, but also for distinctions to be made among physical impairment, functional limitations, and disabilities. This is in line with the *social model of disability,* which posits that society causes disability for those living with impairments or functional limitations by creating barriers to built and social environments that constrain access and participation (Oliver, 1996). The social model of disability can be combined with the capabilities approach to address both individual experiences and structural constraints. As we said at the beginning of this chapter, we do not want AOP social workers to reject any theories outright (i.e., because they are more micro-oriented), but rather consider how adopting a particular lens or perspective enables you to engage with these micro-oriented or direct practice theories differently. As Putnam (2002) recommends, geron- tological social workers should not only make the distinctions among physical impairments, functional limitations, and abilities to better serve older adults aging with disabilities, but they should also consider the person in their environment and the social context of aging.

Culture as a resource and resiliency theory

As a counterpoint to double jeopardy theory (see **Age/ism: age as a category of differ- ence**), Simic (1993) sought to demonstrate that *culture is a resource*, claiming that double jeop- ardy neglects the benefits provided to older people through ethnic group membership, such as adaptive strategies, positive self-image, and "insurance," and citing the involvement of older people in activities, roles, and rituals as evidence of the strength of this argument. This is an important point – ethno-cultural and racialized group membership may result in benefits as well as disadvantages. However, it discounts the facts that structural disadvantage differentially affects minority ethnic and racialized older people and that communities provide their members with resources in the face of inequitable, oppressive, and systemically patterned social conditions. Zubair and Norris (2015) note both the positive or protective factors of ethnic group membership and the multiple and interconnected dimensions of social inequalities and argue that the latter should be the focus of research, rather than ethnic culture per se. This has occurred in social work research on Indigenous aging by pairing resiliency theory with a strengths-based perspective (Baskin & Davey, 2015). Through conducting a sharing circle with 12 older Indigenous women in Toronto, most of whom were residential school survivors, the researchers found "the importance of friendships and community involvement to [be key to] their wellbeing and enjoyment of life" as women growing older together (Baskin & Davey, 2015, p. 84). This is precisely the "insurance" that Simic (1993) refers to in his theory of culture as resource.

Postmodernism and post-structuralism

Postmodern and post-structural thought has not been well developed in the context of aging, particularly within critical gerontology (van Dyk, 2014) as the latter views inequalities as due to relatively fixed or stable categories of difference and systems of domination like capitalism and patriarchy. *Postmodernism* (meaning "after modernism") rejects the belief in and search for one universal truth that was a key trait of modernism, favouring instead partial truths, diversity and difference, and multiple knowledge claims. For example, there is no one "right" way to age or experience being older. Power is thought to be more diffuse by post-structuralists, rather than held by certain groups (e.g., the power elite, the bourgeoisie, the ruling class, the dominant class), and they go farther than postmodernists in challenging the stability of (and deconstructing) categories of difference like gender, race, class, and age. For example, van Dyk (2014) contests the binary constructs and homogenizing tendencies of critical gerontology (e.g., old age and middle age), arguing for the introduction of "concepts that problematize on difference and (age) identity" (p. 101) in order to overcome the positioning of older adults as either the same as or different than the rest of the population.

In reviewing postmodern and post-structuralist (specifically Bourdieu's) views on power, Dumbrill and Yee (2019) argue that "the anti-oppressive social worker needs to be able to think outside simplistic binaries to develop a more nuanced understanding of power struggles" (p. 75). Bourdieu's conceptualization of power as embedded in four different forms of capital – economic, cultural, social, and symbolic – is important for AOP social workers to understand as it moves beyond Marx's view of capital as singular/economic and the associated binary opposition (i.e., ruling class and working class).

Narrative approaches are associated with postmodernism and post-structuralism and hold promise for social work with older adults (Armstrong, 2017; Clark, 2015; Randall, Baldwin, McKenzie-Mohr, McKim, & Furlong, 2015); for this reason, narrative therapy/care is included in our praxis worksheet (see Table 2.2). Randall et al. (2015) connect resilience theory to narrative therapy based on their analysis of interviews with older adults in New Brunswick who received either high or low scores on a resilience scale, concluding that these narratives are best viewed as "first drafts". Thus, the authors suggest that working through narratives with older adults can enhance their resilience. Based on a review of reminiscence work with older adults,

Armstrong (2017) suggests there are benefits to using narrative approaches with iso-lated older adults in particular and calls for specific training in reminiscence, life story work, and/or narrative therapy for those working in aging services. In Clark's (2015) analysis of narratives operating in interprofessional teamwork with older adults, the role of social work is identified as crucial in "ensuring that the patient's story encom-passes the entire context of his or her life, not just those aspects that are more nar-rowly disease-specific" (p. 180) and notes that in light of the stereotypes and ageism in health and social care "convincing counter-stories are needed to challenge the dominant narrative being forced upon an older patient" (p. 180).

Queer theory

Like post-structuralism, queer theory disrupts binaries, particularly those related to sex and gender, calls into question what is considered "normal" with respect to sexuality and gender identity/expression, and challenges both heteronormativity – the presumption that all people are heterosexual – and cissexism – discrimination towards those who transgress gender norms. Look at Table 2.3 and try to identify which categories of difference or groups of people are left out (excluded) when a binary sex/gender system is used.

Although queer theory is increasingly used in social work and social gerontology, it is not well developed theoretically in terms of its application to the aging process and the lives and experiences of older adults. In their recent systematic review of the use of theory in LGBTQ aging research, Fabbre, Jen, and Fredriksen-Goldsen (2019) found the most common theories used to be minority stress, the health promotion equity model, and resiliency theory. Importantly, they note that gerontologists researching LGBTQ aging are "utilizing or developing theories that fill conceptual gaps left by mainstream gerontology" (p. 14), including queer theory. This includes social work scholar Anne Siverskog who states that "a queer lens on gerontology questions the often-taken-for-granted assumptions about "men" and "women" having bodies, iden-tities, and expressions that follow linearity" (2015, p. 16), noting that the term "cisgen-der" is an example of a linear approach. Relying on a post-structural understanding of the body as agential (i.e., having agency), Siverskog (2015) demonstrates through her life story research with six older transgender persons that "bodies are not passive mater-ial" (bodies do, they are not just done to) and suggests that applying this approach to theorizing later life can bridge the divide between a social and discursive (as in dis-course) approach to aging versus a strictly biomedical one. Drawing on queer, feminist, and crip[5] theory, Sandberg and Marshall (2017) illustrate how *successful aging* relies on "narratives of hetero-happiness and of able-bodiedness/able-mindedness" (p. 7), thus foreclosing the possibility of aging well into the future for queer folk and those with life-limiting illnesses and disabilities. They suggest that these critical theories be brought into gerontological theory and research not only to overcome binaries like success and failure, but also to enable a greater range of aging futures to be envisioned.

Table 2.3 Sex and gender binaries

Sex	Male/Female
Gender Identity	Man/Woman
Sexual Orientation	Heterosexual (straight)/Homosexual (gay or lesbian)

Indigenous worldviews

Indigenous worldviews generally present the aging process as cyclical rather than linear, with the starting point being birth, after which the individual moves through youth and adulthood before becoming an Elder and returning to the start of the circle at death, which represents a return to the spirit world from whence the individual came (Grande, 2018; Hulko et al., 2010; Hulko, Wilson, & Balestrery, 2019; Pace & Grenier, 2017). The significance of this cyclical perspective on aging is evident in the similar findings of dementia research conducted with Indigenous Elders in Saskatchewan, BC, and Ontario; most of the Elders from six different First Nations viewed memory loss in later life from this cyclical perspective, as in "back to the baby stage" (SK), "going through the full circle of life" (BC) and "coming full circle" (ON) (Purves & Hulko, 2019, p. 197; see also Hulko et al., 2019). Importantly, Elders implicated colonization in the disruption of this cyclical view of aging (Hulko et al., 2010; Purves & Hulko, 2019).

Searching for an Indigenous counter-narrative of aging that foregrounds relations of responsibility, collectivity, mutuality, and reciprocity, Grande (2018) sees the possibility of a "decolonial option" in the aforementioned dementia research as well as Lewis' (2010) research on successful aging for Alaskan Elders. These counter-narratives hint at the Indigenous elsewhere evoked by Grande's (2018) reflection on her mother's experience of living and dying with dementia, which we include here as a counter-story on Indigenous aging.

It was a privilege to be by Ona's side as she journeyed elsewhere. She reported back on her travels through the spirit world in great and vivid detail. During the Ukrainian crisis, she recounted her visit to the Oval Office and the advice she gave to the President. She often travelled back home to her community and once she went back to school where she recalled working "so hard" to please the nuns. Across all her excursions, she was powerful, instrumental, and ruminative. In her final days, she spoke in multiple languages – English, Spanish, and Quechua – moving effortlessly through her life span, including a visceral and dramatic reliving of her experience of giving birth. As the so-called "disease" of dementia progressed, she gained a deeper sense of herself, becoming ever more cognizant of where she had been and where she was going. Until, she went.

(Grande, 2018, p. 178)

This chapter concludes with the above quote, to leave you pondering its meaning/lesson, consistent with an Indigenous approach to storytelling. We hope that the contents of this chapter will enable you to be conscious and critical about the linkage between theory and practice and perhaps encourage you to consider ways in which other theories (including those yet to be created) shape and explain our social world and the work we do within it.

Exercise

Take a blank piece of paper and make a drawing of the theories discussed in this chapter. This can be a diagram, a map, a flow chart, or any other type of drawing. It should depict one of the following: (1) the relationship between aging theories and social work theories; (2) connections between the theories discussed and social work practice in a particular site or sector of health and social care; or (3) the links between these theories and micro (personal/individual), meso (community/socio–cultural and relational), and macro (societal/structural) levels of social problems/social work practice. After you finish your drawing, discuss it with a classmate. Then compare your drawings with Figure 2.1.

Takeaways

- Like social work theories, theories of aging describe and explain micro, meso, and macro experiences of older adults in relation to themselves, their families and communities, and society at large.
- Some theories of aging are more aligned with AOP social work and include the theories that fall under critical gerontology.
- The theories we use when working with older adults, their families, and communities are informed by our ideological positioning and the practice settings in which we work and may be social work theories, theories of aging, or a blend of these two bodies of knowledge.
- Gerontological social work needs to expand beyond the use of micro- or individual-oriented theories and practice approaches to adopt critical theories of aging and AOP perspectives that focus on the socio-cultural, relational, and political-economic contexts of older adults' lives.

Notes

1 Social determinants of health (SDOH) are the economic and social factors that cause the poor health of individuals, communities, and societies as a whole (Health Canada, 2019; Mikkonen & Raphael, 2010; WHO, 2013). Income and income distribution/social status, housing/physical environments, gender, education, employment and working conditions, Aboriginal status/race and racism and childhood development/experiences are the most commonly cited SDOH which range from 12 to 14 when enumerated (Health Canada, 2019; Mikkonen & Raphael, 2010). Importantly, when Health Canada added race and racism to its list of determinants on June 28, 2019, it also noted that "experiences of discrimination, racism and historical trauma are important social determinants of health for certain groups such as Indigenous Peoples, LGBTQ and Black Canadians" (para. 3). Further, the World Health Organization (CSDH, 2008) identifies negative health experiences as arising from "a toxic combination of poor social policies and programmes, unfair economic arrangements, and bad politics" (as cited in Mikkonen & Raphael, 2010, p. 8), all of which are targets of AOP social work interventions.

2 A genogram is a pictorial display of a person's family relationships (McGoldrick, Gerson, & Petry, 2008) while an ecomap depicts systems with which the family interacts (Hartman, 1978). These tools are commonly used in social work for client personal records and/or to explore family dynamics with the client. Although there have been many adaptations to genograms and ecomaps over the past three decades, they continue to be critiqued for focussing almost entirely on the individual and paying little or no attention to structural and contextual forms of power that influence family dynamics, including impacts of racism, classism, sexism, and other forms of oppression (see Iversen, Gergen, & Fairbanks, 2005 for a fuller accounting of the history, tensions, and uses of the genogram and ecomap from a social constructivist perspective).

3 Order and conflict views of society refer to (1) interest in *conserving* the status quo and use of law and order to maintain it and (2) understanding of (capitalist) societies as necessarily conflictual due to competing interests and structural inequalities (see Mullaly, 2007).

4 Critical race theory (CRT) and by extension critical race feminism (CRT-f) emerged following the Civil Rights era in the United States and draws from several disciplines to examine how race and gender intersect with other categories of difference such as class, dis/ability, and sexual orientation (Bell, Delgado, & Stefancic, 2005; Matsuda, Lawrence, Delgado, & Crenshaw, 1993) and how the experiences of "people of color" are situated within interlocking vectors of power and oppression (Razack, Smith, & Thobani, 2010). To date there have been few attempts to introduce CRT and CRT-f into social gerontology though this has been recommended by feminist gerontologists (Byrnes, 2016).

5 Crip theory shares with queer theory a concern with challenging notions of normalcy *and* the adoption of an intersectionality perspective with the central focus of the former being the body and pleasure. Crip theory asks what makes some bodies "able" and others "disabled" and why the sexuality of disabled and/or queer bodies is deemed deviant (McRuer, 2006). Both queer and crip are words that have been reclaimed by queer and disability activists/ scholars respectively. While it is okay to use these words in relation to theory or a body of knowledge if it is named as such, AOP social workers need to be cautious about adopting words that were (and may still be) used to harm certain groups of people, especially if we are not members of the communities in question.

References

Armstrong, C. (2017). Combining reminiscence therapy with oral history to intervene in the lives of isolated older people. *Counselling Psychology Review, 32*(1), 26–32. Retrieved from https:// dspace.lboro.ac.uk/dspace-jspui/handle/2134/22362

Auger, J., Tedford-Litle, D., & Wallace-Allen, B. (2018). *From the inside looking out: Competing ideas about growing old* (2nd ed.). Halifax, NS: Fernwood Publishing.

Auger, J., & Tedford-Litle, D.(2002). *From the inside looking out: Competing ideas about growing old.* Halifax, NS: Fernwood Publishing.

Bailey, G., & Gayle, N. (2008). *Ideology: Structuring identities in contemporary life.* Toronto, ON: University of Toronto Press.

Baskin, C., & Davey, C. (2015). Grannies, elders, and friends: Aging aboriginal women in Toronto. *Journal of Gerontological Social Work, 58*(1), 46–65. doi:10.1080/01634372.2014.912997

Bell, D. A., Delgado, R., & Stefancic, J. (2005). Race and class. In D. A. Bell, R. Delgado, & J. Stefancic (Eds.), *The Derrick Bell reader* (pp. 369–396). New York: New York University Press.

Bengston, V. L., Burgess, E. O., & Parrott, T. M. (1997). Theory, explanation, and a third generation of theoretical development in social gerontology. *Journal of Gerontology: Social Sciences, 52B*(2), S72–S88. doi:10.1093/geronb/52B.2.S72

Berridge, C. (2012). Envisioning a gerontology-enriched theory of care. *Affilia: Journal of Women and Social Work, 27*(1), 8–21. doi:10.1177/0886109912437498

Bond, J., Briggs, R., & Coleman, P. (1993). The study of ageing. In J. Bond, P. Coleman, & S. Pease (Eds.), *Ageing in society: An introduction to social gerontology* (pp. 19–52). London: Sage.

Brotman, S. (1998). The incidence of poverty among seniors in Canada: Exploring the impact of gender, ethnicity and race. *Canadian Journal of Aging, 17*(2), 166–185. doi:10.1017/ S0714980800009247

Byrnes, M. (2016). Grow old with me! Future directions of race, age, and place scholarship. *Sociology Compass, 10*(10), 906–917. doi:10.1111/soc4.12348/epdf

Calasanti, T. (1996). Incorporating diversity: Meaning, levels of research, and implications for theory. *The Gerontologist, 36*(2), 147–156.

Chambers, P. (2004). The case for critical social gerontology in social work education and older women. *Social Work Education, 23*(6), 748–758. doi:10.1080/0261547042000294518a

CSDH Commission on Social Determinants of Health. (2008). *Closing the gap in a generation: Health equity through action on the social determinants of health. Final Report of the Commission on Social Determinants of Health.* Geneva: World Health Organization. Retrieved from https://apps.who.int/iris/ bitstream/handle/10665/43943/9789241563703_eng.pdf;jsessionid=7C05D49F86FA79 B5657AB84C73ABEC51?sequence=1

Chonody, J., & Teater, B. (2017). Promoting actively aging: Advancing a framework for social work practice with older adults. *Families in Society: The Journal of Contemporary Social Services, 98*(2), 137–145. doi:10.1606/1044-3894.2017.98.19

Clark, P. (2015). Emerging themes in using narrative in geriatric care: Implications for patient centred practice and interprofessional teamwork. *Journal of Aging Studies, 34*, 177–182. doi:10.1016/j.jaging.2015.02.013

Cumming, E., & Henry, W. E. (1961). *Growing old: The process of disengagement.* New York: Basic Books.

Davis, K., Grant, P., & Rowland, D. (1990). Alone and poor: The plight of elderly women. *Generations, 14*(3), 43–47. doi:10.1017/S0714980800008783

Dowd, J. J. (1975). Aging as exchange: A preface to theory. *Journal of Gerontology: Social Sciences, 30*(5), 584–594.

Dressel, P., Minkler, M., & Yen, I. (1997). Gender, race, class, and aging: Advances and opportunities. *International Journal of Health Services, 27*(4), 579–600. doi:10.2190/7XAY-PYBN-AA5L-3DRC

Dumbrill, G. C., & Yee, J. Y. (2019). *Anti-oppressive social work: Ways of knowing, talking, and doing.* Don Mills, ON: Oxford University Press.

Estes, C. (1979). *The ageing enterprise.* San Francisco, CA: Jossey-Bass.

Estes, C. (1993). The ageing enterprise revisited. *The Gerontologist, 33*(3), 291–298.

Estes, C. L., Biggs, S., & Phillipson, C. (2003). *Social theory, social policy and ageing: A critical introduction.* Maidenhead: Open University Press.

Fabbre, V., Jen, S., & Fredriksen-Goldsen, K. (2019). The state of theory in LGBTQ aging: Implications for gerontological scholarship. *Research on Aging,* 1–24. doi:10.1177/0164027518822814

Ferrer, I., Brotman, S., Grenier, A., & Koehn, S. (2017). Understanding the experiences of racialized older people through an intersectional life course perspective. *Journal of Aging Studies, 41,* 10–17. doi:10.1016/j.jaging.2017.02.001

Freeden, M. (2003). *Ideology: A very short introduction.* Don Mills, ON: Oxford University Press.

Funk, L. (2016). *Sociological perspectives on aging.* Don Mills, ON: Oxford University Press.

Ginn, J., & Arber, S. (1995). 'Only connect': Gender relations and ageing. In S. Arber & J. Ginn (Eds.), *Connecting gender and ageing: A sociological approach* (pp. 1–14). Milton Keynes: Open University Press.

Grande, S. (2018). Aging, precarity, and the struggle for Indigenous elsewheres. *International Journal of Qualitative Studies in Education, 31*(3), 168–176. doi:10.1080/09518398.2017.1401145

Grenier, A. (2012). *Transitions and the life course: Challenging the constructions of "growing old".* Chicago, IL: Policy Press.

Grenier, A. M., & Guberman, N. (2009). Creating and sustaining disadvantage: The relevance of a social exclusion framework. *Health and Social Care in the Community, 17*(2), 116–124. doi:10.1111/j.1365-2524.2007.00804.x

Gubrium, J. F. (1972). Toward a socio-environmental theory of aging. *The Gerontologist, 12*(3, Pt. 1), 281-284. doi:10.1093/geront/12.3_Part_1.281

Gurbrium, J. F. (1973). *The myth of the golden years: A socio-environmental theory of aging.* Springfield, IL: Thomas.

Gubrium, J. F., & Wallace, B. (1990). Who theorises age? *Ageing & Society, 10,* 131–149. doi:10.1017/S0144686X00008047

Hartman, A. (1978, reprinted 1995). Diagrammatic assessment of family relationships. *Families in Society: The Journal of Contemporary Human Services, 76*(2), 111–122.

Havighurst, R. J. (1961). Successful aging. *The Gerontologist, 1,* 8–13. doi:10.1093/geront/1.1.8

Health Canada. (2019, June 28). *What determines health.* Retrieved from www.canada.ca/en/public-health/services/healthpromotion/populationhealth/what-determines-health.html

Healy, K. (2014). *Social work theories in context: Creating frameworks for practice* (2nd ed.). Houndsmills: Palgrave Macmillan.

Holstein, M. B., & Minkler, M. (2003). Self, society and the "new gerontology." *The Gerontologist, 43*(6), 787–796. doi:10.1093/geront/43.6.787

Hooyman, N., Browne, C. V., Ray, R., & Richardson, V. (2002). Feminist gerontology and the life course. *Gerontology & Geriatrics Education, 22,* 3–26. doi:10.1300/J021v22n04_02

Hulko, W. (2009). The time and context contingent nature of intersectionality and interlocking oppressions. *Affilia: Journal of Women and Social Work, 24*(1), 44–55. doi:10.1177/0886109908326814.

Hulko, W., Brotman, S., & Ferrer, I. (2017). Counter-storytelling: Anti-oppressive social work with older adults. In D. Baines (Ed.), *Doing anti-oppressive practice: Social justice social work* (3rd ed., pp. 193–211). Halifax, NS: Fernwood Publishing.

Hulko, W., Camille, E., Antifeau, E., Arnouse, M., Bachynksi, N., & Taylor, D. (2010). Views of First Nation Elders on memory loss and memory care in later life. *Journal of Cross-Cultural Gerontology*, *25*(4), 317–342. doi:10.1007/s10823-010-9123-9.

Hulko, W., Wilson, D., & Balestrery, J. (Eds.). (2019). *Indigenous peoples and dementia: New understandings of memory loss and memory care*. Vancouver, BC: UBC Press.

Iversen, R. R., Gergen, K. J., & Fairbanks, R. P., II. (2005). Assessment and social construction: Conflict or co-creation? *British Journal of Social Work*, *35*(5), 689–708. Retrieved from https://repository.upenn.edu/spp_papers/27

Katz, S. (1996). *Disciplining old age: The formation of gerontological knowledge*. Charlottesville, VA and London: University Press of Virginia.

Katz, S. (2000). Busy bodies: Activity, aging, and the management of everyday life. *Journal of Aging Studies*, *14*(2), 135–152. doi:10.1016/S0890-4065(00)80008-0

Krekula, C. (2007). The intersection of age and gender reworking gender theory and social gerontology. *Current Sociology*, *55*(2), 155–171. doi:10.1177/0011392107073299

Lewis, J. P. (2010). Successful aging through the eyes of Alaska natives: Exploring generational differences among Alaska natives. *Journal of Cross-Cultural Gerontology*, *25*(4), 385–396. doi:10.1007/s10823-010-9124-8

Lorde, A. (2001). Age, race, class, and sex: Women redefining difference. In M. L. Andersen & P. Hill Collins (Eds.), *Race, class, and gender: An anthology* (4th ed., pp. 177–184). Belmont, CA: Wadsworth.

Manis, J. G., & Meltzer, B. N. (Eds.). (1967). *Symbolic interaction: A reader in social psychology*. Boston, MA: Allyn and Bacon.

Matsuda, M. J., Lawrence, C. R., Delgado, R., & Crenshaw, K. M. (1993). *Words that wound: Critical race theory, assaultive speech, and the first amendment*. Boulder, CO: Westview Press.

McCullough, H. B. (2017). *Political ideologies* (2nd ed.). Don Mills, ON: Oxford University Press.

McGoldrick, M., Gerson, R., & Petry, S. (2008). *Genograms: Assessment and intervention* (3rd ed.). New York: W.W. Norton & Company.

McRuer, R. (2006). *Crip theory: Cultural signs of queerness and disability*. New York: New York University Press.

Mikkonen, J., & Raphael, D. (2010). *Social determinants of health: The Canadian facts*. Toronto, ON: York University School of Health Policy and Management.

Minkler, M., & Estes, C. (Eds.). (1991). *Critical perspectives on aging: The political and moral economy of growing old*. Amityville, NY: Baywood.

Mullaly, B. (2007). *The new structural social work* (3rd ed.). Toronto, ON: Oxford University Press.

Netting, E. (2011). Bridging critical feminist gerontology and social work to interrogate the narrative on civic engagement. *Affilia: Journal of Women and Social Work*, *26*(3), 239–249. doi:10.1177/0886109911417689

Neysmith, S. M., & Reitsma-Street, M. (2009). The provisioning responsibilities of older women. *Journal of Aging Studies*, *23*, 237–244.

Oliver, M. (1996). *Understanding disability: From theory to practice*. Basingstoke: Palgrave.

Olshansky, S. J., Carnes, B. A., & Butler, R. N. (2015). If humans were built to last. *Scientific American*, *24*, 106–111.

Pace, J., & Grenier, A. (2017). Expanding the circle of knowledge: Reconceptualizing successful aging among North American older Indigenous peoples. *The Journals of Gerontology. Series B, Psychological Sciences and Social Sciences*, *72*(2), 248–258. doi:10.1093/geronb/gbw128

Payne, M. (2014). *Modern social work theory* (4th ed.). Chicago, IL: Lyceum Books.

Phillipson, C. (1998). *Reconstructing old age: New agendas in social theory and practice*. London: Sage.

Purves, B., & Hulko, W. (2019). Adapting CIRCA-BC in the post residential school era. In W. Hulko, D. Wilson, & J. Balestrery (Eds.), *Indigenous peoples and dementia: New understandings of memory loss and memory care* (pp. 196–214). Vancouver, BC: UBC Press.

Putnam, M. (2002). Linking aging theory and disability models: Increasing the potential to explore aging with physical impairment. *The Gerontologist, 42*(6), 799–806. doi:10.1093/geront/42.6.799

Randall, W., Baldwin, C., McKenzie-Mohr, S., McKim, E., & Furlong, D. (2015). Narrative and resilience: A comparative analysis of how older adults story their lives. *Journal of Aging Studies, 34*, 155–161. doi:10.1016/j.jaging.2015.02.010

Ranzijn, R. (2010). Active ageing – Another way to oppress marginalized and disadvantaged elders? *Journal of Health Psychology, 15*(5), 716–723. doi:10.1177/1359105310368181

Razack, S., Smith, M., & Thobani, S. (2010). *States of race: Critical race feminism for the 21st century.* Toronto, ON: Between the Lines.

Riley, M. W. (1971). Social gerontology and the age stratification of society. *The Gerontologist, 11* (1 part 1), 79–87. doi:10.1093/geront/11.1_part_1.79

Robeyns, I. (2005). The capability approach: A theoretical survey. *Journal of Human Development, 6*(1), 93–117. doi:10.1080/146498805200034266.

Rowe, J. W., & Kahn, R. (1987). Successful aging. *The Gerontologist, 37*(4), 433–440. doi:10.1093/geront/37.4.433

Rudman, D. L. (2015). Embodying positive aging and neoliberal rationality: Talking about the aging body within narratives of retirement. *Journal of Aging Studies, 34*, 10–20. doi:10.1016/j.jaging.2015.03.005

Saleebey, D. (1996). The strengths perspective in social work: An extension and a caution. *Social Work, 41*(3), 297–305. doi:10.1093/geront/37.4.433

Sandberg, L., & Marshall, B. (2017). Queering aging futures. *Societies, 7*(21), 1–11. doi:10.3390/soc7030021

São José, J. M., Timonen, V., Filipe Amado, C., & Pereira Santos, S. (2017). A critique of the active ageing index. *Journal of Aging Studies, 40*, 49–56. doi:10.1016/j.jaging.2017.01.001

Simic, A. (1993). Aging and ethnic identity: A refutation of the double-jeopardy theory. *Journal of Case Management, 2*(1), 9–13.

Siverskog, A. (2015). Ageing bodies that matter: Age, gender and embodiment in older transgender people's life stories. *Nordic Journal of Feminist and Gender Research, 23*(1), 4–19. doi:10.1080/08038740.2014.979869

Townsend, P. (1981). The structured dependency of the elderly: A creation of social policy in the twentieth century. *Ageing & Society, 1*(1), 6–28. doi:10.1017/S0144686X81000020

van Dyk, S. (2014). The appraisal of difference: Critical gerontology and the active-ageing paradigm. *Journal of Aging Studies, 31*, 93–103. doi:10.1016/j.jaging.2014.08.008

Vincent, J. A. (1995). *Inequality and old age.* London: UCL Press.

Walker, A. (1981). Towards a political economy of old age. *Ageing & Society, 1*(1), 73–94. doi:10.1017/S0144686X81000056

WHO. (2013, May 7). *What are social determinants of health.* Retrieved April 17, 2014 from www.who.int/social_determinants/en

Wilson, G. (1997). A postmodern approach to structured dependency theory. *Journal of Social Policy, 26*(3), 341–350. doi:10.1017/S0047279497005047

Zarb, G., & Oliver, M. (1993). *Aging with a disability: What do they expect after all these years?* London: University of Greenwich.

Zubair, M., & Norris, M. (2015). Perspectives on ageing, later life and ethnicity: Ageing research in ethnic minority contexts. *Ageing & Society, 35*(5), 897–916.

Chapter 3

Sites and sectors of health and social care

Questions to consider as you read this chapter

- What factors distinguish each sector?
- How are older adults perceived and received in these sectors?
- How is "partnership" operationalized in each sector? Who counts as a "partner"?
- What power/agency do older people have in these sectors? (what constrains/supports older people's opportunities for agency in each sector)?

The challenges of accessibility across sites and sectors: my (Shari's) story of social work practice

My first job after I graduated with my MSW was at a culturally specific, non-profit, community-based agency providing assessment, homecare, and caregiver support services in the Jewish community. I was eager to begin my career within my own cultural community supporting older adults and their caregivers. I met many older people who shared their stories and advice about living and aging, and I drew inspiration from their courage in the face of significant challenges. One of the things I most appreciated from working in the community sector for an organization arms-length from government was that, as an organization, we were not as restricted in the way we operated. For example, we had more time to both assess situations and provide interventions and were not as limited by the large caseloads and waitlists when compared with those in public sector health centres. We also had time to engage in research to inform practice. The research on caregiver experiences I undertook led to innovative programming, including support groups for caregivers designed to be open-ended (not time limited).

As a non-profit community-based agency, our mandate was to complement and supplement public sector services. In other words, we worked to ensure that clients were first receiving the homecare services to which they were entitled from the public sector before being eligible for services from our agency. This meant that we did a lot of referrals to the public sector health centre as a first step in meeting the needs of our clients. Time and again, I heard the same story repeated. Older adults, particularly those who spoke very little English or French and/or were Holocaust survivors were told by the intake workers at the health centre that they would be better served by our agency and referred them back to us. This led me to question the fundamental principle of universal access. Universal access for whom? Only those who represented the majority population? Why were public sector services not being adapted to reflect the realities of diverse marginalized communities? Rather, culturally specific agencies, with smaller and less stable budgets were being required to fill these gaps.

In addition, several of our clients who were receiving services from the local health centre were frustrated by the lack of understanding of their unique issues and realities and so returned to us with complaints and requests for help in advocating on their behalf. This reality seemed an extension of the problem of neoliberalism and familism, whereby families were relied upon to fill the care gap of the retreating public health care sector – with the extension of the definition of "family", in our case, to also include "the larger cultural community". What about communities with no infrastructure or institutional completeness/readiness to pick up the slack due to the unwillingness of the public sector to adapt services to make them more accessible? What happened to older adults and their (chosen)[1] families from those communities without any voice, power, or financing to enact support? In my community, we were lucky to have been able to provide some supports through our community organizations.

I also began to question the reality that referrals were made to our organization with little communication between us and those from public sector services in an organized or formal fashion. Front-line workers exchanged information on clients when necessary, but little planning, organization, and training were undertaken across sites and sectors. We, as a culturally specific community-based organization were rarely asked to provide training to workers in the public health and social care system so that they could better serve marginalized older adults, such as Holocaust survivors, from within their own health care agencies. Nor were we called upon to proactively serve as advisors or advocates to evaluate processes and policies using an equity, diversity, and inclusion (EDI) lens.

*The silos in operation between the organizations and institutions across the health and social care continuum were quite significant when I graduated in the early 1990s. Unfortunately, these issues are still prevalent in the system today. Coordination of care between sites and sectors continues to be problematic, as are the constraints (both financial and programmatic) that shape structures and relationships within the system. Older adults and their (chosen) families and communities bear the ultimate cost of these gaps and silos that exist largely as a result of neoliberalism and eurocentrism (see **Introduction** for a textbox definition of this term). This is essentially what took me back to school to study the state of readiness of public sector homecare agencies to address issues of race and racism in the design and delivery of services (see Brotman, 2000).*

This chapter describes the different sites and sectors of health and social care older adults must navigate as they age and where social work practitioners most often work. We introduce a continuum model to situate the spaces and contexts in which older people come into contact with health and social care service delivery systems. In this chapter, we not only explain the linkages between sectors, but also illuminate the discourses shaping their mandates, philosophies, and practice principles, whether explicitly or implicitly and call attention to the relative power or voice that older people have in shaping priorities and claiming ownership over services.

The objectives of this chapter are to

- Identify the main sites and sectors that provide services and supports to older people and the types of organizations and institutions that make up these sectors;
- Expose the dominant discourses that inform how services are designed and delivered within each sector;

- Explore the main role of social workers in each sector; and
- Identify counter-discourses that can support social workers to enhance AOP within these sectors.

Setting the stage: the impact of social discourse on the design and delivery of services

As we highlighted in **Age/ism: age as a category of difference**, social views on aging influence how society treats older people. In turn, the way we treat older people reinforces and confirms our social views on aging. For example, if we think of older people as valued members of society with much accumulated knowledge and experience, then we are more likely to create opportunities for older people to contribute and feel included (social inclusion). If, however, we consider older people to be a burden or resistant to change, then we are more likely to exclude them from participation in social and economic life (social exclusion). Social views reflect complex relationships of power that exist within social systems and between social actors in society. How these views (and corresponding values) manifest in social institutions and in everyday interactions represents a set of *discourses*. Discourses are more than a form of communication between social actors; they constitute knowledge in a given society (Foucault, 1989). Social discourse calls attention to the power relationships that operate in the way knowledge is created and what gets counted as "truth" (Foucault, 1980) (see textbox 3.1). Discourses are more than ways of thinking and producing meaning, they are also forms of social practice – how we think, communicate, relate, and disseminate knowledge (Weedon, 1987). Discourses are not fixed; they are shifting and are based upon the ways in which power is both created and contested. Dominant discourses are shaped by the views and values of dominant institutions, such as government, and dominant actors who exert power, authority, and control in a given society (see textbox 3.1). Those in power hold privilege rooted in intersecting dominant identity categories such as gender (cis/male), race (white), class (wealthy), sexual orientation (heterosexual), and ability (able-bodied). Dominant discourses can also be contested through the application of counter-discourses that operate at the margins and serve to displace and challenge dominant ideas about what counts as truth. Analyzing how social discourses operate can help us to understand how they influence multiple aspects of social life, including sites and sectors of health and social care.

In her popular textbook on social work theories in context, Healy (2014) examines how discourses operate in social work to shape both the context in which we work and professional priorities and practices. She quotes Taylor (2013) to describe critical discourse analysis as a tool to better understand

> how language use contributes to the dominance of certain truth claims and the privileging of particular actors within any practice context and what if anything other actors such as social workers, care providers, or service users can do to disrupt these truth claims to allow for alternative meanings including different ways of understanding need and responding to problems.
>
> (Taylor, 2013 in Healy, 2014, p. 4)

Healy (2014) describes the concept of *"competing discourses"* as the ways in which both dominant and alternative interpretations shape "the nature of client needs, expert knowledge, the nature of the social work role and specifically the kinds of 'help' or interventions that will best address the concerns and issues facing service users" (p. 4). Although there is variability in the (in)visibility of "competing discourses" across the various sites and sectors in which social workers find themselves, they are, nevertheless present (see textbox 3.1). As Healy (2014) explains, "In these contexts, one discourse, or set of compatible discourses, has gained dominance in determining the official practices of the institution" (p. 6). It is important to remember that social workers can, and often do, actively contest and resist dominant discourses within their work, whether individually through their interactions with clients, collectively within their professional associations, departments, and interdisciplinary teams, or by engaging in systemic-level advocacy and policy development.

Healy's articulation of the three sets of discourses influencing practice can be helpful to gerontological social workers seeking to better understand how and why their work/places are constrained to particular tasks and perspectives over others, which at times, can seem to put into conflict their social work values and the actual work they can perform. These discourses are dominant, disciplinary, and alternative. Dominant discourse is the most influential in shaping power and knowledge relations in the various sites and sectors of health and social care. Disciplinary discourses emerge from the social and behavioural sciences and have "traditionally provided the knowledge and theory base for the social work profession" (p. 6). These include systems and ecological theories, which have been central to social work education for several decades. These disciplinary discourses, while influential, have been the site of considerable tension within the profession with significant variations across different fields of practice. In the context of social gerontology, particularly in health and social care services, bio-medicalization (at the macro level) and risk/decline (at the practice level, as is highlighted in **Deconstructing risk and frailty**) still function as the most common dominant discourses shaping contemporary practice.

Alternative discourses are described by Healy as "existing outside the other two discourses but nonetheless exert a powerful influence on the construction of our purpose and practices as social workers" (2014, p. 6). As explained in **Theorizing later life and social work praxis,** approaches to practice identified by social workers in the field of social gerontology have included systems, strengths-based, and problem-solving approaches. These approaches can look very different depending on the discourses constraining or influencing them across and within different sectors and sites of practice. This is why understanding how competing discourses operate in our work is key to operationalizing our chosen approach. We suggest that replacing "alternative discourses" with the concept of "counter-narratives" or "counter-discourses", a term more common to AOP, helps social workers to more explicitly embed resistance, social justice, and advocacy into both critical consciousness and social action.

Textbox 3.1

Discourse

Social discourse calls attention to the power relationships that operate in the way knowledge is created and what gets counted as "truth" (Foucault, 1980).

Discourses are forms of social practice: how we think, communicate, relate, and disseminate knowledge. Discourses are based upon the ways in which power is both created and contested.

Dominant discourses are shaped by the views and values of dominant institutions (e.g., government) and dominant actors (those who exert power, authority, and control in a given society). Those in power hold privilege due to belonging to dominant groups related to categories of difference including gender (cis-male), race (white), class (wealthy), sexual orientation (heterosexual), and ability (able-bodied).

Competing discourses operate at the margins and serve to displace and challenge dominant and mainstream ideas about what counts as truth.

As stated above and discussed in **Age/ism: age as a category of difference**, the dominant social discourse of aging is one of decline, dependence, risk, and frailty (Marques, Lima, Abrams, & Swift, 2014). This plays out significantly in the way health and social care services are designed and delivered. For social workers working in the field of aging, understanding sectors and sites of care from an AOP perspective requires us to be aware of the impact of this dominant social discourse of aging on how our institutions are funded and shaped, how terms such as partnership in care are operationalized, and how our work is structured. Understanding these multiple impacts will also help us to identify counter-discourses and to engage in strategies to resist practices that reinforce this dominant discourse in our work (Fook, 2002).

In our society, people tend to view aging as a process of becoming increasingly incapable of doing for oneself and of needing help from others (National Centre for the Protection of Older People, 2009). As one ages, the capacity for productivity is assumed to decline, and this assumption was used in the past to justify exclusionary practices such as mandatory retirement. The cause of such decline is understood to be situated in the individual and as a function of the process of aging. Alongside and interconnected to this phenomenon is the belief that older people's need for increasing support to deal with health care issues and to help them function in their daily lives is a "personal problem" (Brossoie & Chops, 2015); that is, the social and support needs of older people is largely a private matter, best addressed by the individual themselves and/or their family. These beliefs are rooted in the interconnected social discourses of neoliberalism, medicalization, and familism (see textbox 3.2).

Textbox 3.2

Familism is an ideology that identifies the (nuclear) family as the most appropriate and valued form of care, regardless of the realities, needs, and/or desires of individual family members or the functionality of the family unit. Familism is characterized by hetero-patriarchy in that women are assumed to be the natural care providers (Hulko et al., 2017).

Textbox 3.3

Neoliberalism is a set of economic and social policies that favour free-market capitalism and individualism.

Neoliberal ideology underpins much of what we do as social workers because it shapes the institutions in which we work and creates parameters through which we interact with older people, their families, and communities (see textbox 3.3). Neo-liberal ideology tells us who is responsible for problems in our society and how we, as a society, address them. Productivity and self-reliance are primary cornerstones of neo-liberalism, thus shaping our perceptions and values regarding those deemed no longer "productive" (through reduced capacity or opportunity) (Carr & Batlle, 2015). The target of this social discourse – the old and retired – are thus perceived and treated as the "problem". Social beliefs regarding productivity and capacity in Global North societies are so predominant that, by their very existence, older people are conceptualized as a problem to be managed and a burden to society. The overlapping social discourse that reinforces this idea of decline and frailty is called bio-medicalization (see textbox 3.4). Bio-medicalization of aging refers to a social process in which older adults are reduced to aging bodies and minds in need of surveillance and treatment by the medical system, as they degenerate and ultimately fail (Hulko et al., 2017; see also Kaufman, Shim, & Russ, 2004). This social construct of aging as frailty works together with neoliberal ideas of aging as decline and dependence to reinforce paternalistic practices across sites and sectors of care that emphasize and prioritize the role of experts and professionals as decision-makers.

Textbox 3.4

Bio-medicalization refers to the focus on bio-medical explanations for the aging process whereby it is understood largely through the lens of "disease".

In reality, very few older people require any kind of support. The vast majority live independently in their own homes their entire lives. It has been estimated that only 7.9% of older people require long-term-care services (Statistics Canada, 2011), but we have this impression that older people are a significant problem and use up the vast majority of public dollars. Growing older can increase the risk of chronic and acute health conditions and disability (The American Psychological Association, 2017). How we understand and respond to this reality is a key question. Both health (medical) and allied health professionals (including social workers) have an important part to play in working with older adults to address disability, health, and illness management. We must not forget that many health concerns faced by older adults are exacerbated by social conditions beyond the particular health situation of any individual person. These *social determinants of health (SDOH)* play an important role in shaping how and why we face particular states of vulnerability as we age.

The following counter-story is presented as an illustration of how discourses shape our interventions. As you read, think about the different assumptions that are made by Jill, the nurse, regarding the overall level of functioning and informal support available to the patient, Les. How are the dominant discourses of neoliberalism and bio-medicalization operating in Jill's assessment of what services can, and need to, be put in place for Les? Then consider how Franca pushes back against these assumptions in their intervention. Can you identify which specific SDOH are present in this story and how they operate? (e.g., gender, culture, race and racism, income, education, homophobia: see endnote 1 in **Theorizing later life and social work praxis** for more information on SDOH).

The lonely old lady emerges as the community pioneer

Les, a 78-year-old Franco-Ontarian, fell and broke her hip. After two weeks of rehabilitation, it was determined that Les could be discharged from hospital. Franca, the discharge planner (and a social worker), was asked to meet with her to determine if a long-term care placement was necessary. The file was already flagged by the floor nurse, Jill, indicating that Les had no husband or children to provide support, so social isolation was a concern. Les had increasing challenges with mobility and required a walker to get around. The nurse was also concerned about the capacity of Les to maneuver in her small apartment and get in and out of the bath on her own. Due to recent cutbacks to community health services, Les was only eligible to receive homecare support twice per week and help with a bath once per week, grossly inadequate according to Les who was used to daily baths. Les did not have any savings so could not afford to supplement homecare privately. It was the nurse's opinion that Les would be best off moving into a nursing home where proper care could be provided.

Franca was already concerned about some of the assumptions Jill was making about Les, and in particular that, without a husband or children, Les was isolated and alone. As a gender non-conforming queer person, Franca had witnessed many times in their practice how heterosexist assumptions can render invisible the identities and experiences of queer older adults. Franca kept this thought in their mind when they went to see Les in her room, and decided to try a narrative approach to interviewing in order to give space for Les to talk about her reality. After introducing themselves, Franca asked Les to talk about her life. Les remarked that no one had asked this before. Les told Franca that Annabelle, Les' friend with whom she spent 35 years, had died two years ago. After Anabelle's death, Les moved to the city because she could no longer drive and, with complications from diabetes, found living in the country difficult. Les had not accumulated much savings to pay for private help because of lifelong experiences of workplace discrimination. Having been a teacher most of her life, Les had some trouble finding employment because, as she described "in my day, being out as a lesbian made finding work in schools more difficult". Franca asked what life was like back in the country and Les brightened. Les spoke about a strong sense of community – Les and Anabelle had had a close group of friends in the small local Francophone lesbian community and they had taken care of each other for over 50 years. Les spoke of her early activism and pride in how the "lesbian brigade" had managed to overcome a lot of prejudice and plan activities for the younger folks. In the big city, and with a circle of friends aging and unable to travel, Les was more or less alone. Franca knew of a local LGBTTsIQ organization and asked Les for permission to speak to them about the situation. Within a week, the community had rallied volunteers to provide home support and friendly visiting. They asked Les to join their documentation project, which was collecting life stories of queer pioneers in the province. The act of counter-storytelling made room to re-vision Les from a "lonely old lady with no visitors" to an "engaged community activist and pioneer". Rethinking notions of family from nuclear to "chosen" kin models enabled Les to go home with support and feel a sense of belonging in her new city. Franca was pleased that they were able to use their personal knowledge and experience to help them connect with Les, build trust, and create an opportunity to counter heterosexist assumptions and re-think responses.

(adapted from Hulko et al., 2017, p. 207)

This story highlights the difference in outcomes between when a discourse of neo-liberalism, familism and bio-medicalization dominates intervention and when AOP principles are used to explore unique identities, strengths and resilience.

Understanding the structural causes of exposure to health and social problems as we age is key and goes largely unrecognized within state and institutional policies and practices. Asking why this is the case and how things can be challenged and changed is an important starting point for social workers in the field of aging. The vast majority of social workers will find work in public health and social care services (i.e., hospital, community health, social services, and residential care). As such, the predominance of concomitant discourses of bio-medicalization and neoliberalism will shape the framework within which many social workers will spend our working lives. Over time, these ideologies of the everyday can easily become internalized as the only acceptable reality of professional practice. Because we have contact with older people, mostly as patients/clients of the health and social care system, we tend to see them in this totalizing vacuum of sickness, decline, incapacity, isolation, and dependence. Because older people often present with complex chronic health issues, we also see them as "unfixable", thus entrenching ideas of age as decline, dependence, and frailty. Bio-medical and neoliberal ideology puts the blame on the individual person but also tells us that the solution to caring for older people is a private matter, resting primarily with the biological family, referred to as familism. Since our health care system prioritizes cure and rehabilitation, anyone presenting with an "incurable" condition is viewed with caution, treated with some mix of pity and disdain, and required to supplement the limited availability of formal care services with family support or personal funds.

An additional challenge is that social workers in the health and social care system tend to work in isolation from those outside the health care sector, in voluntary, community-based, or activist organizations, for example. The response to patient need is so fixed in the body and the mind that our main goal is often reduced to managing immediate problems without accounting for the entire person and their environment. Losing this vision of a person in their entirety, across their life course and embedded within a community, decontextualizes the individual, thereby jeopardizing our understanding of their unique history and realities – and risks losing the value of connection and strength, both with respect to how we understand that person and how we intervene with them.

Social workers work with older people in many different contexts and across many different sites. The proliferation of bio-medicalization as the context of care in the formal health and social care system and the extent to which "health" dominates both public and professional discourses has an important impact on how we see social work with older people and where jobs are available. When we think about the sectors (main systems) and sites (places) of care in which social workers work with older people, we tend to only think about those related to health and long-term-care services. In fact, as aging is far more dynamic and diverse, so are the sites and sectors of care in which social workers work! Understanding sites and sectors of care across a continuum helps us to see older people as engaged actors and places critical attention on the ways in which systems are set up to encourage inclusion, voice, and recognition or exclusion, reductionism, and medicalization. Social workers "meet up" with older people along this continuum in a variety of ways that can connect easily with our professional values of social justice and self-determination or that can challenge us to use these values to help confront systemic discrimination, paternalism, bio-medicalization, familism, and neoliberalism.

The continuum of care

Figure 3.1 outlines the main sectors predominant in the provision of services and supports to older people in Canada. The remainder of the chapter will describe these sectors, paying particular attention to how these sectors operate, what types of organizations and institutions make up these sectors, what discourses underlie how services are delivered within each sector, and the main role of social workers in these

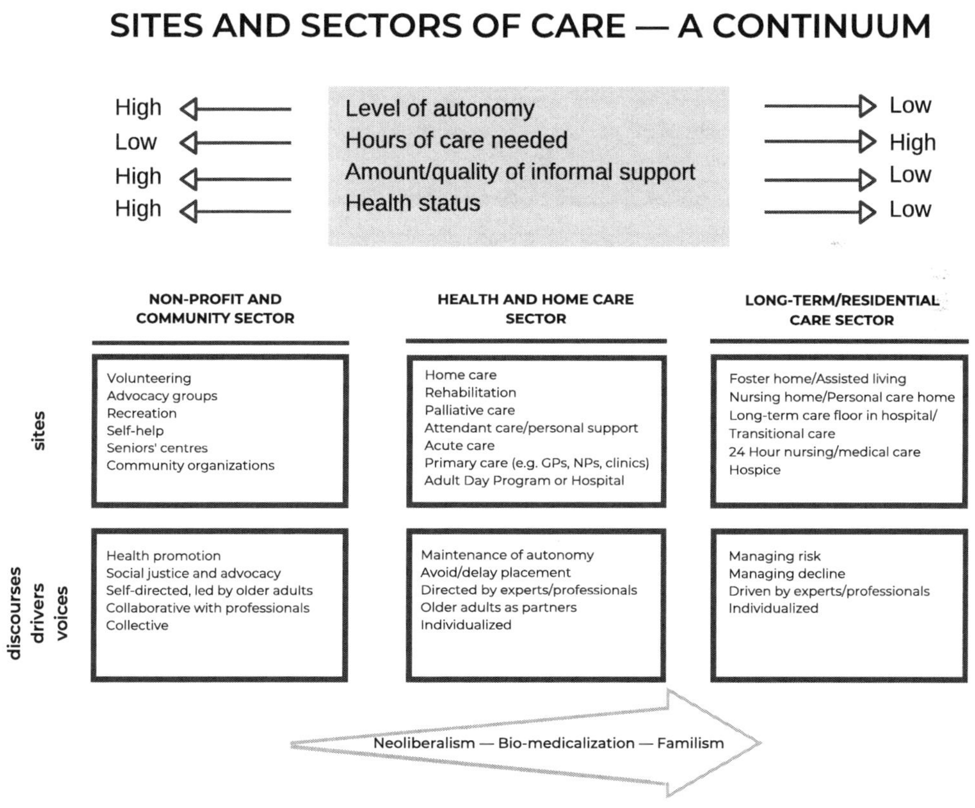

SITES AND SECTORS OF CARE — A CONTINUUM

High ◁———	Level of autonomy	———▷ Low
Low ◁———	Hours of care needed	———▷ High
High ◁———	Amount/quality of informal support	———▷ Low
High ◁———	Health status	———▷ Low

	NON-PROFIT AND COMMUNITY SECTOR	HEALTH AND HOME CARE SECTOR	LONG-TERM/RESIDENTIAL CARE SECTOR
sites	Volunteering Advocacy groups Recreation Self-help Seniors' centres Community organizations	Home care Rehabilitation Palliative care Attendant care/personal support Acute care Primary care (e.g. GPs, NPs, clinics) Adult Day Program or Hospital	Foster home/Assisted living Nursing home/Personal care home Long-term care floor in hospital/ Transitional care 24 Hour nursing/medical care Hospice
discourses drivers voices	Health promotion Social justice and advocacy Self-directed, led by older adults Collaborative with professionals Collective	Maintenance of autonomy Avoid/delay placement Directed by experts/professionals Older adults as partners Individualized	Managing risk Managing decline Driven by experts/professionals Individualized

Neoliberalism — Bio-medicalization — Familism ▷

Figure 3.1 Sites and sectors of care – a continuum

sectors. We will also highlight several tensions that exist in each sector, identifying challenges and opportunities that emerge in the daily work of social workers. In **Deconstructing risk and frailty**, we will focus specifically on how these discourses shape ideas of frailty and risk in the context of the mandate and daily work of social workers and how we can learn to counter, protest, or push against policies and ways of working in order to enhance AOP social work and enact our fundamental values of self-determination, inclusion, and social justice.

The continuum of care can generally be understood as made up of three sectors of care within which there are many different sites (organizations or institutions geospatially located) and programs. While described here as distinct, it is important to note that there is overlap between and within sectors, with particular sites having features that place them at the intersection of sectors across the continuum. In addition, some sites have programs that link within or across sectors, and while social workers themselves may work primarily in one sector, they may refer to, or engage in, tasks that are associated with another sector, site, or program. Although sectors are described as having specific conceptual boundaries, the reality is that distinctions can be more nuanced, depending on the actual site. Figure 3.1 provides a pictorial description of the continuum of care services.

The three sectors along the continuum can be described as (1) non-profit and community care, (2) health and homecare, and (3) long-term/residential care. They are placed from left to right to demonstrate the shift along four axes of assessment in which health professionals, most notably social workers, engage to determine eligibility (level of autonomy, hours of care needed, amount/quality of informal support, and health status). The continuum also reflects another kind of critical shift in ideology and assumptions regarding the capacity of older people for self-determination, authority, and agency and of the integration of *citizenship* as a fundamental aspect of care. So, for example, as we move from left to right along the continuum, the opportunity for older adults, their families, and communities to shape programs, choose what services they receive, and engage as active agents in care diminishes, and the authority and voice of experts and professionals increases.

The non-profit and community care, health and homecare, and long-term/residential care sectors are not equal in size or shape. This has much to do with both who is involved in their creation (community members or professionals/government) and in the size and source of funding. Financing has an important impact on how sites are organized and operate. There also exist regional variations in the overall availability and diversity of services, which can result in significant inequities in access to appropriate and culturally/linguistically relevant health and social care depending on region, community, or group. For example, although the provision of health and social care is the responsibility of provinces and territories, there are exceptions. Health and social care for specific populations, such as Indigenous people living on reserves, refugee claimants, and veterans is the responsibility of the federal government (a more detailed discussion of this issue is located in **Policy and planning for an aging society**). These jurisdictional issues, historic and current governmental priorities, and localized histories and traditions of community-based alternative service-delivery and advocacy initiatives result in variability in the availability (and sustainability) of options across sites and sectors. Financial capacity (whether through public or private funding sources) and population density are also factors influencing the availability and accessibility of health and social care services across Canada. In rural and remote communities, as well as language minority communities, for example, there may be fewer public sector options, requiring older people and their families to travel long distances to receive public sector and specialized health services or to relocate altogether in order to have access to appropriate health or long-term/residential care. This is especially problematic given the lack of attention to adapting services to ensure their relevance in the context of regional and cultural diversity. At best, a "cultural competence" framework is used (see textbox 3.5), thereby limiting responses to the level of the individual interaction, while simultaneously ignoring structural, regional and other forms of in/equity. With respect to Indigenous peoples for whom cultural safety (see textbox 3.6) is not a guarantee or even commonplace within mainstream health and social care sectors, this reality represents a significant barrier to care (Brascoupe & Waters, 2009; Halseth, 2018).

Textbox 3.5

Cultural competency includes an awareness of cultural differences and ability to be sensitive to these differences in direct practice, as well as having sufficient knowledge and skills to intervene in a competent fashion with those who are from cultures different than one's own.

Textbox 3.6

Cultural safety, a concept created by a Maori nurse (Ramsden, 1990), refers to both the process (how we work with people) and the outcome (service user or patient feeling safe) of care that intentionally acknowledges racism and other forms of discrimination and shifts power away from the service provider and towards service users, supporting their agency and voice.

In rural and remote contexts, the non-profit sector, including volunteer-exchanges between neighbours, often fills the gap in available services in creative and personalized ways. By doing so, rural and remote communities demonstrate a sense of solidarity, belonging, and connection not common in urban settings (Kulig & Williams, 2011). Rural older adults caution against applying a "cookie-cutter" approach (i.e., designing and/or delivering primary and community care services to rural and small rural towns based on large urban or small city models). At the same time, better homecare, transportation, and more knowledgeable doctors ("proper" doctors) were found in a recent study to be top priorities for the restructuring of primary and community care regardless of small city or rural residency and cultural background (Hulko, Mirza, & Seeley, in press).

The sectors described

The *non-profit and community care sector* is community-based and encompasses both direct service and advocacy organizations that are designed and delivered in response to need, interest, and solidarity principles. These sites are largely community-driven with older adults themselves playing a major part in development and direction in many cases. Professionals like social workers play a supporting role under the direction of advisory boards and committees. This is the sector in which we are most likely to work collaboratively, where older adults are perceived as actors and agents with full autonomy and voice. In fact, many non-profit and community care organizations engage older adults as workers, largely volunteers, who not only receive but supply services. Think about meals on wheels, friendly visiting, mutual aid, ethno-cultural support groups, and other programs in which older people participate as visitors and drivers, and perform other acts of engagement and support to their peers such as accompaniment and personal advocacy. Here we will also find recreational and social groups that represent a plethora of agencies and activities such as retirement and veterans' associations, adult learner societies, YWCAs, faith-based organizations, ethno-cultural community groups, councils on aging, and municipal programs in which recreational, support, and social activities are offered. There are self-help and mutual aid organizations on a wide variety of subjects run by older people like support groups for caregivers or isolated seniors and also advocacy and rights based organizations, like associations of retired persons or caregiver associations, and lobby groups that address policy-related and economic issues, with older people and their allies organizing for the rights of older people, their families and communities to government and within society. General rights-based organizations like anti-poverty groups and social housing groups also often direct specific attention to the issues facing older people with respect to poverty, homelessness, and food and income security. Here we would find rights-based and service organizations for people from equity seeking groups like LGBTTsIQ, immigrant, refugee, Indigenous, and disability groups that either consider older people within a larger mandate, or older adults have created their own groups.

The non-profit and community care sector is dynamic, fluid, and localized. A broader discussion of this sector will be developed in **Building inclusive communities**. The shape and nature of work within the non-profit and community care sector can be flexible and shifting for a number of reasons, including such factors as funding instability and local priorities. We introduce this sector here for the purposes of understanding how it fits along the continuum of care. Rights-based work within this sector can "spring up" in the context of new legislation or targeted funding opportunities; older adults and/or allies identify concerns, realities, and/or needs within local communities that require immediate attention. The term "partnership" or "ally" is often used within this sector to refer to the relationship between citizens, volunteers, or service users and experts/professionals, including social workers. Where there is interaction with social workers and other service providers, this is often on a collaborative basis so even when volunteer organizations or community organizations engage paid staff, this is most often done in collaboration with older adults and their communities through advisory groups and boards of directors in which older people take an active decision-making role.

The non-profit and community care sector enacts counter-discourses of social justice and self-determination more commonly than any other sector. Two approaches that underlie services and programs are (1) advocacy and rights and (2) health promotion (Milne et al., 2014) (see textbox 3.7). Social workers undertake a variety of tasks including community organizing, program development, group work, and advocacy. Social workers also undertake assessment, evaluation, and referral, particularly in the context of direct service programs and services.

Textbox 3.7

Health promotion refers to the process of enabling people to increase control over and improve their health. It moves beyond a focus on individual behaviour to include a wide range of social and environmental factors that are implicated in the health status of individuals and populations (World Health Organization, 1998).

With respect to work with older people, non-profit and community care sector organizations, particularly those with a support or direct service function, often incorporate a "health" agenda, as "health" is a basic indicator of need for service. Yet within this sector, health is operationalized more broadly to include holistic aspects of health and well-being including approaches more directly tied to health promotion and SDOH and consistent with the World Health Organization definition of health as more than the absence of disease. For example, social engagement and social inclusion are considered rights that contribute to overall promotion of health and well-being for older people and their families (Baer, Bhushan, Abou Taleb, Vasques, & Thomas, 2016). Health promotion, at its best, takes into account social justice, social inclusion, and agency. At its worst, health promotion is articulated as an individualist approach predicated on the idea of "successful aging" in which the responsibility for good health and social participation rests squarely on the shoulders of individuals through the maintenance of "healthy habits" and decisions, irrespective of the SDOH affecting them.

Health promotion (and SDOH), although recognized theoretically as an important area of health and well-being, still gets little attention by government and within funding structures. Ironically as dynamic and self-driven as the non-profit and community care sector is, it actually cannot count on or rely upon as much stable basic financial support from government as somewhat is the case within the public sector. There are pluses and minuses to this. Alternative funding can mean less interference in values and philosophy and daily activities within these sites, allowing organizations to work more on advocacy or to have broader latitude in the design of services. On the negative side, this can limit the long-term planning capacity of those sites that cannot accurately determine, from year to year, how much money will be available to hire staff or run certain programs. What this also means is that there may be fewer opportunities for social workers to find employment within these sites, and when they do, they are not paid as well or have little guarantee of permanence, relying as they are on short-term contract funding or donations. Only in communities that have adequate infrastructure (largely through non-profit funding channels) can social workers engage in a long-term context.

The *health and homecare sector* is largely driven, not self-directed, by experts and professionals. Older adults and families are perceived predominantly as clients or patients in the context of service delivery; however, an emphasis is still placed upon the idea of partnership between service users, families, and professionals. How partnership is defined and operationalized can vary considerably from one site to another. Sites within the health and homecare sector include homecare, rehabilitation services, primary and acute care and short-term stay in hospital settings in the case of patients who will return home after a health crisis, and attendant care within independent living retirement homes. The basic function of health and homecare is to support older adults with some loss of autonomy, disability or health concerns to continue to live at home (Siegler, Lama, Knight, Laureano, & Carrington, 2015). So, for example, an older adult who has a fall and breaks their hip might have a short-term stay in hospital, spend a few weeks in a rehabilitation centre with the goal of regaining functional autonomy, and then return home with some homecare support. The social worker's role here varies and includes individual case management, discharge planning, and resource referral. Attention to the voices of older adults is more typically focussed upon the incorporation of their wishes and choices with respect to what types of support resources to put in place, with the social worker working to balance these wishes and choices against eligibility criteria and available community supports.

The fundamental discourse in health and homecare is "maintenance of autonomy" in which there exists a tension between medical and social models of care. This often presents as a challenge for social workers whose values reflect self-determination and social justice, but whose professional priority is to manage functioning within the constraints of available services. The role of the case manager is threefold: assessment, monitoring, and referral. The client is most often the older person and most work is individually based. This is a highly regulated field of practice, particularly with respect to public sector services in which workers must contend with high caseloads and substantial formalized reporting and documentation. This aspect of the work of social workers in publicly funded homecare, for example, has been conceptualized as "street level bureaucracy," which is identified by its focus on automation, bureaucratization, strict regulation of eligibility and performance, and standardization (Lipsky, 2010).

Daily life on the front line includes such activities as home visits, interdisciplinary communication, and referral, program planning, and evaluation. Still, there is potential within this sector for meaningful partnership work at the individual level with older people, family members, and caregivers and for the actualization of agency in the individual encounter between workers and clients. These anti-oppressive moments of individual intervention can facilitate acts of engagement in trust building and advocacy with clients and the development of a deeper understanding of clients' lived experiences. Home visits represent one of those "intervention moments" that are ripe with possibility. Social workers undertaking home visits have a significant opportunity to get up from behind their desks and to pay witness to older people's lives within their own home and community, to uncover how people live and discover what has meaning for them. During home visits, social workers can move beyond the required focus on paperwork to engage in counter-storytelling with clients during assessments for example, providing opportunity for older people to tell their stories in their own words and to shape the conversation. As Les' counter-story describes, this opportunity is also possible in other health care encounters.

Finally, the *long-term/residential care sector* refers to the range of institutions in which older people with significant limitations in their capacity to live independently reside. This includes assisted living, nursing or personal care homes, or transitional care, which refers to such spaces as long-term-care floors/beds in acute care hospitals in which older adults might await placement in a more permanent setting.

Social workers within this sector work to develop placement plans through assessment and referral, coordinate transfer, and engage with residents and their families to support adaptation during times of transition (particularly for those who have recently moved into a long-term/residential care setting) (Solomon, 2004). They are also involved in end-of-life care, although this aspect of their work is significantly challenging given the combined factors of time constraints, regulation, and a lack of training on end-of-life intervention among social workers (Janssen, 2019) (see **Moral legal and ethical issues**). The long-term/residential care sector is largely dominated by a medical model. This has been identified as a particular challenge, as there is an inherent tension in creating a sense of "home" within an institutional environment that is largely focussed upon managing symptomatology and behaviour. The long-term/residential care sector is dominated by expert and professional discourses with a significantly reduced opportunity to include older adults as partners in decision-making and planning. Residents' or caregivers' committees or family councils are often the spaces in which residents and their families can act to influence the design and delivery of services to some extent, but the work of these committees varies, particularly across sites and sectors. Here in the long-term/residential care sector the dominant discourse is about managing risk and decline, which places older people in the position of the object, rather than the subject of care services. Standardized reporting is also a distinct feature in these settings. Although sometimes challenging, particularly given the reality that only a small number (1–2) of social workers, if any, are typically hired within a single residence (and so must manage a potentially large caseload), there are many opportunities to engage with older people in ways that enhance people's opportunities for agency and voice. In the long-term/residential care sector, the social worker's role is primarily managing the admissions process, transitions, risk management, and family work. Social workers are part of an interdisciplinary team, and their specific role centres on individual assessment and evaluation, integration of new residents, interdisciplinary meetings and communication, intervention with individuals, group work, and communication with family members and caregivers. Here, advocacy might centre on communicating concerns of family members and residents to other members of the team and developing programs to better meet the needs and reflect the desires of residents. The important and meaningful role of supporting older people during the preliminary transition period cannot be over-stated, with social workers being key to building trust, providing emotional support, and creating cultural safety for both the new resident and their family. This role can be a powerful articulation of AOP.

There is a fundamental shift across the continuum from older people as driving, with social workers working in collaboration (non-profit and community care sector), to spaces in which the social and medical sit in uneasy tension with older people received as individuals (health and homecare sector) to a model driven by attention to frailty and risk in which expert voices are predominant (long term/residential care sector). The ways in which older adults access these sectors and sites within them varies according to these same principles. It is important to remember that social workers have an important gatekeeping function across sites and sectors of health and social care. The continuum of care diagram highlights the factors that play into the determination of access across four axes: health status, level of autonomy, hours of care needed, and the quality and level of social support. The interplay of these axes influence the professional gatekeeping function inherent to older people's access to one sector or another along this continuum with the non-profit and community care sector sites largely open to older adults to choose for themselves, and those in the health and homecare and long term/residential care sectors shaped by professional, expert gatekeepers and operationalized through "functional" assessments of various kinds.[2]

As stated previously, social workers in the health and social care system tend to work in isolation or in silos from those outside the health care sector, in voluntary, community-based, or activist organizations. This has led to some significant challenges for older people and for social workers for whom a *holistic approach* to understanding problems is a central component of professional values and identity. The silo effect limits the capacity for us to exchange information, knowledge, and expertise across sites and sectors. It also represents a significant challenge for those older adults who occupy a liminal space in and between sectors, such as those within acute care sites in hospitals, who are in transition from one sector to another, or who have complex chronic disease (CCD) which requires simultaneous, ongoing multi-sector intervention (see textbox 3.8).

Textbox 3.8

Complex chronic disease (CCD) is a medical term used to categorize those who have "multi-morbidities" or the presence of two or more chronic health conditions. CCD affects older adults in particular with common conditions including diabetes, arthritis, heart disease, dementia, osteoporosis, chronic obstructive pulmonary disease, depression, Parkinson's disease, and hypertension.

Occupying a liminal space may produce greater risks of falling between the cracks, either because of being assessed as not eligible for certain services, being excluded from participation, or being identified as having too many complex needs to be given access to specific targeted services. In this context, and more generally, social workers have a pivotal role to play in pushing back against rigid boundaries and criteria in order to enhance inclusion, to activate attention to the whole person, to ensure consideration of principles of social justice, and to share decision-making power with older people and their families across the continuum of care. Our role as change agents means that we are uniquely positioned to call attention to and name the structural constraints that arise from the imposition of dominant discourses such as neoliberalism and bio-medicalization on the policies and practices that shape our interventions and relationships with older people, their families, and communities and to engage in efforts to transform them, through our individual and collective work.

Exercises

- Think about your practicum and work experiences and situate your workplace within the sites and sectors continuum. What is your main role as a social worker?
- What discourses are operationalized in your organization and in your direct practice? Can you identify counter-discourses?

- Who are your partners? How are older people and their (chosen) families involved in decision-making regarding care plans and access to resources?
- What is your and/or your organization's relationship to other sites within your sector and across sectors? How do you facilitate communication and transitions across sites and sectors?
- As a group, name as many sites (organizations, institutions, programs) as you can in your urban centre, small city, or rural town (i.e. the place where you all study and/or work) and place each of them in one of the three sectors.

Takeaways

- Discourses of neoliberalism and bio-medicalization dominate health and social care policies and professional practices across the continuum of sites and sectors; critical reflection is required in order to expose them.
- There is a significant shift in the relative influence of older adults on the design and delivery of services across the continuum, with older adults more likely to have a central role in decision-making in the non-profit and community sector and professionals more likely to be driving decisions in both the health and home-care and long term/residential care sectors.
- Silos that exist across sectors limit our capacity to address older adults' realities within context and across the life course.
- Counter-discourses can serve to challenge taken-for-granted assumptions in the design and delivery of health and social care services.
- Social workers play a pivotal role across sites and sectors, with both challenges and opportunities for enacting counter-discourses, in both their individual practice and within and across organizations.

Note

1 The term chosen is placed in brackets here to indicate both chosen families and families of origin/biological families.
2 These functional assessment tools often include the Mini-Mental Status Exam (MMSE) used to screen for cognitive impairment (Folstein, Folstein, & McHugh, 1975) and the Geriatric Depression Scale (GDS) (Greenberg, 2019; Yesavage et al., 1983) used to detect symptoms of depression in older adults. Other tools are used to determine an older adult's eligibility for home health services and/or residential care (The Resident Assessment Instrument-Home Care (RAI-HC, 2010), readiness for discharge (RHDS-OP), and transitions in care (CTM-15)).

References

The American Psychological Association. (2017). *Older adults' health and age-related changes: Reality versus myth*. Retrieved from www.apa.org/pi/aging/resources/guides/myth-reality.pdf

Baer, B., Bhushan, A., Abou Taleb, H., Vasques, J., & Thomas, R. (2016). The right to health of older people. *The Gerontologist, 56*(2), 206–217. doi:10.1093/geront/gnw039

Brascoupe, S., & Waters, C. (2009). Cultural safety: Exploring the applicability of the concept of cultural safety to aboriginal health and community wellness. *International Journal of Aboriginal Health, 5*(2), 6–41.

Brossoie, N., & Chops, W. C. (2015). Social gerontology. In R. H. Robnett & W. C. Chops (Eds.), *Gerontology for the health care professionals* (pp. 17–50). Burlington, MA: Jones & Bartlett Learning.

Brotman, S. (2000). An institutional ethnography of eldercare: Understanding access from the standpoint of ethnic and "racial" minority women. Book, whole. UMI Dissertation Services, ProQuest Information and Learning, Ann Arbor, MI.

Carr, S., & Batlle, I. C. (2015). Attachment theory, neoliberalism, and social conscience. *Journal of Theoretical and Philosophical Psychology*, *35*(3), 160–176. doi:10.1037/a0038681

Folstein, M. F., Folstein, S. E., & McHugh, P. R. (1975). Mini-mental state: A practical method for grading the cognitive state of patients for the clinician. *Journal of Psychiatric Research*, *12*(3), 189–198.

Fook, J. (2002). *Critical theories and practice*. Oakland, CA: Sage.

Foucault, M. (1980). *Power/knowledge: Selected interviews and other writings 1972–1977*. C. Gordon (Ed.). Brighton: Vintage.

Foucault, M. (1989). *Archaeology of knowledge*. London and New York: Routledge Classics.

Greenberg, S. (2019). The Geriatric Depression Scale (GDS). Try this: Best practices in nursing care to older adults. Retrieved July 30, 2019 https://consultgeri.org/try-this/general-assessment/issue-4.pdf

Halseth, R. (2018). *Overcoming barriers to culturally safe and appropriate dementia care services and supports for Indigenous peoples in Canada*. Prince George, BC: National Collaborating Centre for Aboriginal Health.

Healy, K. (2014). *Social work theories in context: Creating frameworks for practice* (2nd ed.). London: Palgrave Macmillan.

Hulko, W., Brotman, S., & Ferrer, I. (2017). Counter-storytelling: Anti-oppressive social work with older adults. In D. Baines (Ed.), *Doing anti-oppressive practice: Social justice social work* (3rd ed., pp. 193–211). Halifax, NS: Fernwood Publishing.

Hulko, W., Mirza, N., & Seeley, L. (in press). Older adults' views on the repositioning of primary and community care. *Canadian Journal of Aging*.

Janssen, J. S. (2019). Hospice social work in nursing homes. *Social Work Today*, *17*(6), 20. Retrieved from https://www.socialworktoday.com/archive/ND17p20.shtml

Kaufman, S. R., Shim, J. K., & Russ, A. J. (2004). Revisiting the biomedicalization of aging: Clinical trends and ethical challenges. *The Gerontologist*, *44*(6), 731–738. doi:10.1093/geront/44.6.731

Kulig, J., & Williams, A. (2011). *Health in rural Canada*. Vancouver, BC: UBC Press.

Lipsky, M. (2010). *Street level bureaucracy: Dilemmas of the individual in public services*. New York: Russell Sage Foundation.

Marques, S., Lima, M. L., Abrams, D., & Swift, H. J. (2014). Will to live in older people's medical decisions: Immediate and delayed effects of aging stereotypes. *Journal of Applied Social Psychology*, *44*, 399–408. doi:10.1111/jasp.12231

Milne, A., Sullivan, M., Tanner, P., Richards, S., Ray, M., Lloyd, L., … Phillips, J. (2014). *Social work with older people: A vision for the future*. The College of Social Work. Retrieved from www.bl.uk/collection-items/social-work-with-older-people-a-vision-for-the-future

National Centre for the Protection of Older People. (2009). *Public perceptions of older people and ageing: A literature review*. Dublin: UCB. Retrieved from www.academia.edu/2867848/Public_Perceptions_of_Older_People_and_Ageing_A_Literature_Review_November_2009

Ramsden, I. (1990). Cultural safety. *The New Zealand Nursing Journal Kai Tiaki*, *83*(11), 18–19.

Resident Assessment Instrument-Home Care (RAI-HC). (2010, September). *User's manual, Canadian version*. Retrieved from https://secure.cihi.ca/estore/productSeries.htm?pc=PCC130

Siegler, E. L., Lama, S. D., Knight, M. G., Laureano, E., & Carrington, R. M. (2015). Community-based supports and services for older adults: A primer for clinicians. *Journal of Geriatrics*, *2015*, 1–6. doi:10.1155/2015/678625

Solomon, R. (2004). The role of the social worker in long-term care. *Journal of Gerontological Social Work*, *43*(2/3), 187–202. doi:10.1300/J083v43n02_13

Statistics Canada. (2011). *Living arrangements of seniors*. Retrieved from www12.statcan.gc.ca/census-recensement/2011/as-sa/98-312-x/98-312-x2011003_4-eng.pdf

Taylor, S. (2013). *What is discourse analysis?* London: Bloomsbury.

Weedon, C. (1987). *Feminist practice and poststructuralist theory*. Oxford: Blackwell.

World Health Organization. (1998). *Health promotion glossary*. WHO/HPR/HEP/98.1. Geneva: Division of Health Promotion, Education and Communications (HPR), Health Education and Health Promotion Unit (HEP). Retrieved July 23, 2019 www.who.int/healthpromotion/about/HPR%20Glossary%201998.pdf

Yesavage, J. A., Brink, T. L., Rose, T. L., Lum, O., Huang, V., Adey, M. B., & Leirer, V. O. (1983). Development and validation of a geriatric depression screening scale: A preliminary report. *Journal of Psychiatric Research*, *17*, 37–49.

Part 2

Doing AOP social work with older adults

Chapter 4

Deconstructing risk and frailty

Questions to consider as you read this chapter

- What are your own attitudes to risk and risk-taking? How could this influence your approach to working with older adults?
- Consider the last time you supported a person to make a decision that involved an element of risk. Did you empower or disempower them? How? What would you do differently?
- What specific social work skills do you see as essential to supporting older adults like Eleanor (see below)?
- What challenges do you see as preventing older adults like Eleanor from living with an "acceptable level of risk"?

You are a social worker in a hospital who receives the following referral at weekly inter-professional rounds:

> Eleanor is an 85-year old widow living in her own small home that she has owned for the last 51 years. She was admitted to the hospital after a fall at home where she was found by a neighbour who comes in to check on her once in a while. When Eleanor came to the hospital, she was described as being, "a frail, elderly woman with poor cognition and insight into her situation". Now that she has been medically stabilized, the care team feel that she is too "high risk" to return to her own home and want the social worker to follow up with her regarding long-term care placement.

The sites and sectors of health and social care where gerontological social workers practice, such as hospitals, long-term care facilities, and community health units, have become increasingly "risk averse". This leads to problematic implications for social work practitioners and disempowering outcomes for the older adults with whom they work. The social work referral received for Eleanor represents a common occurrence in social work practice with older adults. That is, the diagnosis or categorization of older adults as "frail" and "at-risk" and the directive for the social worker to manage and eradicate the potential for risky behaviours and incidents from occurring in the future. Chronological age itself is enough to initiate a social work referral/intervention; anyone over the age of 80 who is admitted to hospital often automatically receives a visit from a social worker. The main expression and measure of risk in older adults is frailty, a bio-medically constructed label and condition that focusses on individual deficits associated with aging such as cognitive and physical decline and their resulting limitations, vulnerabilities, and deficits (Grenier, 2007; Rush, Kvorjen, & Hole, 2016). Looking critically at how risk and frailty are constructed for older adults is important for social workers because they are actively involved in the processes and practices of constructing, assessing, and managing risk, often in ways that are not compatible with professional values such as social justice, empowerment, and self-determination. This in turn impacts relationships and the ways that social workers engage with older adults, the evidence used to understand their experiences, and the interventions applied to resolve their "problems".

In this chapter, the stories of practitioners and older adults like Eleanor who are negotiating the aging process will be used to critically explore how designations of frailty and risk are used to manage their experiences and what social workers can do to address the challenges of AOP social work within these sites and sectors of care where tensions between self-determination/social justice and managing risk and frailty run quite high.

The objectives of this chapter are to

- Define and deconstruct risk and frailty as they are problematically constructed and managed through the lived experiences of older adults;
- Situate these experiences in the larger structural forces of organizational practices such as the emergence of risk management and neoliberalism and their relationship to the bio-medicalization of aging in health and social care for older adults;
- Explore the role of self-determination and the rights of older people to live at-risk and how social workers can support this; and
- Reflect on ways that social workers can challenge and resist practices (push back) that support and reinforce individual and structural risks.

As a new social worker, I (Louise) began my practice 25 years ago, at a small community agency that supported older adults to live independently in their own homes. The agency was located in an ethno-culturally diverse working-class community, where many of the older adults had been living their lives and dealing with inequitable social and structural factors like poverty due to inter-secting categories of difference such as gender, race, and ethnicity. Many of the people I worked with were what could be described as living "at-risk", with a wide range of physical and cognitive challenges like dementia, mental illness, addictions, and other chronic illnesses that, while not specific to the aging process, were exacerbated by it. Their living conditions would be considered by some (including the authorities) as problematic, unsafe, and unhygienic and they were often described as being "hoarders", "cat ladies", or "hermits". They had limited social, economic, political, and material supports, and they were often mistrustful of, and resistant to, interference from traditional sites and sectors of health and social care.

All together, this meant that supporting them to keep living on their own terms was often a challenge, but because of a lifetime of challenges, they were also particularly resilient to both the conditions of aging and living in circumstances that others may deem "problematic" or "risky". Age and the aging process may have exacerbated the precarious nature of their abilities to live independently in their own homes, but these individuals remained determined to be in control of their own lives.

We were able to work with these clients to keep them in their homes safely, while reducing the potential for harm. This could be as simple as having meal delivery once a day, or having a "home maker" [personal support worker] take them grocery shopping once a week, or even agreeing to have us touch base and build relationships with them on their doorsteps. Unfortunately, once a crisis or tipping point happened, they came under the gaze and control of the more mainstream care sectors, specifically the mental health and health care system – even the police or the public health department. Once engaged in these systems, the ability to make "risky" decisions and control their own lives was considerably diminished. The nature of these interventions tended to decontextualize older adults' lives and focussed on their so-called pathologies and deficits – like their cognitive or physical functioning – rather than on their strengths and capacity to live at the "margins".

The "official" assessment and intervention process did little to identify and address factors such as poverty, ageism, racism and sexism that created and facilitated structural risk such as social isolation and inadequate access to resources and services. Risk as applied to their living circumstances, their decision-making capacities, and their choices were often seen as a "problem" to be fixed and changed rather than as a circumstance to work with and around. I used to call this, "getting sucked into the system and disappearing" rather than "falling through the cracks". The latter implicates the individual for not being careful enough, while the former identifies the system as the source of the problem.

This chapter starts with an overview of a social worker reflecting back on how risk came to be constructed and embedded in their early practice experiences. It points to the fact that there has been an incremental and increasingly problematic shift happening in social work generally and with older adults specifically. This is described by Hardy (2015) as

a notable shift from approaches to social work which take the welfare of the individual service user as their principle concern and rationale for practice, to systems which seek to assess and manage risk which service users pose, either to themselves or others.

(p. 1)

The social worker initially saw themselves as an advocate and ally of the older adults with whom they were working, helping them to navigate complex and disempowering systems and co-creating with them the least intrusive interventions that took into account safety and professional, ethical, and legal responsibilities. The shift to risk management has increasingly become the central organizing principle of most gerontological social work practice. More often, social workers are being directed to intervene in ways that tend to emphasize protection of and vigilance over older adults with roles that become primarily managerial, consisting of "a series of short term investigatory, crisis management or surveillance related tasks" (Carey, 2016, p. 344). This shift is to the detriment of the professional values of advocacy, empowerment, and social justice, the roles and relationships held with the clients, and the increasing accountability to sites and sectors of care rather than to people. Most importantly, this shift has influenced the rights, choices, and quality of life and well-being of the older adults with whom social workers are involved.

Defining risk

How "risk" is defined and understood has implications for its application to both the practice and policy on which social workers draw (Waugh, 2009). For AOP social workers, this means it is important to explore not only the concept of "risk" through the academic and practice literature, but also how it is applied to the lives of older adults as they navigate the aging process. Lupton (1999) posits two very different ways in which risk is currently understood and practiced. The first is a *technico-specific approach* (p. 27) that positions risk as a set of objective realities that can be identified, measured, and managed or controlled. Experts are able to measure the potential of hazard and danger facing individuals through scientific methods, such as assessment tools, risk analysis, and standardized practice. In turn, individuals are considered conscious and rational actors who make decisions based on these realities and their potential outcomes. Standardized methods of risk appraisal and probability are seen as viable because of the objective nature of "risk", where it is viewed as independent from an individual's socio-cultural context. This approach closely aligns with neoliberalism (see textbox 3.3) and governmentality that has facilitated the rise of risk management in the sites and sectors of health and social care that work with client groups deemed particularly "vulnerable" and in need of "protection" and oversight, like older adults.

Lupton (1999) describes a second approach to risk: a *socio-cultural approach* that situates risk in specific socio-cultural contexts by focussing on how it is understood, lived, embodied, and negotiated (p. 36). Specifically, risk is described as a socially and politically constructed concept that is used to organize, monitor, and regulate individuals, groups, and institutions. Mitchell and Glendinning (2008) capture the socially constructed nature of this concept and define risk as "complex and multidimensional, the definitions of which vary across and within different cultural contexts and settings, and that are historically and event specific" (p. 2). This means that what is defined as "risk" is open to interpretation within the context in which it is constructed. What is "risky" to one person may be completely normal to another. This extends beyond the individual to include the perceptions of professional and social structures such as institutions, the media, policies, and laws. Perceptions about tolerable and intolerable risks for older adults have become embedded in the systems, structures, and practices of care that many older adults find themselves interacting with as they age (Ballinger & Payne, 2002). Because of this, defining and assessing risk can never be a neutral act and are susceptible to a number of dominant societal and professional discourses (see textbox 3.1 in **Sites and sectors of health and social care**) around choice, aging, individual responsibility, danger, autonomy, and decision-making, amongst others.

Risk and "being at-risk", then, are labels that are commonly articulated and used when discussing older adults (as seen in the referral for Eleanor), yet there are critiques about whether there is an universally accepted definition of what it is (MacLeod & Stadnyk, 2015), and it remains to many an "ambiguous social construct" (Vyvey, Roose, De Wilde, & Roets, 2014, p. 760). AOG social workers should have a critical understanding of both approaches because while they may naturally be drawn to the socio-cultural approach because of its emphasis on context and environment, they are often working in sites and sectors of care that adhere to a technico-specific approach. This means that their practice may be dominated by one approach, with little room for the other unless it is championed and made explicit. In the next section, we will deconstruct how risk is understood in practice with older adults. As you read this, consider what approach informs the following practices.

Situating risk in older adults' lives

As it applies to older adults, risk reflects the discourses of successful aging and the bio-medicalization of aging, where older adults who are considered "at-risk" are portrayed as "frail", incapacitated, passive, morally problematic, and in need of special oversight and protection (see Table 4.1). This conceptualization is further enabled by external factors and influences such as professional socialization, organizational mandates, and the policies and legislation that attempt to prevent and curtail risk and risk-taking. Finally, it is important to note that there is a particularly ageist slant to these discourses, in that somehow older people should not be able to or cannot take the same risks as younger people (Carey, 2016). Even within the context of disability, older adults are seen as frail and vulnerable people who need to be protected from risk, while younger individuals with disabilities accept risk as the price of full social participation (Kane, Priester, & Neumann, 2007, p. 271).

Risk is essentially "future focused" and predicated on the *potential* that an action, activity, or decision may lead to an undesirable or negative outcome (Browne, Blake, Donnelly, & Herbert, 2002; MacLeod & Stadnyk, 2015). To illustrate, let's look at the case of Charlene:

> *Charlene is a 68-year old Inuit woman who has come down south for three months from Nunavut for cancer treatment at an Ottawa hospital. Charlene also has arthritis and uses a four-wheeled walker. She is slow but prides herself on her mobility and her ability to get out and "enjoy life". The nurses make a referral to the social worker because Charlene wants to leave the hospital, which reminds her too much of residential school. She wants to go visit family that live in the Ottawa area and plans to get there on the public bus as she is used to getting around on her own back home. The care staff feel she should not leave the building unaccompanied because something might happen to her, especially because of her complex chronic disease (CCD, see textbox 3.6) and the fact that she is not used to being in a "big city".*

The suggested restrictions in Charlene's case may be framed as the potential for her to fall, exacerbate her CCD, or even get lost while outside of the hospital. The reality is that any of these outcomes and events could happen to her regardless of

Table 4.1 How risk is constructed in relation to older adults

Risk

- Is future focussed;
- Situates the problem (and the solution) in the individual;
- De-contextualizes older adults' lived experiences;
- Ignores the structural risks, like poverty, that older adults face;
- Implies it is the moral responsibility of individuals to avoid risk;
- Focusses on risk as something to be avoided and problematized; and
- Proposes it should be defined and managed by experts.

where she was residing – but the assumption is that the formalized care setting of the hospital should be "safer" and should "protect" her from risk. Risk is a part of any individual's life, but in this case, the focus is only on the present and the future, rather than the past. As it relates to Charlene's story, for example, her arthritis has been part of her life for a long time, and it is safe to assume that she has specific strategies to cope with and manage it. In this context, there is limited exploration of how risk has been managed across the life course, specifically with a focus on strengths and strategies, and a discounting of the cultural and historical dimensions of risk knowledge (Clarke, 2000).

Another consideration of Charlene's case is the perceived potential for an undesirable future outcome for the care staff – the assumption that she will be "safer" and "protected" in care settings. Health care professionals (some more than others) are compelled to have a "duty to protect/care" and may feel "liable" and responsible if harm occurs to Charlene. The professional "duty to protect or care" that focusses on protecting vulnerable individuals from foreseeable harm is often at cross-purposes with self-determination and individual autonomy (Mitchell & Glendinning, 2008). Taylor's (2006) research in long-term care, for example, found that risk-based policies and legislation, along with a fear of litigation, influenced professionals to focus more on maleficence (do no harm) rather than beneficence (duty to do good). This is a fear-based and "defensive approach to care" (Ibrahim & Davis, 2013) where professionals err on the side of caution, without necessarily recognizing the impacts on personal factors such as an individual's quality of life and well-being. Stripping Charlene of the ability to actively participate in her world outside of the hospital "just in case" may not be the intention of the care staff, but these practices have the ability to do just that.

As evident in the cases of Charlene and Eleanor, risk is conceptualized as something *negative or undesirable*, a problem that needs to be avoided, prevented, or managed (Tanner, 1998). The current everyday language used to describe risk, for example, uses terms that emphasize risk as being related to *threat, hazard, or danger*. This is particularly evident in the professional practice of those involved with caring for "vulnerable populations". Research shows that when talking about risk and older adults, professionals tend to describe risk exclusively in terms of its negative outcomes (MacLeod & Stadnyk, 2015). This "negative lens" used to understand risk is at once constructed by a societal fear of liability and blame and reinforced and embedded in the policies, practices, and professional socialization and training in the sites and sectors of health and social care where these professionals work (MacLeod & Stadnyk, 2015). To illustrate this, let's follow up on Eleanor's case.

> *The team talks about Eleanor's case at rounds in more depth. The shared consensus is that if she goes back home, then she will be at the same risk as before she came in. One person describes it as "another disaster waiting to happen". The team decides it would be better for Eleanor to have round-the- clock care to build up her strength and keep her safe than to allow her to go home.*

Living alone at home with risk is described as "*another disaster waiting to happen*" and "*unsafe*". Even the care team's description or labelling of Eleanor as "high risk" infers immediate and serious threats to her safety. This lens primarily focusses on Eleanor's deficits and problems, with little emphasis or discussion about strengths, capacities, and resources. There is little to no emphasis on "positive risk-taking" in the gerontological practice and research literature (Croft, 2017; Robertson & Collinson, 2011). Because it is viewed in such a negative light, social and health care professionals have been charged with avoiding and diminishing potential harms and poor outcomes relating to risk and risk-taking. This leads to a number of challenges for AOG social workers relating to their professional values, roles, and responsibilities and the types of relationships they may develop with the older adults with whom they work.

Risk as frailty

Risk is situated in the individual and is often linked to contributing or causal factors such as physical and cognitive impairments that are considered age specific. Eleanor's diagnosis of "being high risk" is based primarily on her diagnosis of "frailty" (on the referral form) – specifically her physical and cognitive status and functioning. According to Grenier (2007), the dominant expression of risk as it relates to aging bodies and minds is *frailty*. Frailty is a bio-medical term that attempts to measure functional (physical, medical, and cognitive) loss; it is considered a strong predictor of mortality, institutionalization, loss of autonomy, falls, and fractures (St. John, Montgomery, & Tyas, 2013). This means that for older people, risk or being at-risk is understood using a medicalized categorization that focusses primarily on the inabilities and limitations of their aging bodies and minds. This narrow and medicalized category of frailty and the situating of risk primarily in the individual renders invisible the many social and structural factors that create and facilitate risk. The assessment and intervention process, therefore, will focus primarily on the specific individual without identifying inequalities that contribute and facilitate "risk" such as social isolation, socio-economic status, gender, ethno-cultural identity, racism, and ageism (Tanner, 1998). Going back to Eleanor's case, the focus is on her falls, her nutritional state, and her poor memory and insight, ignoring the risks inherent in other factors (social determinants of health) such as her social isolation, poverty, or lack of access to support services and resources. Eleanor may have been like many older adults living in the community, who are not eligible for increasingly scarce subsidized homecare services and may not have the material means to afford private care. Also, her social isolation may have prevented her from accessing help before the fall.

Risk as a moral lapse

There is a moral tone attributed to the discourse of risk as it applies to older adults, especially in how it stigmatizes those who are perceived to be living "at-risk". Hardy (2015) states that "being 'at-risk' is a manifestation of a failure to fulfil one's responsibility to function capably within society, or a moral lapse of a flawed identity" (p. 30). Eleanor's case reflects the idea that at-risk older adults are often described as unable to "cope" or successfully manage the aging process – to be active agers – and for that reason, intervention and protection are required.

When you (the social worker) go visit Eleanor, she states to you that there is absolutely no way she will move to a long-term care facility. She is adamant that she wants to return home. This frustrates the team because they believe that she has no real insight into her coping abilities and limitations. They wonder if they should assess her capacity to make decisions.

This moral tone can be linked to the discourse of *successful aging*, discussed in **Theorizing later life and social work praxis**, which posits that some people age more successfully than others and are in turn less likely to require support or help or rely on scarce resources. Rowe and Kahn (1997) describe successful aging as "low probability of disease and disability, high cognitive and physical capacity, and an active engagement with life" (p. 433) through the facilitation of an appropriate lifestyle. Interventions therefore are centred on maintaining positive functioning and activity for as long as possible. The moral tone of this discourse is the premise that it is the individual's responsibility to age successfully and to avoid risk by being physically and cognitively well and active. It also assumes that aging can be measured as either successful or a failure – and that those who are not aging "successfully" are problematic (Katz, 2000; Katz & Calasanti, 2015; Katz & Marshall, 2004).

If aging successfully is an individual choice and one that is valued culturally, then it is one's duty and moral obligation to make choices that will facilitate it. An example of this is Ballinger and Payne's (2002) exploration of the construction of risk and falling for older adults. The authors found that in health care, falls are constructed as objective reality, with a focus on managing physical risks that can be predicted and prevented. A resistance to or a denial of the objective realities of their "unsuccessful aging" through falling and its inherent risks results in victim blaming (p. 309). Victim blaming is evident in Eleanor's case, where the team is frustrated with her resistance and non-compliance with their assessment (the objective reality of risk) and attribute this to her lack of "insight" or cognitive ability. The successful aging paradigm is also problematic because of a lack of systemic or structural exploration on how un/successful aging may occur, and the impacts of personal biography and lifetime experiences on the aging process including cumulative disadvantages such as poverty and poor health, which are related to gender, ethnicity, and race (Rubinstein & de Medieros, 2015).

Expert management of risk

Perceptions of risk and the ways in which it is assessed and determined are managed by "experts". In settings such as hospitals, care facilities, and community health units, expertise about the threat of harm of risk is often located in the assumed knowledge base of the medical professional (or expert) rather than in the preferences or experiences of the older adults themselves. Research shows that there are perceptible differences between professionals, family members, and older adults (clients) in defining "risk" and being "at-risk" (Taylor, 2006; Waugh, 2009). Hospital discharge planning is a good example of how different perceptions and definitions of risk are played out between health care professionals and older adults, specifically as it relates to power.

As a practice, discharge planning has been identified as primarily driven by a discourse of risk management (Huby, Stewart, Tierney, & Rogers, 2004). In the culture of risk management, "being at risk" is almost always classified by the system/

expert the client is engaged with, rather than by the client themselves (Clancy, Happell, & Moxham, 2015; Clarke, 2000). Research on the process of discharge planning, decision-making, and risk has found that older adults are often completely left out of the process. In Huby et al.'s (2004) study, practitioners justified a lack of involvement of older adults in the discharge planning process as having to do with their assessment of declining mental and physical abilities. The authors also found that the older adults who were excluded from the process occupied a place of reduced social standing because of their lower socio-economic status and limited education (including literacy), which impeded their skills to negotiate with "experts" (p. 126). The ability to execute autonomous decision-making as it relates to risk has therefore been found to be severely limited by age, economic status, language and literacy, diagnosis (such as dementia), gender, and the availability of resources for older adults to advocate for themselves.

In the decision-making process, older adults are guided towards what Hicks, Sims-Gould, Byrne, Khan, and Stolee (2012) describe as "decisions that suit both normative health goals and social ordering" (p. 141). That is, practitioners controlled and defined the decisions, while believing they were actually offering the patients a choice. Mac-Court and Tuokko (2010) found that the ratings of risk and safety (both through standardized and informal assessments) that health care practitioners use about decision-making and risk are value laden and differ from those articulated by older adults. Practitioners underestimated the importance of quality of life when assessing risk for older adults, by using their own personal and professional values to assess whether the older adults could and should make "risky" decisions. Clancy, Happell, and Moxham (2015) also found a difference between the language and terminology used to describe risk between older adults and health care practitioners. As it relates to risk, older adults would focus on their own safety, including the security and confidence in themselves to manage their risk – rather than measures that would be used to avoid potential harm. These findings infer that the perspectives, values, and interests of older adults and health care practitioners are often in conflict when determining service plans and interventions, and that the nature and extent of these conflicts are rarely acknowledged.

Pushing back

The social work referral to "see" Eleanor presented at the beginning of this chapter illustrates that many health and social care professionals experience complex tensions relating to the practice and management of risk in older adult's lives. This includes anxiety about who is responsible when harm occurs and how it would be addressed legally and professionally (Gilmour, Gibson, & Campbell, 2003); the tension experienced when meeting professional and organizational responsibilities, while attempting to adhere to person-centred principles of empowerment and autonomy (de Witt & Ploeg, 2016); and addressing competing "best interests" by care professionals, family members, and the older person themselves (Waugh, 2009). These findings infer that the organizational and systemic contexts where social workers practice create environments that disempower both the social worker and older adults. As AOG social workers, part of our practice should be to critically reflect on these tensions and to *push back* against them.

Subverting definitions of risk

AOG social workers should be willing to challenge and subvert the reliance on systemic, technico-specific definitions and appraisals of "risk" and risk-taking that dominate sites and sectors of practice. This includes challenging the *exclusive* use of standardized measurements, screening tools, and assessments that de-contextualize the lives of older adults, and working to include and prioritize older adults' understanding and conceptualizations of risk. The current language of risk adopted by health and social care professionals does little to reflect the concerns of older adults (Browne et al., 2002), such as how it can represent a loss of independence, loss of autonomy, and the disruption of life as they have known it (Rush et al., 2016). This can be done through the exploration of each individual's narrative and lived experience and by identifying dominant discourses that inform and impact them. In Eleanor's case, this may mean exploring with her how she perceives risk, how she has handled adversity and risk throughout her life course, and identifying strengths and strategies that can be used to address risks that could make returning home tenable. It also requires social workers to consider how "risk" has been constructed as problematic in her life – for example, as a single, older woman. In translating these conversations to team members, social workers should emphasize the importance of quality of life and the emotional context of these "decisions", as well as the potential to reframe how "risk" is perceived and understood.

Least intrusive practices

AOP social workers should attempt to focus on least intrusive practices in addressing risk with older adults. This means that interventions should be guided by principles (both social work practice ethics and guardianship legislation) that balance the responsibility to intervene, support, and protect vulnerable older adults *along with* the ethical responsibility to respect and protect their rights of autonomy and self-determination. Browne et al. (2002) posit that "interference" with older adults as it pertains to "risk" should follow specific principles such as

- Freedom is the rule.
- Interference always needs justification.
- The onus of justification lies on those wanting to interfere.

Central to this type of approach is that an older adult's capacity (the ability to make informed decisions) must be presumed until proven otherwise (see **Dementia, personhood, and citizenship as practice**). For example, in Eleanor's case, her capacity to make informed decisions is questioned by the team, but with limited formal or legally assessed evidence. Even when it is assessed, capacity must be seen as a multidimensional concept that encompasses a number of different domains of functioning that cannot be applied globally to all decision-making processes and abilities (Ibrahim & Davis, 2013). So, for example, while a person may be deemed "incapable" of managing their finances, it does not mean that they cannot make decisions about their daily activities. Social workers must be aware of the legislative parameters and checks and balances relating to professional responsibilities around capacity/competency in their own jurisdictions. This will help guide their practice and ability to educate other professionals and stakeholders on the rights of older people to make decisions.

Emerging research and practice literature have pointed to the adoption and integration of harm reduction principles in addressing risk and aging in place (Whitfield, Daniels, Flesaker, & Simmons, 2012). While used mainly as it applies to alcohol and substance mis/use, a harm reduction approach can be applied to "risk" and "risk-taking" in general. A more fulsome exploration of the harm reduction philosophy can be found in **Mental illness, mental wellness and substance mis/use**. As a philosophy of care, it conceptualizes risk on a continuum. This means that not all risks have the same potential impacts or outcomes, and they should be treated differently. An integration of harm reduction principles such as pragmatism, human rights, maximizing intervention options, starting where the person is at, and involvement of the person can be a useful approach to addressing risk. It detracts from paternalism and attempts to mitigate problems or structural factors that have contributed to older adults being "at-risk" such as poverty, racism, and social isolation. This becomes most essential when working with older adults who have impaired cognition and abilities such as Eleanor and Charlene whose "voices" and "experiences" are silenced or constructed as problematic within a bio-medical context. Instead, social workers should work to integrate advocacy and collaboration with older adult clients into their practice, by recognizing and respecting their decision-making capabilities and rights and integrating them into planning and intervention processes. A better approach with Eleanor would be to engage with her to prioritize her preferences. Rather than asking the question: "Do you want to go home or to a nursing home?" it may be more useful to reframe the question as: "Where do you see yourself going from here and how can that happen?"

Positive risk-taking

As noted earlier in this chapter, risk and risk-taking have been constructed as dangerous, negative, and to be avoided or heavily managed. A positive risk-taking approach starts with the assumption that living with risk is a normal part of everyday life, that it can be minimized but never eradicated, and that it is constantly evolving according to changing individual, structural, and contextual circumstances (Morgan, 2004). Bornat and Bytheway (2010) state that risk in everyday life for older adults should be viewed as an "ongoing process" of "managing in relation to different types of adversity and changed circumstances" (p. 1132). This approach opens up the opportunity and space to begin to work collaboratively with older adults where the social worker can work to

- Identify potential risks;
- Develop plans and actions that reflect the positive potentials and stated priorities of the older adult; and
- Use available supports and resources to achieve desired outcomes and minimize potential harmful outcomes (Morgan, 2004, p. 18).

If we again go to Eleanor's case, the social worker would work collaboratively with Eleanor and the team to identify potential risks that could be present in her home setting by including her in meetings with the team to plan for discharge. This would be an opportunity for both the team and Eleanor to collaboratively identify strengths, supports, and resources that she could access and draw upon.

Recognizing and changing structural risks

An important role that AOG social workers can take is to make visible and change the structural factors that create and facilitate risk in older adults' lives. For example, in Eleanor's case, this includes how social isolation and lack of accessibility to services and supports may have created conditions where her ability to cope with physiological or cognitive changes were compromised. She had no family members and no community supports to help advocate for her, and so she was left to cope on her own, resulting in a medical crisis. Research shows that older adults, especially older women who live alone and who have some form of cognitive impairment, are at greater risk for placement than any other individuals or groups (de Witt & Ploeg, 2016). Repositioning risk *outside* of the individual helps to detract from a singular focus on physical and cognitive functioning (and decline) through the assessment and intervention process. Recognizing and reducing the impacts of these structural factors may allow for clients like Eleanor to return home with appropriate supports and services in place. This is especially important when working with groups and individuals who have traditionally experienced discrimination and disadvantage across the life course due to gender, race, and class and their intersection with age. As noted earlier, the ability to participate in these types of professional negotiations in health and social care settings are often limited for older adults where the power of professional expertise and a focus on risk management encroach on their autonomy.

Clarity in roles and responsibilities

Social work roles and responsibilities relating to "risk" and older adults will vary according to where their practice is located. Hospital-based social workers are often involved in discharge planning; community-based social workers are mostly focussed on case management or community development; and long-term care social workers are involved in admissions and transition, family issues, and end-of-life care. Regardless of where they work, there are essential roles and responsibilities that social workers applying AOG principles can take to ensure that the ways in which they work with older adults are strengths-based and anti-oppressive; these include an understanding of the physical and mental health problems older people may experience within the context of economic, social, cultural, and environmental influences.

First is the acknowledgement, development, and maintenance of relationship as the fulcrum of what Ray et al. (2015) describe as creative practice, where the social worker is as focussed on the process of their work as on its potential outcomes. Second is the importance of knowledge acquisition and education on issues and systems relevant to older adults, the conditions that create and maintain risk in their lives, and how these conditions are constructed for older adults by sites and sectors of care and sustained by them. This includes the need to be critically reflective of our own (and those of the sites and sectors we work in) ageist attitudes, biases, and assumptions that we hold about older adults and risk-taking and how that may impact the work we do with older adults like Charlene and Eleanor. Finally, we need to de-centre the dominant "knowledge and expertise" of professionals and make room for older adults' perspectives, wishes, and experiences relating to risk-taking.

Exercise

Social workers are often asked to assess and evaluate risk in the lives of older adults. For this exercise, choose and identify a tool that has been developed to assess risk. This tool can be situated in a number of different settings (long-term care, hospitals, day programs, community care) and for different kinds of risks (falls, cognition, decision-making, medication, safety). As you examine this tool, consider the following questions:

- What is this tool looking to measure or understand?
- What are some underlying assumptions about aging that informs this tool?
- How is the tool to be administered?
- How does this tool include the perspectives of older adults (or not)?
- What do the outcomes of the assessment tool help to facilitate?
- What are some of the pros and cons of this tool? What does it value and what does it "miss"?
- What social work skills would you draw on to complement the use of this tool?
- How could you make the use and application of this tool more anti-oppressive?

Takeaways

- The management and eradication of risk have become a central organizing principle of gerontological social work practice within neo-liberal and bio-medical contexts.
- Defining, assessing, and intervening in risk are never neutral acts.
- Anti-oppressive approaches to addressing risk in older adults' lives should include practices that are least intrusive, focussed on positive risk-taking, and the reduction of harm, rather than its complete eradication.
- Social workers should be willing to "push back" against the dominance of risk aversion and management in their AOG work with older adults and the practices that increase or reinforce structural and socially situated risks and the disempowerment of older adults who wish to live "with risk".
- Risk should be explored using a life course perspective that takes into account individual and structural risks across an individual's life as well as resilience and coping strategies.

References

Ballinger, C., & Payne, S. (2002). The construction of risk of falling among and by older people. *Aging and Society, 22*, 305–324. doi:10.1017/S0144686X02008620.

Bornat, J., & Bytheway, B. (2010). Perceptions and presentations of living with everyday risk in later life. *British Journal of Social Work, 40*(4), 1118–1134. doi:10.1093/bjsw/bcq001.

Browne, A., Blake, M., Donnelly, M., & Herbert, D. (2002). On liberty for the old. *Canadian Journal of Aging, 21*(2), 283–293. doi:10.1017/S0714980800001537.

Carey, M. (2016). Journey's end: From residual service to newer forms of pathology, risk aversion and abandonment in social work with older adults. *Journal of Social Work, 16*(3), 344–361. doi:10.1177/1468017315578639.

Clancy, L., Happell, B., & Moxham, L. (2015). Perception of risk for older people living with a mental illness: Balancing uncertainty. *International Journal of Mental Health Nursing, 24*, 577–586. doi:10.1111/inm.12175.

Clarke, C. L. (2000). Risk: Constructing care and care environments in dementia. *Health, Risk and Society, 3*(1), 83–93. doi:10.1080/136985700111477.

Croft, J. (2017). Enabling positive risk-taking for older people in care homes. *Nursing and Residential Care, 19*(9), 515–519. doi:10.12968/nrec.2017.19.9.51.

de Witt, L., & Ploeg, J. (2016). Caring for older people living alone with dementia: Health care professional's experiences. *Dementia, 15*(2), 221–238. doi:10.1177/1471301214523280.

Gilmour, H., Gibson, F., & Campbell, J. (2003). Living alone with dementia: A case study approach to understanding risk. *Dementia, 2*(3), 403–420. doi:10.1080/02650533.2017.1397612.

Grenier, A. (2007). Constructions of frailty in the English language, care practice and the lived experience. *Ageing & Society, 27*, 425–445. doi:10.1017/S0144686X06005782.

Hardy, M. (2015). *Governing risk: Care and control in contemporary social work.* Houndmills, Basingstoke: Palgrave Macmillan.

Hicks, E., Sims-Gould, J., Byrne, K., Khan, K. M., & Stolee, P. (2012). "She was a little bit unrealistic": Choice in health care decision making for older people. *Journal of Aging Studies, 26*, 140–148. doi:10.1016/j.jaging.2011.10.004.

Huby, G., Stewart, J., Tierney, A., & Rogers, W. (2004). Planning older people's discharge from acute hospital care: Including risk management and patient participation in decision making. *Health, Risk and Society, 6*(2), 115–132. doi:10.1080/1369857042000219797.

Ibrahim, J. E., & Davis, M. C. (2013). Impediments to applying the dignity of risk principle in aged care services. *Australasian Journal of Aging, 32*(3), 188–193. doi:10.1111/ajag.12014.

Kane, D. L., Priester, R., & Neumann, D. (2007). Does disparity in the way disabled older adults are treated imply ageism? *The Gerontologist, 47*(3), 271–279. doi:10.1093/geront/47.3.271.

Katz, S. (2000). Busy bodies: Activity, aging, and the management of everyday life. *Journal of Aging Studies, 14*(2), 135–152.

Katz, S., & Calasanti, T. (2015). Critical perspectives on successful aging: Does it "appeal more than it illuminates"? *The Gerontologist, 55*(1), 26–33.

Katz, S., & Marshall, B. (2004). Is the functional "normal"? Aging, sexuality and the bio-marking of successful living. *History of the Human Sciences, 17*(1), 53–75.

Lupton, D. (1999). *Risk.* London: Routledge.

MacCourt, P., & Tuokko, H. (2010). Marginal competence, risk assessment, and care decisions: A comparison of values of health care professionals and older adults. *Canadian Journal of Aging, 29*(2), 173–183. doi:10.1017/S0714980810000097.

MacLeod, H., & Stadnyk, R. L. (2015). "Risk: I know it when I see it": How health and social practitioners defined and evaluated living at risk among community dwelling older adults. *Health, Risk and Society, 17*(1), 46–63. doi:10.1080/13698575.2014.999749.

Mitchell, W., & Glendinning, C. (2008). Risk and adult social care: Identification, management and new policies: What does UK research evidence tell us? *Health, Risk and Society, 10*(3), 297–315. doi:10.1080/13698570802163677.

Morgan, S. (2004). Positive risk taking: An idea whose time has come. *Health Care Risk Report, 10* (10), 18–19. Retrieved from http://static1.1.sqspcdn.com/static/f/586382/9538512/1290507680737/OpenMind-PositiveRiskTaking.pdf?token=hM8ijWso%2Bb1TnttcfN4%2B49wcYd4%3D.

Ray, M., Milne, A., Beech, C., Phillips, J. E., Richards, S., Sullivan, M. P., … Lloyd, L. (2015). Gerontological social work: Reflections on its role, purpose and value. *British Journal of Social Work, 45*(4), 1296–1312. doi:10.1093/bjsw/bct195.

Robertson, J. P., & Collinson, C. (2011). Positive risk taking: Whose risk is it? An exploration in community outreach teams in mental health and learning disabilities services. *Health, Risk and Society, 13*(2), 147–164. doi:10.1080/13698575.2011.556185.

Rowe, J. W., & Kahn, R. L. (1997). Successful aging. *The Gerontologist, 37*(3), 433–440.

Rubinstein, R., & De Medeiros, K. (2015). "Successful aging," gerontological theory and neoliberalism: A qualitative critique. *The Gerontologist, 55*(1), 34–42.

Rush, K. L., Kvorjen, M., & Hole, R. (2016). Older adult's risk practices from hospital to home: A discourse analysis. *The Gerontologist, 56*(3), 454–503. doi:10.1093/geront/gnu092.

St. John, P. D., Montgomery, P. R., & Tyas, S. L. (2013). Social position and frailty. *Canadian Journal of Aging, 32*(3), 250–259. doi:10.1017/S0714980813000329.

Tanner, D. (1998). The jeopardy of risk. *Practice, 10*(1), 15–28.

Taylor, B. (2006). Risk management paradigms in health and social services for professional decision making in the long-term care of older people. *British Journal of Social Work, 36*(8), 1411–1429. doi:10.9013/bjsw/bch406.

Vyvey, E., Roose, R., De Wilde, L., & Roets, G. (2014). Dealing with risk in child and family social work: From an anxious to a reflexive professional? *Social Sciences, 3*, 758–770. doi:10.3390/socsci3040758.

Waugh, F. (2009). Where does risk feature in community care practices with older people with dementia who live alone? *Dementia, 8*(2), 205–222. doi:10.1177/1471301209103255.

Whitfield, K. Y., Daniels, J. S., Flesaker, K., & Simmons, D. (2012). Older adults with hoarding behaviour aging in place: Looking to a collaborative community-based planning approach for solutions. *Journal of Aging Research, 2012*. doi:10.1155/2012/205425.

Chapter 5

Moral, legal, and ethical issues

Questions to consider as you read this chapter

- What does consent mean in the context of illness and end of life? Should decision-making be autonomous (individual) or shared (collective)?
- How do we balance the care and control dynamic in social work practice with older adults?
- What are our legal and ethical responsibilities as social workers? How does the jurisdiction in which we practice relate to this?
- What are your personal and cultural beliefs about invasive treatments, Medical Assistance in Dying (MAiD) and other moral, legal, and ethical issues? How do Eurocentrism, familism, and neo-liberalism play into these issues?

Mrs. P is an 81-year-old woman who was recently admitted to hospital in downtown Halifax due to "failure to thrive". The social worker who receives the referral for discharge planning has been assigned to oncology and general surgery for over a year and is unsurprised to see a possible diagnosis of colon cancer in the chart notes, as "failure to thrive" often precedes a diagnosis of cancer.

Mrs. P lives in a social housing apartment with her 53-year-old son Miles who has intellectual and developmental disabilities, a form of neuro-diversity.[1] She has two other adult children and five grandchildren and has been a widow for over 30 years. Her daughter lives close by in Dartmouth with her partner and their three children, and her other son and his family live about two hours east of Halifax in Antigonish. Both are concerned about their mother's ability to manage at home due to her recent memory problems and their brother's need for assistance and question whether the current living situation is safe due to the "trillions of cockroaches" the daughter has seen there.

After probing Mrs. P's understanding of why she is in hospital and what the doctors think might be wrong with her, it becomes clear to the social worker that Mrs. P is unaware of her possible cancer diagnosis. Further, while she denies any problems with cognitive functioning, she displays memory loss and disorientation. When asked about how well she manages at home and what supports she has in place, Mrs. P discloses that she had continuing care services (nursing, home support) and Meals on Wheels, but cancelled all of these services through the care coordinator six months ago, as they were "too much up in her business". As the referral is for discharge planning, the social worker discusses the possibility of long-term care (i.e., a nursing home) with Mrs. P, should the doctors determine that she is unable to return home. She is open to alternate living arrangements, so long as she and her son Miles can remain together as they "look after each other".[2] *Her primary concerns are cooking and cleaning. The two adult children feel it is unsafe for Mrs. P and their brother Miles to return to their own apartment, though both are reluctant to look after the two of them in their own homes as each has a young family. Complicating the situation further, they do not want either Mrs. P or Miles to know about their mother's cancer diagnosis, and the daughter has been liaising with the health care team.*

Although the social work referral was for Mrs. P, Miles cannot live independently; thus, he too is in need of social work services. The doctors are respecting the family's desire for non-disclosure of the cancer diagnosis as long as possible and have been seeking the daughter's consent rather than that of Mrs. P as her capacity has been called into question. The social worker is tasked with navigating this complexity, and their first step is to determine who the client is in this scenario and who should be the **substitute decision-maker (SDM)** *if informed consent cannot be given by the client(s). In order to wade through the moral, legal, and ethical issues raised by this case, the social worker also needs to be clear on their ethical and legal responsibilities.*

This chapter focuses on ethical and moral issues that relate to social work with older adults and that have a legal dimension. It builds on **sites and sectors of health and social care** as well as **deconstructing risk and frailty** and provides context for the more practice-focused chapters to follow. Specific topics and pieces of legislation addressed in this chapter include social work codes of ethics and standards of practice; health care consent, assent, and capacity; advance care planning, substitute decision-making, and adult guardianship; and end of life care and Medical Assistance in Dying (MAiD), also known as physician-assisted suicide. We address the ethical requirement to respect autonomy and self-determination as well as the limitations of bio-medical models that treat individuals as separate from their families and communities for decision-making purposes, unless their capacity to consent is compromised, in which case the individual is often neglected/side-lined, as seen in the opening case study.

In the case of Mrs. P and her son Miles, the capacity of each individual has been called into question, and the social worker should start by determining the reason for this and the accuracy of the assessment. When we talk about capacity, we are referring to capacity to consent to health or personal care decisions, including admission to a residential care home or a life-sustaining treatment such as a feeding tube. Capacity to consent to financial decisions is separate, and while this distinction is made clear in this chapter, it is not discussed in depth. Miles may be capable of determining what he would like to eat or do on any given day and express a wish that he prefers to live with his mother rather than with other family members yet be incapable of deciding amongst various alternatives in terms of housing and care arrangements. Alternatively, he may be capable of making decisions about his health and personal care but not about his finances. It is for this reason that we do not say that a person is "incapable", rather that they lack the capacity to make a (specific) decision. The person for whom a treatment is intended must always be asked for their consent first (i.e., before approaching a SDM and before providing treatment). Further, health care providers cannot rely upon advance directives, as "wishes are not decisions. Even if a patient has done advance care planning, health practitioners MUST talk to the patient or the incapable patient's SDM to get an informed consent before treatment" (Advocacy Centre for the Elderly, 2016).

Contemporary issues like first available bed policies,[3] MAiD, austerity measures, and decisions related to the rationing of health and social care represent debates within direct and indirect practice that have ethical, legal, and moral dimensions. This chapter addresses these emerging issues and applies them to the context of social work practice and anti-oppression gerontology (AOG) guidelines. Counter-storytelling highlights the need to recognize in practice that being ethical is challenging in a neo-liberal and managerialist context; definitions of quality of life of persons living with life-limiting illnesses may be markedly different than those of their care partners; decision-making is not always autonomous, rather it can be shared and occur in a collective context; and views on and approaches to end of life are culturally constructed and mediated.

The objectives of this chapter are to

*   Review ethical guidelines and regulatory practices for social work in Canada;
*   Clarify legal concepts like consent, capacity, guardianship, and substitute decision-making;
*   Describe and critically analyze legislation on health care consent (HCC) and substitute decision-making across Canada as well as social work guidance and roles; and
*   Highlight MAiD as an example of a moral, legal, and ethical issue that social workers need to be prepared to address in practice.

Social work codes of ethics and standards of practice

This chapter starts with an overview of the codes of ethics that govern our profession and the standards of practice that guide our work as social workers. Social work is a regulated health profession in most provinces and one of 30 health professional groups in Canada; there are more social workers per capita (143: 100,000 people) than any other health care provider group except for physicians and nurses (Canadian Institute for Health Information, 2017). As regulation of the profession is a provincial responsibility, social workers need to be familiar with the ethical standards of practice for their specific province or territory. Regulation of Social Work in Canada happens through provincial colleges (BC, AB, MB, ON, NS), associations (SK, QC, NB, NF), or other regulatory bodies (PEI and Northern Canada); while being a member is not always mandatory to practice social work, becoming a member of a regulatory body requires holding a degree from an accredited BSW or MSW program and/or successfully passing a licensure exam. Most provinces require both criteria be met; the exception is Quebec, where a licensure exam is not part of the registration process.

In terms of the relationship between federal and provincial professional association guidelines and provincial professional and regulatory body guidelines, the extent to which one supersedes the other also varies. For example, in BC the Code of Ethics and Standards of Practice jointly adopted by the BC Association for Social Workers (BCASW) and the BC College of Social Workers (BCCSW) in 2003 guide social workers, with the Canadian Association of Social Work (CASW) (2005a, 2005b) Code of Ethics being referred to as a valuable resource. There are six core values in the CASW Code: (1) Respect for Inherent Dignity and Worth of Persons; (2) Pursuit of Social Justice; (3) Service to Humanity; (4) Integrity of Professional Practice; (5) Confidentiality in Professional Practice; and (6) Competency in Professional Practice.

While the BCASW/BCCSW code contains 11 principles, none explicitly addresses social justice. The closest is number 11, which states: "A social worker shall advocate change in the best interest of the client, and for the overall benefit of society". This is significant for AOP social workers for whom the social justice mandate of our profession is key; in fact, this is often what drew us into the profession. The draft version of the new BCCSW standards of practice addresses this oversight by including a clear statement on the need for social workers to "demonstrate a commitment to economic and social justice and human rights" (BCCSW, 2018, p. 5).

When the 2005 version of the CASW Code of Ethics was released, it was heavily critiqued as it was seen to be far less progressive than the 1994 version and indicative of a "liberal-humanist" social work approach "that seeks to comfort victims of social problems, rather than a critical approach that seeks fundamental social change or transformation" (Mullaly, 2006, p. 145). Further, rather than the client's best interests being "primary", they were now to be "a priority", which allows the state's interests to supersede those of the service user. In effect, this shifted the care and control dynamic (Dominelli, 1997) towards control (by the state) and away from care (by the social worker and for the service user). Social work scholars who have been critical of the revised Code are more likely to be "skeptics" than "believers", according to Fine and Teram's (2009) categorization of social workers' orientations to the Code. Based on their interviews and focus groups with 71 social workers in Ontario, Fine and Telman concluded that "believers" follow the Code, seeing it "as the best representation of what the social work profession embodies" while "skeptics" question the Code's ability to serve the best interests of clients, specifically to "address the particular, the local, and the contextual" (Fine & Telman, 2009, p. 73). Seeking to return social work to its social justice roots and mandate, alternative Codes have been developed/promoted, including the Code of Ethics for Progressive Social Workers by Australian social work academics (Fraser & Briskman, 2004), adopted by AOP social workers in Canada. Two ways in which the Progressive Code is different is that it (1) does not recognize jurisdictions, believing that the welfare of all humanity should be the concern of progressive social workers, and (2) directly challenges global capitalism, seeing this political–economic system as incommensurate with social work values and beliefs.

It has also been argued that the globalized, neo-liberal, and managerialist context in which social workers in the Global North practice is impeding our ability to do "ethics work" (Weinberg & Banks, 2019). Yet, "this work is second nature to social workers [as] they are educated and socialised to see moral injuries and social injustices and are generally motivated to be people of integrity, who care for others and work for social change" (p. 14). This new practice context of austerity measures and precarity (see textbox 0.5) poses challenges for social workers wanting to adhere to their code of ethics, especially for those who belong to regulatory colleges for whom the code of ethics supersedes any other policy or guidelines. For example, if the nursing/personal care home in which we work decides to require residents to complete an advance directive upon admission, then we would have to refuse to take on this task not only because the mandatory completion of an advance directive is illegal (ACE, 2016; BC Centre for Elder Advocacy and Support, 2014), but this practice also contravenes our ethical responsibility to act in the best interests of the client. The connection to austerity and precarity is that care homes likely implement policies such as this one in order to expedite care (and perhaps save the cost of an ambulance trip or a long-distance phone call) in the event that a resident's capacity to give informed consent is compromised. Wahl and colleagues (2016) note the "pressures in the health system to deliver health care faster, cheaper, and more efficiently" and link this to "the ability of health practitioners to adhere to the best HCC [health care consent] and ACP [advance care planning] processes" (pp. 46–47).

As members of our provincial and national associations, social workers are also members of the International Federation of Social Workers (IFSW). IFSW underwent an extensive consultative process in updating its Global Definition of Social Work (IFSW, 2014) and Statement of Ethical Principles and adopted the latter in June 2018 (IFSW, 2018). The intent of the Statement was to challenge Western hegemony/Eurocentrism in social work and support decolonization efforts. The Statement recognizes the need/desire for national and local adaptations or refinements and allows for this as long as the spirit of the Global Statement is respected. That is to say that national and provincial codes and statements should reflect "a commitment to doing no harm, social justice, recognition of the inherent dignity of humanity, and to the universal and inalienable rights of people" (IFSW, 2018, p. 2); social workers are advised that the Statement is most useful when it "reflects the moral impulse on the part of the social worker" (IFSW, 2018, p. 2). This suggests a need for congruency between our personal moral codes and our professional ethics and values. Hence, the focus in this chapter is on moral, legal, and ethical issues in relation to social work with older adults, their families, and communities.

Returning to Mrs. P and Miles, let's consider our ethical requirement to "advocate change in the best interest of the client". Who is our client in this scenario? Is it only Mrs. P because she is the person who was admitted to the hospital? Is it also Miles as he is unable to live independently, or is Miles the responsibility of a social worker in the community? Do we have any responsibility for the other family members? The answers to these questions depend on whether or not we are considering our legal, ethical, or moral responsibilities and accountabilities. **Legally**, we are responsible for Mrs. P; **ethically**, we are responsible for her and her son Miles; and **morally**, we may feel that it is our role to ensure the best interests of the family as a whole.

Health care consent (HCC) and substitute decision making (SDM)

Consent must be voluntary and relate to the proposed treatment, and the adult to whom the treatment pertains must be capable of giving informed consent. This includes appreciating what it means to accept or to refuse the treatment offered. If the adult is unable to provide informed consent on their own behalf, then the social worker should not only seek to determine who should be the SDM, but they should also attempt to gain the assent of the adult. Assent means agreement, and while it is not legally required, it is morally and ethically advisable. Keep in mind that consent is decision-specific (e.g., Do you want to have a bath today? Do you agree to take this medication?) Note that there is no such thing as a blanket lack of consent. Social workers may have a formal role to play as capacity assessors, but more often than not their role is to ensure the rights of the older adult are protected and that they are provided information on the process of appointing an SDM and that the health care team abides by the written, stated, or inferred wishes of the older adult. BC Seniors' First (n.d.) developed a continuum model of capacity to guide social workers and other health care professionals in their assessments of whether an individual is capable of making a particular health or personal care decision (see Figure 5.1).

The state has a role to play if there is no one available to provide proxy or substitute consent, the individual is under the care of the state, or there is a conflict and the state needs to step in. The state's role is referred to as guardianship, and it applies to both financial and health care decisions; this is distinct from the role played by family or friends who serve as SDMs by virtue of their placement in the hierarchy of consent or being legally appointed through a power of attorney or representation agreement. As communication is central and stated wishes supersede any previously written ones (i.e., advance directives) the process of advance care planning (ACP) is recommended. There are essentially two types of advance directives (ACP tools): one that outlines the kind of care a person wishes or does not wish to receive in the future and one that is used to appoint a person to make decisions on one's behalf should one be incapable of giving informed consent (see Table 5.1).

For their commissioned report on tools related to HCC, ACP, and goals of care in Ontario, Wahl et al. (2016) located and analyzed 100 different tools with a screening survey and held interviews and focus groups with various stakeholders. They found there to be "numerous issues noted across tools, in particular, very few contextualized these [ACP] processes appropriately, typically omitting the connection to the law, and

Capacity continuum (Seniors First BC)

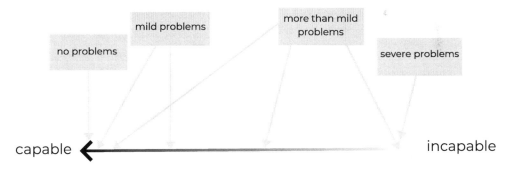

Figure 5.1 Capacity as a continuum

Table 5.1 Types of advance directives

Statement of wishes for future care	Appointment of SDM
• DNR (do not resuscitate) order	• Power of attorney
• Living will	• Representation agreement
• Goals of care	• Protection mandate

often lacking key definitions" (Wahl et al., 2016, p. iv) and noted that language, culture, and health literacy played a role in the variable awareness and understanding of these tools amongst the various stakeholder groups (p. 34).

The process is more important than the tool: my (Wendy's) story of working on ACP

I was hired by the Ontario Seniors' Secretariat (OSS) in January 2000 to work as a policy advisor on the implementation of Ontario's Alzheimer strategy after working at Mount Sinai Hospital as a social worker. I remained at OSS until starting my PhD in October 2001 and my main responsibility was Initiative #7 – Advance Care Planning (ACP). After reviewing the literature on ACP, I developed a survey instrument (far too long and detailed for busy practitioners to complete) for an external firm to administer on behalf of OSS, conducted an environmental scan – or cross-jurisdictional review – on ACP, and consulted with stakeholders, including Judith Wahl of the Advocacy Centre for the Elderly (ACE), a lawyer, and Dr. Kerry Bowman of the University of Toronto's Centre for Bioethics, a former social worker. We shared a commitment to what is now referred to in policy circles as equity, diversity, and inclusion (EDI), and I learned a great deal from these two "thought leaders". All of this research and planning work led to OSS offering ACP education and training sessions to physicians and other health professionals across the province in conjunction with two of the other Alzheimer Strategy initiatives and developing a booklet on ACP for public distribution. What OSS did not do was endorse, promote, and distribute Dr. William Molloy's widely publicized ACP tool called "Let Me Decide", which had been the expectation of some stakeholders as to how the funds for this initiative would be spent. As a result, I was called to the Assistant Deputy Minister's (ADM's) office more than once to answer the question "Why are we not promoting a tool?", as the ADM had to answer the Deputy Minister (of Health and Long Term Care), the Minister (Responsible for Seniors), and their office staff as well as external stakeholders. This is an example of evidence-based and AOP social work – the evidence had indicated to me that the process of ACP is more important than the tool and that tools create more problems than they solve, particularly for ethno-cultural minority older adults. I was able to convince my supervisor and the ADM of this and then further use my AOP knowledge, skills, and values to make change from within the system to benefit older adults, their families, and communities.

Health care is largely a provincial responsibility in Canada. Similarly, support services for older neuro-diverse adults like Miles are coordinated at the provincial level, and as such there is significant variation across the country. Services are geared more towards younger populations, and the needs and realities of older adults are often overlooked (Dickson, 2016) from Halifax to Victoria. Neither aging-related services nor disability-related services have adapted adequately to the increasing prevalence of neuro-diversity in the older adult population (Bigby, 2002), with the possible exception of dementia in aging services, which is a form of neuro-diversity though not often characterized as such. Frequently neuro-diverse individuals are presumed to lack capacity to consent to health care; however, it is not always the case that they are unable to make decisions on their own behalf. The type of decision to be made is an important consideration, as we discussed earlier in relation to Miles. Family members are also often unaware of their rights in the context of decision-making (Bigby, Bowers, & Webber, 2011).

Further, at times, our own discomfort may prevent us from maximizing the involvement of persons with dementia and/or neuro-diverse individuals; if so, then we should seek assistance from a colleague or a supervisor in the moment and incorporate this into our professional development plans. At the same time, the particular issue to be discussed – rather than or in addition to the type of client – may be a challenge for social workers. This is often the case with respect to death and dying and may relate more to our own fears than to those of the older adults with whom we work.

> Robin is a hospital social worker who works with the palliative care team and often has conversations with older adults about end-of-life care. At first, they were worried about upsetting people by raising the topic of death but quickly discovered that most older adults are comfortable talking about death and dying. Now that medical assistance in dying (MAiD) is legal in Canada, these conversations have taken on an added dimension. Older service users are curious about what this will mean for their care, should they become seriously ill, and some have expressed concern that they will be pressured to end their lives early.

Legislation across Canada and implications for social work practice

Legislation related to HCC, SDM, and adult guardianship as well as the promotion of ACP and associated tools varies by province or territory in Canada as Tables 5.2 and 5.3 indicate. While there is no legal structure for advance directives in Nunavut, April 16th is recognized as National Advance Care Planning Day in Newfoundland and Labrador. There is also a fair amount of uniformity across the country, however. For example, the presumption of capacity is standard across all jurisdictions as is the ability for consent to be given orally or writing or inferred by conduct. Endnotes for each jurisdiction (provinces and territories) listed in the headings at the top of Table 5.2 provide the references for the information contained in Tables 5.2 and 5.3.

The language used to refer to those who are authorized to make decisions on behalf of another person lacking capacity to give informed consent varies, with SDM and/or proxy being the most common designations and other terms including representative (BC), agent (AB and NWT), delegate (NS), mandatory (QC), and attorney for personal care (ON). The idea of a co-decision-maker in Saskatchewan, that is someone who is provided with information about the health care matter but does not have the final say, is potentially a more empowering or inclusive way of involving neuro-diverse individuals like Miles and older adults with cognitive impairment like Mrs. P in HCC. This would be a form of "supported decision-making" (Browning, Bigby, & Douglas, 2014), which recognizes "the interdependent nature of decision making and the concept of shared capacity" (p. 34) and is thus recommended for persons with disabilities. Guardianship is generally more formal or restrictive with respect to financial decisions than it is for health or personal care decisions, as is SDM for finances, both of which are detailed in Table 5.3.

The earliest legislation in Canada was New Brunswick's Infirm Persons and Mental Health Act of 1973 (revised in 2016), and the most recently passed legislation was Alberta's Adult Guardianship and Trusteeship Act of 2008 (revised in 2013). Quebec is unique in that the Civil Code of Quebec guides much of the policy and practice on

Table 5.2 Health care consent (HCC) and substitute decision-making (SDM) across Canada

Province/ Territory	BC[4]	AB[5]	SK[6]	MB[7]	ON[8]	QC[9]	NS[10]	NB[11]	PEI[12]	NF & LB[13]	NWT[14]	YK[15]	NVT[16]
Title of health care consent (HCC) legislation	HC Consent & Care Facility Admission (CFA) Act	Alberta Health Services Consent to Treatment/ Procedure(s) Policy	HC Directives & Substitute HC Decision-makers Regulations	HC Directives Act	HC Consent Act	Civil Code of Quebec	Hospitals Act	Infirm Persons Act; Mental Health (MH) Act	Consent to Treatment & HC Directives Act	Advance HC Directives Act	Personal Directives Act	Care Consent Act	Guardianship & Trusteeship Act; MH Act
Year enacted/ revised	1996/2019 (CFA not in force)	2008/2013	1997/2017	1993	1996/2018	1989/2019	1989/2014	1973/2016	1988/2010	1995/2011	1994/2015	2003/2018	1997/2012; 1988/2018
Separate legislation for SDM?	Yes – Representation Agreement Act	Yes – Personal Directives Act	No	No	No	Yes – Act Respecting End of Life Care	Yes – Personal Directives Act	Yes – Advance HC Directives Act	No	No	No	No	No legal recognition of SDM for personal care
Title of SDM (for personal care)	Representative	Agent	Personal co-decision-makers (assistance) or proxy (full control)	Proxy	Attorney for personal care	Mandatory	Delegate	Proxy	SDM/Proxy	SDM	Agent	Associate (assistance) or proxy (full control)	N/A
Allowance for advance directive	Yes – below SDMs and	Yes – to be interpreted by SDM/Guardian	Yes – to be interpreted by SDM/Guardian	Yes-AD given priority though HC	Yes – to be interpreted by	Yes – can choose to name SDM	Yes - given priority though HC	Yes – taken as consent, but SDM/	Yes – to be interpreted by SDM/Guardian	Yes – to be interpreted by SDM/Guardian	Yes – given priority though HC	Yes – to be interpreted by SDM/Guardian	No – not officially recognized

	SDM/Guardian			(protection mandate) or procedures (advance care directive)		Guardian's interpretation of AD given priority			
(AD) tools, e.g. living will?	Guardians in hierarchy of consent	Mentioned & promoted	Mentioned & promoted	providers not required to ask or search for AD	providers not required to ask or search for AD	Mentioned & promoted	Mentioned & promoted	providers not required to ask or search for AD	Neither mentioned nor promoted
Advance care Planning (ACP) process mentioned/promoted in government healthcare information?	Mentioned on government websites, but less promotional content for ADs than others	Mentioned & promoted	Only SDMs mentioned and promoted; ADs only promoted by advocacy sites	Mentioned & promoted	Mentioned & promoted	Mentioned & promoted	Mentioned & promoted & April 16 is National Advance Care Planning Day in NF & LB	Not prevalent on NWT health information websites (general lack of HC info for the North)	Mentioned & promoted

Table 5.3 State appointed guardians and SDM (financial) across Canada

Province/ Territory	BC	AB	SK	MB	ON	QC	NS	NB	PEI	NF & LB	NWT	YK	NVT
Title of guardianship/ trustee-ship legislation	Adult Guardianship Act	Adult Guardianship & Trusteeship Act	Adult Guardianship & Trusteeship Co-Decision-Making Act	The Vulnerable Persons Living with a Mental Disability Act	The Substitute Decisions Act	Public Curator Act	Adult Capacity & Decision-Making Act	Infirm Persons Act; Mental Health (MH) Act	MH Act; Public Trustee Act	Mentally Disabled Persons' Estate Act; Advance HC Directives Act	Guardianship & Trusteeship Act	Care Consent Act	Guardianship & Trusteeship Act; MH Act
Hierarchy of decision-makers (top 3 or more)	Spouse, Child, Parent	None. HC provider selects nearest adult & available relative who has seen patient in last year	Spouse, Adult Son or Daughter, Parent or Legal Custodian	None. HC providers usually follow this order: Spouse, Child, Parent	Guardian, Attorney for Personal Care, Rep. of Consent & Capacity Board, Partner, Child, Parent	Mandatary, Tutor, Curator, Spouse, Close Relative	Spouse, Adult Child, Parent	Any family member who applies to be Attorney, Public Trustee	Proxy, Guardian, Spouse	Spouse, Children, Parents	Spouse, Eldest Adult Child, Eldest Parent	Guardian, Proxy, Spouse	Spouse, Eldest Adult Child, Eldest Parent
Separate legislation for SDM (financial)?	Power of Attorney (POA) Act	POA Act	POA Act	POA Act	POA Act	No	POA Act	Mix of info from Infirm Persons Act & Property Act create legal grounds for POA	POA Act	POA Act	POA Act	POA Act	POA Act

Title of SDM – Financial	Attorney	Attorney	Attorney	Attorney	Attorney for property	Mandatary (named in Protection Mandate)	Attorney	Attorney	Attorney	Attorney	Attorney	Attorney	Attorney
Title of state-appointed Guardian (personal care)	Adult Guardian	Adult Guardian	Personal Co-decision-makers (assistance); Personal Guardians (full control)	SDM (Personal Care)	Guardian of Personal Care	Curator (assistance); Tutor (temporary control); Adviser (full control)	Guardian	Attorney for Personal Care	Guardian	Guardian of the Person	Guardian	SDM	Guardian
Title of state-appointed Guardian (financial)	Statutory Property Guardian	Trustee	Personal Co-decision-makers (assistance); Property Guardians (full control)	SDM (Financial)	Guardian of Property	Curator (for adults with permanent incapacity); Tutor (temporary control)	Guardian	Trustee	Trustee	Guardian of the Estate	Trustee	Trustee	Trustee

HC: Health Care, SDM: Substitute Decision Maker, POA: Power of Attorney, MH: Mental Health

HCC and SDM. Not every jurisdiction has a full suite of legislation: New Brunswick, Newfoundland and Labrador, and Nunavut all lack legislation specific to HCC and Alberta has a policy (Alberta Health Services Consent to Treatment/Procedures Policy) rather than legislation. HCC in Quebec is covered by the Civil Code and there are three different titles for state-appointed guardians for personal care (curator, tutor, advisor) depending on the degree of incapacity to consent and the decision-making authority granted.

Medical assistance in dying (MAiD)

In June 2016, the Criminal Code of Canada was amended through Bill C-14 to allow for MAiD (Government of Canada, 2019). Since that time, the social work profession has been grappling with the implications for practice and guidelines have been produced by both professional associations (Saskatchewan Association of Social Workers, 2017a; 2017b) and regulatory bodies (Nova Scotia College of Social Work (NSCSW), 2018; Ontario College of Social Workers and Social Service Workers, 2016). The guidelines from NSCSW are unique in stressing the importance of self-care due to the strong emotional reactions MAiD can provoke (2018, p. 4). MAiD is arguably more concerning for AOP social workers, who not only uphold the rights of older adults to live in dignity until the end of their lives, but also are critical of austerity measures and aware of their impact on the provision of health and social care. Thus, we approach MAiD with caution as we do not want its legalization to create pressure for older adults – or persons living with disabilities – to hasten their deaths. We welcome guidance from professional and regulatory bodies on the role of social workers with MAiD.

Table 5.4 provides information on the role of the social worker and guidance from provincial regulatory and professional bodies with respect to HCC and SDM in general and MAiD in particular and Table 5.5 in the additional resources section includes the full references to the guidelines used to create this table.

MAiD is included in Quebec's 2019 Act Respecting End of Life Care and addressed in Ontario; both provinces prohibit the inclusion of MAiD in advance directives or substitute decisions; this is not part of legislation in Ontario, however. Even though legislation in BC and Yukon was revised in 2019 and 2018 respectively, MAiD was not included. Social workers in BC may not assess for MAiD eligibility or suggest it, but they can support clients through the MAiD process. Not only is MAiD not addressed in legislation outside Quebec, but – as of the writing of this text – none of the provinces or territories include information on MAiD on their government webpages that have other ACP and SDM resources.

The role of the social worker with respect to consent, capacity, and decision-making is most clearly articulated in Alberta, Quebec, and Ontario where social workers serve as capacity assessors. With appropriate training, social workers in Nova Scotia will be able to serve as capacity assessors once the Adult Capacity and Decision-Making Act comes into effect. In Quebec, social workers are responsible for the psycho-social portion of the evaluation of capacity to consent while doctors and nurse practitioners complete the medical section, thus they play a much greater role than social workers in other provinces and territories, and there are a number of regulations they must follow regarding determination of capacity. We were unable to locate any statements regarding the role of social workers in consent,

Table 5.4 MAiD in HCC and SDM legislation and social work roles/guidelines across Canada

	BC	AB	SK	MB	ON	QC	NS	NB	PEI	NF & LB	NWT	YK	NVT
MAiD	No mention in act; info on MAiD & SW role on BCCSW website (SWers may not suggest MAiD nor assess eligibility but can support client's MAiD process)	No mention in act or in SDM resource material online; responsibility of SWers to allow for MAiD outlined by ACSW	No mention in act or on health info pages for proxies; SASW supports service users' rights to access MAiD	No mention in act or on pages relevant to proxies or SDM; MCSW supports service users' rights to access MAiD	No mention in acts, but neither SDM nor AD can be used for MAiD	Yes, in act – cannot be done by AD, must be done orally by the person, not by SDM	No mention in relevant legislation or in online info on ADs & SDMs	No mention in relevant legislation or in online info on advance directives & SDMs.	No mention in relevant legislation or in online info on ADs & SDMs	Not in provincial legislation, but advanced consent/SDM consent for MAiD is not permitted	Not addressed	Not addressed	Not addressed.
Professional/regulatory guidelines	No specific guidelines other than BCCSW mandating that social workers get informed consent	Nothing specific, but ACSW practice guidelines allow for some discretion in attaining	Nothing specific, but SASW standards of practice allow for discretion in attaining	Nothing specific	SWer can evaluate capacity of client to consent; if do not believe can provide	SWers complete psychosocial half of capacity evaluation (physician or NP does	Capacity assessment training is forthcoming; guidelines developed by NCSW	Nothing specific	None	No explicit policies, but NLASW site considers education & assistance in	None	No (no regulatory body for SW)	No (no regulatory body for SW)

(Continued)

Table 5.4 (Cont.)

	BC	AB	SK	MB	ON	QC	NS	NB	PEI	NF & LB	NWT	YK	NVT
	from clients	deter-mining capacity to consent	informed consent		informed consent, can refer to per-son's SDM	medical half) so there are several regula-tions				ACP to be within the scope of Swers			
Social Work (SW) role	Members of College must remain up-to-date on relevant acts, including those related to HCC & decision-making	SWers can become desig-nated capacity asses-sors, i.e., assess ability of clients to make own decisions (in AB & ON only)	None stated	Service pro-viders cannot be SDMs	Capacity Assessor	Respon-sible for psycho-social evalu-ation to help deter-mine capacity to make decisions & for "protec-tion of incapable adults"	Soon will be able to assess for cap-acity with appropri-ate train-ing under Adult Capacity & Deci-sion-Making Act	None stated	None stated	Provide educa-tion & support for people inter-ested in ACP	None stated	None stated	None stated

Table 5.5 The death box

We use different words and phrases to talk about death, many of which are euphemisms that allow us to deny that death is happening, avoid being direct, and protect either ourselves or those with whom we are talking (Heerema, 2019). The words we choose may be related to our care and concern for the dying person or our own emotions and fears about death. Think about the words you would use to talk about death. Which questions can you see yourself asking? And how might you react to each of the questions below?

- How do you feel about *passing on*?
- What do you need to do to prepare for your *death*?
- Are you ready to *cross over* to the other side?
- *How long* has the doctor given you?
- Are you seeking *release* from the pain you've been living with?
- Would you like to talk about *death and dying*?
- Have you made any *arrangements*?
- Tell me how you feel about this *stage of your life*?
- How is your *spirit*?

capacity, and decision-making for 3/10 provinces (AB, NB, PEI) or any of the territories (NWT, YK, NVT). This is understandable for the latter, as social work is not as well developed as a profession in the North as it is in the South, though it is rather surprising for Alberta given how heavily regulated social work is in Alberta with social work diploma holders and those teaching social work needing to be members of the College, not only those with degrees in social work who are currently practicing, as is the case in other provinces.

The results of our jurisdictional review detailed in Table 5.4 support the findings of a scoping review by Fujioka, Mirza, and McDonald (2018) that determined there is a need for clear guidelines for health care professionals on MAiD and that little attention has been paid to social work in comparison to medicine and nursing. Those articles included in their review that addressed social work (n=3) identified four key roles for social workers: providing consultation/support to patients, providing consultation/support to other providers, assessing eligibility, and policy advocacy (Fujioka et al., 2018, p. 1568). An additional significant role for social workers identified by Antifaeff (2019) is facilitating family meetings and resolving conflicts that may arise over an individual's decision to seek MAiD.

It should be noted that there has been resistance to MAiD from disability rights groups, as MAiD (or "dying with dignity" more generally) rests on an assumption that the quality of life of those living with severe disabilities, particularly life-limiting illnesses, is necessarily poor, and therefore they should be allowed to end their lives with a physician's assistance. Both older adults and health care providers fear that in the context of neo-liberalism and accompanying austerity measures, MAiD will be used as a rationale to reduce health and social care for older adults, including quality palliative care. At the same time, those living with life-limiting illnesses and/or severe disabilities that are accompanied by significant pain and/or functional limitations may choose to "die with dignity", and it is now their right to do so provided they are competent to make this decision at the time they request MAiD.

MAiD may compel social workers to engage in discussions about death and dying more often than in the past or with a greater range of service users, and doing this work requires "advanced skills in rapport building and communication" (Antifaeff, 2019, p. 3). As indicated by the scenario with Robin earlier in the chapter, social workers may be less comfortable talking about the dying process and end-of-life care than the older adults with whom we work. This could be due to lack of familiarity with appropriate terminology, discomfort with discussing death, and other reasons (Heerema, 2019). Table 5.5 – the "death box" – helps students determine a suitable form of questioning and consider what response various questions might elicit. Think of how you as an AOP social worker can promote the dignity and autonomy of older adults while recognizing interdependency.

Conclusion

This chapter has addressed moral, legal, and ethical issues in gerontological social work. While the focus has mainly been on the **sites and sectors of health and social care**, moral, legal, and ethical issues permeate the daily lives of older adults as you will observe in **Everyday lives and realities**. While legal discourse permeates some practice settings more than others, law governs our social work practice regardless of whether we work in a hospital, a social assistance office, a food bank, or a seniors centre. Our knowledge and application of the law is balanced with our adherence to social work codes of ethics and standards of practice, and any policy and practice guidelines in our practice settings should accord with this legal and ethical framework. That is to say that if there is a conflict between the discourse of our social work profession and the managerial discourse of our agency, then it is the former that we should heed as much as possible.

Further, while it is critical to be cognizant of our own moral code, we need to guard against this influencing our practice. While it is impossible to be purely objective, we have a responsibility to be non-judgmental and non-discriminatory as members of the social work profession. We cannot let our personal views on moral, legal, and ethical issues such as MAiD allow us to impede older adults' right to die with dignity or to pressure older adults to consider life-limiting treatment options. Autonomy and self-determination must be safe-guarded. AOG social workers should respect and support interdependency and collective decision-making as much as possible, however, provided this is consistent with the cultural beliefs and practices and/or the stated, written, or implied wishes of our clients.

Exercise

- Using what you have learned in this chapter about **Moral, legal, and ethical issues**
    a   Develop an intervention plan for Mrs. P and her son Miles;
    b   Ensure that you address the following at the personal, cultural/relational, and structural levels:
        - Agency (resilience and resistance);
        - Access (ensuring that people are able to receive services);
        - Equity (ensuring that people are adequately represented); and
        - Anti-discrimination (ensuring that forms of interlocking oppressions are addressed).

Takeaways

- Social work codes of ethics and standards of practice guide our practice in all settings in which we work, as do the laws of the jurisdiction in which we practice.
- Consent is a process, not an event, and fostering communication is key. Social work skills in biopsychosocial assessments, rapport building, communication, and family meetings are critical.
- Older adults whose legal capacity to consent is compromised still can and should be involved as much as possible in ACP and SDM processes.
- Social workers need to be familiar with HCC and SDM legislation in their province and comfortable talking about death and dying.
- The role of social workers is to provide information and support to older adults and their families with respect to moral, legal, and ethical issues, which may include assessing their capacity to consent and advocating for their wishes to be respected.

Additional resources

- Advocacy Centre for the Elderly: www.advocacycentreelderly.org/
- Seniors First BC (formerly known as the BC Centre for Elder Advocacy & Support): http://seniorsfirstbc.ca/
- Medical Assistance in Dying Resource hub: www.casw-acts.ca/en/resources/medical-assistance-dying-resource-hub

Table 5.6 Social work guidelines for ethical practice and MAiD (as referenced in Table 5.4)

Canada	Canadian Association of Social Workers. (2005b). *Guidelines for ethical practice.* Retrieved from https://www.casw-acts.ca/sites/default/files/attachements/casw_guidelines_for_ethical_practice.pdf
British Columbia	British Columbia College of Social Workers. (2009). *Code of ethics and standards of practice.* Retrieved from http://www.bccollegeofsocialworkers.ca/wp-content/uploads/2016/09/BCCSW-CodeOfEthicsStandardsApprvd.pdf
	British Columbia Association of Social Workers and British Columbia College for Social Work. (2003). *Code of ethics.* Retrieved from www.bcasw.org/aboutbcasw/casw-code-of-ethics/
Alberta	Alberta College of Social Workers. (n.d.). *Information sheet: Medical assistance in dying.* Retrieved from http://acsw.in1touch.org/uploaded/web/website/ACSW_MAID_%20Info.pdf
	Alberta College of Social Workers. (2019). *Standards of practice.* Retrieved from https://acsw.in1touch.org/document/2487/FINAL%20ACSW%20Standards%20of%20Practice%2003282019.pdf
Saskatchewan	Saskatchewan Association of Social Workers. (2017a). *Guidance for social workers on medical assistance in dying.* Retrieved from https://www.casw-acts.ca/sites/default/files/attachements/sk_paper_on_maid_for_social_workers_-_2017_jan_13_r1873193_0.pdf
	Saskatchewan Association of Social Workers. (2017b). *Standards of practices for registered social workers in Saskatchewan.* Retrieved from https://www.sasw.ca/document/4577/SASW%20Standards-of-Practice-%20June%201%202017%20Approved.pdf

(*Continued*)

Table 5.6 (Cont.)

Manitoba	Manitoba College of Social Workers. (2016). *Medical assistance in dying (MAID) information summary.* Retrieved from https://mcsw.ca/wp-content/uploads/2015/06/MAID-Information-Summary.pdf
	Manitoba College of Social Workers. (2015). *Standards of practice.* Retrieved from https://mcsw.ca/wp-content/uploads/2015/06/Standards-of-Practice-WEB.pdf
Ontario	Ontario College of Social Workers and Social Service Workers. (2016). *Medical assistance in dying: Guidance for members of the OCSWSSW.* Retrieved from http://www.ocswssw.org/2016/09/14/medical-assistance-in-dying-guidance-for-members-of-the-ocswssw/
	Ontario Ministry of the Attorney General. (2016). *The capacity assessment office: Questions and answers.* Retrieved from https://www.attorneygeneral.jus.gov.on.ca/english/family/pgt/capacityoffice.php#eligible
Quebec	Act respecting end-of-life care, Revised Statutes of Quebec (2016, c. S-32.0001). Retrieved from http://canlii.ca/t/52t5r
	Educaloi. (2019). *Incapacity (being unable to care for yourself or your affairs).* Retrieved from https://www.educaloi.qc.ca/en/capsules/incapacity-being-unable-care-yourself-or-your-affairs
Nova Scotia	Government of Nova Scotia. (2017). *Adult capacity and decision-making act.* Retrieved from https://novascotia.ca/just/pto/adult-capacity-decision.asp
Newfoundland and Labrador	Newfoundland and Labrador Association of Social Workers. (2019). *Enduring power of attorney, substitute decision-maker: What is the role of social work?* Retrieved from https://nlasw.ca/sites/default/files/inline-files/Substitute%20Decision-Making%20%28Final%29_0.pdf
Northwest Territories	Government of the Northwest Territories. (2011). *Northwest Territories standards of practice for social workers.* Retrieved from https://www.hss.gov.nt.ca/sites/hss/files/nwt-standards-practice-social-workers.pdf

Notes

1 "Neuro-diversity" is a term developed by disability rights communities that has started to gain recognition in sites and sectors of health and social care. Neuro-diverse people include (but are not limited to) those living with intellectual and developmental disability, autism spectrum disorder, fetal alcohol spectrum disorder, and Down syndrome. Neuro-diversity is characterized by early aging, and the prevalence of neuro-diversity amongst older adults is increasing due to improvements in health and health care, which has lowered rates of mortality for these populations. Since reaching old age is a relatively recent reality for some neuro-diverse people, we still know little about the impact of neuro-diverse challenges on aging, although there has been some research on the links between Down syndrome and dementia (Janicki, Henderson, Rubin, & The Atlanta Charrette Study Group, 2008; Janicki, Zendell, & DeHaven, 2010).

2 The majority of neuro-diverse adults rely to a great extent on care provided by immediate family members; most either live at home well into their adulthood or in long-term/residential housing while still relying on family (e.g., parents and siblings) for care and support (Janicki et al., 2010). A significant reliance on reciprocal forms of care between aging parents and their adult neuro-diverse children, combined with fears about the future, is resulting in family units like Mrs. P and Miles being subject to intervention by sites and sectors of health and social care.

 3 In some jurisdictions, health authorities/districts have implemented policies whereby an older adult who is admitted to an acute care hospital and is unable to return to their own home (i.e., continue to live independently) must accept the first bed that becomes available in a nursing/personal care home, regardless of where the care home is located and whether or not it is one they would choose for themselves.
 4 Health Care (Consent) and Care Facility (Admission) Act, Revised Statutes of British Columbia, 1996. Representation Agreement Act, Revised Statutes of British Columbia, 1996. Government of British Columbia, 2019.
 5 Alberta Health Services, 2010. Personal Directives Act, Revised Statutes of Alberta, 2000. Government of Alberta, 2019.
 6 The Health Care Directives and Substitute Health Care Decision Makers Regulations, Revised Regulations of Saskatchewan, 2017. Saskatchewan Health Authority, 2017. *Advance care directive (living will).*
 7 The Health Care Directives Act, Continuing Consolidation of the Statutes of Manitoba, 2014. Government of Manitoba, 2017.
 8 Health Care Consent Act, Statues of Ontario, 1996. End of Life Planning Canada, 2016. Ontario Medical Association, n.d.
 9 Civil Code of Québec, Compilation of Québec Laws and Regulations, 1991. Act Respecting End-of-Life Care, Revised Statutes of Québec, 2016, Act Respecting End of Life Care, Revised Statutes of Québec, 2019. Curateur Public Québec, 2002. Régie de l'Assurance Maladie Québec, 2003.
10 Hospitals Act, Revised Statutes of Nova Scotia, 1989. Personal Directives Act, Statues of Nova Scotia, 2008. Government of Nova Scotia, 2013.
11 Infirm Persons Act, Revised Statutes of New Brunswick, 1973. Mental Health Act, Revised Statutes of New Brunswick, 1973. Advance Health Care Directives Act, Revised Statutes of New Brunswick, 2016. Government of New Brunswick, n.d. Public Legal Education and Information Service of New Brunswick, 2019.
12 Consent to Treatment and Health Care Directives Act, Revised Statues of Prince Edward Island, 1988. Health PEI. (n.d.). Government of Prince Edward Island, 2019.
13 Advance Health Care Directives Act, Statutes of Newfoundland and Labrador, 1995. Government of Newfoundland and Labrador, n.d. Speak Up, 2019.
14 Personal Directives Act, Statutes of the Northwest Territories, 2005. Government of the Northwest Territories, 2015.
15 Care Consent Act, Statutes of the Yukon, 2003. Government of the Yukon, 2017.
16 Guardianship and Trusteeship Act, Statutes of the Northwest Territories (Nunavut), 1994. Mental Health Act, Revised Statutes of the Northwest Territories (Nunavut), 1988.

References

Act Respecting End-of-Life Care, Revised Statutes of Québec (2016, c. S-32.0001). Retrieved from http://canlii.ca/t/52t5r.

Act Respecting End-of-Life Care, Revised Statutes of Québec (2019, c. S-32.0001). Retrieved from http://canlii.ca/t/52t5r.

Advance Health Care Directives Act, Revised Statutes of New Brunswick (2016, c. 46). Retrieved from http://canlii.ca/t/52wbb.

Advance Health Care Directives Act, Statutes of Newfoundland and Labrador (1995, c. A-4.1). Retrieved from http://canlii.ca/t/528xr.

Advocacy Centre for the Elderly (ACE). (2016, April). *Advance care planning – Ontario – Summary – Health Care Consent Act.* Toronto, ON: ACE.

Alberta College of Social Workers. (2019). *Standards of practice.* Retrieved from https://acsw.in1touch.org/document/2487/FINAL%20ACSW%20Standards%20of%20Practice%2003282019.pdf.

Alberta College of Social Workers. (n.d.). *Information sheet: Medical assistance in dying.* Retrieved from http://acsw.in1touch.org/uploaded/web/website/ACSW_MAID_%20Info.pdf.

Alberta Health Services. (2010). *Consent to treatment/procedure(s)* (Report No. PRR-01). Retrieved from https://extranet.ahsnet.ca/teams/policydocuments/1/clp-consent-to-treatment-prr01-policy.pdf.

Antifaeff, K. (2019). Social work practice with medical assistance in dying: A case study. *Health and Social Work*, 1–8. doi:10.1093/hsw/hlz002.

Bigby, C. (2002). Ageing people with a lifelong disability: Challenges for the aged care and disability sectors. *Journal of Intellectual & Developmental Disability*, 27(4), 231–241.

Bigby, C., Bowers, B., & Webber, R. (2011). Planning and decision making about the future care of older group home residents and transition to residential aged care. *Journal of Intellectual Disability Research*, 55(8), 777–789. doi:10.1111/j.1365-2788.2010.01297.x.

British Columbia Association of Social Workers and British Columbia College for Social Work. (2003). *Code of Ethics*. Retrieved from www.bcasw.org/aboutbcasw/casw-code-of-ethics/.

British Columbia Centre for Elder Advocacy and Support. (2014). *Legal issues in residential care: An advocates manual*. Retrieved from https://wiki.clicklaw.bc.ca/prerender/pdfs/Legal_Issues_in_Residential_Care.pdf.

British Columbia College of Social Workers. (2009). *Code of Ethics and standards of practice*. Retrieved from www.bccollegeofsocialworkers.ca/wp-content/uploads/2016/09/BCCSW-CodeOfEthicsStandardsApprvd.pdf.

British Columbia College of Social Workers. (2018, June). *Standards project*. Retrieved from www.bccollegeofsocialworkers.ca/standards-project/.

Browning, M., Bigby, C., & Douglas, J. (2014). Supported decision making: Understanding how its conceptual link to legal capacity is influencing the development of practice. *Research and Practice in Intellectual and Developmental Disabilities*, 1(1), 34–45. doi:10.1080/23297018.2014.902726.

Canadian Association of Social Workers (CASW). (2005a). *Code of Ethics*. Ottawa: CASW. Retrieved from www.caswacts.ca/sites/default/files/attachements/casw_code_of_ethics.pdf.

Canadian Association of Social Workers (CASW). (2005b). *Guidelines for ethical practice*. Retrieved from www.casw-acts.ca/sites/default/files/attachements/casw_guidelines_for_ethical_practice.pdf.

Canadian Institute of Health Information (CIHI). (2017). *Canada's health care providers: Provincial profiles, 2008 to 2017 – Data tables*. Retrieved from www.cihi.ca/en/social-workers.

Care Consent Act, Statutes of the Yukon (2003, c. 21, Sch. B). Retrieved from http://canlii.ca/t/53l15.

Civil Code of Québec, Compilation of Québec Laws and Regulations (1991, c. CCQ-1991). Retrieved from http://canlii.ca/t/53k4f.

Consent to Treatment and Health Care Directives Act, Revised Statues of Prince Edward Island (1988, c. C-17.2). Retrieved from http://canlii.ca/t/kt4b.

Curateur Public Québec. (2002). *Mandatary*. Retrieved from www.curateur.gouv.qc.ca/cura/en/majeur/client/representant/mandataire/index.html.

Dickson, D. (2016). *The Governance of developmental disability supports for older adults in Ontario and Quebec*. Dissertation. Public Policy and Administration. Montreal, QC: Concordia University.

Dominelli, L. (1997). Care and control dynamics in caring relationships. In J. Campling (Eds.), *Sociology for Social Work* (pp. 138–150). London: Palgrave.

Educaloi. (2019). *Incapacity (being unable to care for yourself or your affairs)*. Retrieved from www.educaloi.qc.ca/en/capsules/incapacity-being-unable-care-yourself-or-your-affairs.

End of Life Planning Canada. (2016). *Advance care planning kit: Ontario edition*. Retrieved from www.canadianhealthadvocatesinc.ca/pdf/Ontario_Advance%20Care%20Planning%20Kit_-_Final.pdf.

Fine, M., & Teram, E. (2009). Believers and skeptics: Where social worker situate themselves regarding the Code of Ethics. *Ethics & Behavior*, 19(1), 60–78. doi:10.1080/10508420802623682.

Fraser, H., & Briskman, L. (2004). Through the eye of a needle: The challenge of getting justice in Australia if you're Indigenous or seeking asylum. In I. Ferguson, M. Lavalette, & E. Whitmore (Eds.), *Globalisation, global justice and social work* (pp. 109–123). London: Routledge.

Fujioka, J. K., Mirza, R. M., & McDonald, P. L. (2018). Implementation of medical assistance in dying: A scoping review of health care providers' perspectives. *Journal of Pain and Symptom Management*, 55(6), 1564–1576.

Government of Alberta. (2019). *Advance care planning*. Retrieved from https://myhealth.alberta.ca/alberta/Pages/advance-care-planning-topic-overview.aspx.

Government of British Columbia. (2019). *Advance care planning*. Retrieved from www2.gov.bc.ca/gov/content/family-social-supports/seniors/health-safety/advance-care-planning.

Government of Canada. (2019). *Medical assistance in dying*. Last updated April 25, 2019. Retrieved from www.canada.ca/en/health-canada/services/medical-assistancedying.html.

Government of Manitoba. (2017). *The Manitoba health care directive*. Retrieved from www.gov.mb.ca/health/livingwill.html.

Government of New Brunswick. (n.d.). *Advance health care directives*. Retrieved from www2.gnb.ca/content/gnb/en/departments/health/patientinformation/content/advance_health_care_directives.html.

Government of Newfoundland and Labrador. (n.d.). *How to make an advance health care directive*. Retrieved from www.cssd.gov.nl.ca/publications/pdf/seniors/ahcd_booklet.pdf.

Government of Nova Scotia. (2013). *Personal directives in Nova Scotia*. Retrieved from https://novascotia.ca/just/pda/.

Government of Nova Scotia. (2017). *Adult capacity and decision-making act*. Retrieved from https://novascotia.ca/just/pto/adult-capacity-decision.asp.

Government of Prince Edward Island. (2019). *Advance care planning*. Retrieved from www.princeedwardisland.ca/en/information/health-pei/advance-careplanning?utm_source=redirect&utm_medium=url&utm_campaign=advance-care-planning.

Government of the Northwest Territories. (2011). *Northwest Territories standards of practice for social workers*. Retrieved from www.hss.gov.nt.ca/sites/hss/files/nwt-standards-practice-social-workers.pdf.

Government of the Northwest Territories. (2015). *Health information act guide*. Retrieved from www.hss.gov.nt.ca/sites/hss/files/hia-guide.pdf.

Government of the Yukon. (2017). *Adult protection and decision-making*. Retrieved from www.hss.gov.yk.ca/adultdecisionmaking.php.

Guardianship and Trusteeship Act, Statutes of the Northwest Territories (Nunavut). (1994, c. 29). Retrieved from http://canlii.ca/t/52143.

Health Care (Consent) and Care Facility (Admission) Act, Revised Statutes of British Columbia. (1996, c. 181). Retrieved from http://canlii.ca/t/520ts.

Health Care Consent Act, Statues of Ontario (1996, c. 2, Sch A). Retrieved from http://canlii.ca/t/5354b.

The Health Care Directives Act, Continuing Consolidation of the Statutes of Manitoba. (2014, c. H27). Retrieved from http://canlii.ca/t/k998.

The Health Care Directives and Substitute Health Care Decision Makers Regulations, Revised Regulations of Saskatchewan. (2017, c. H-0.002 Reg 1). Retrieved from http://canlii.ca/t/52wht.

Health PEI. (n.d.). *Advance care planning workbook*. Retrieved from www.princeedwardisland.ca/sites/default/files/publications/advance_care_planning_workbook.pdf.

Heerema, E. (2019, July). *Euphemisms for dead, death, and dying: Are they helpful or harmful?* Retrieved from www.verywellhealth.com/euphemisms-for-dead-death-or-dying-1131903.

Hospitals Act, Revised Statutes of Nova Scotia. (1989, c. 208). Retrieved from http://canlii.ca/t/52pkf.

IFSW. (2014, July). *Global definition of social work.* Retrieved from www.ifsw.org/what-is-social-work/global-definition-of-social-work/.

Infirm Persons Act, Revised Statutes of New Brunswick. (1973, c. I-8). Retrieved from http://canlii.ca/t/52r4x.

International Federation of Social Work (IFSW). (2018, July 2). *Global social work statement of ethical principles.* Retrieved from www.ifsw.org/global-social-work-statement-of-ethical-principles/.

Janicki, M., Henderson, C., Rubin, L., & The Atlanta Charrette Study Group. (2008). Neurodevelopmental conditions and aging: Report on the Atlanta Charrette study group on neurodevelopmental conditions and aging. *Disability and Health Journal, 1*(2), 116–124.

Janicki, M., Zendell, A., & DeHaven, K. (2010). Coping with dementia and older families of adults with down syndrome. *Dementia,* 9(3), 391–407. doi:10.1177/1471301210375338.

Manitoba College of Social Workers. (2015). *Standards of practice.* Retrieved from https://mcsw.ca/wp-content/uploads/2015/06/Standards-of-Practice-WEB.pdf.

Manitoba College of Social Workers. (2016). *Medical assistance in dying (MAID) information summary.* Retrieved from https://mcsw.ca/wp-content/uploads/2015/06/MAID-Information-Summary.pdf.

Mental Health Act, Revised Statutes of New Brunswick. (1973, c. M-10). Retrieved from http://canlii.ca/t/531fv.

Mental Health Act, Revised Statutes of the Northwest Territories (Nunavut). (1988, c. M-10). Retrieved from http://canlii.ca/t/52l46.

Mullaly, B. (2006). Forward to the past: The 2005 CASW Code of Ethics. *Canadian Social Work Review, 23*(1–2), 145–150.

Newfoundland and Labrador Association of Social Workers. (2019). *Enduring power of attorney, substitute decision-maker: What is the role of social work?* Retrieved from https://nlasw.ca/sites/default/files/inline-files/Substitute%20Decision-Making%20%28Final%29_0.pdf.

Nova Scotia College of Social Workers (NSCSW). (2018, July 19). *Medical assistance in dying: NSCSW guidelines.* Halifax, NS: Nova Scotia College of Social Workers.

Ontario College of Social Workers and Social Service Workers (OCSWSSW). (2016). *Medical assistance in dying: What are my professional obligations? Guidance for members of the OCSWSSW.* Toronto, ON: OCSWSSW.

Ontario Medical Association. (n.d.). *Advance care planning.* Retrieved from www.ontariosdoctors.com/advance-care-planning/.

Ontario Ministry of the Attorney General. (2016). *The capacity assessment office: Questions and answers.* Retrieved from www.attorneygeneral.jus.gov.on.ca/english/family/pgt/capacityoffice.php#eligible.

Personal Directives Act, Revised Statutes of Alberta. (2000, c. P-6). Retrieved from http://canlii.ca/t/53321.

Personal Directives Act, Statues of Nova Scotia. (2008, c. 8). Retrieved from http://canlii.ca/t/kv9f.

Personal Directives Act, Statutes of the Northwest Territories. (2005, c. 16). Retrieved from http://canlii.ca/t/52g46.

Public Legal Education and Information Service of New Brunswick. (2019). *Advance Health Care Directives.* Retrieved from www.legal-info-legale.nb.ca/en/uploads/file/pdfs/Advance_Health_Care_Directives_EN.pdf.

Régie de l'Assurance Maladie Québec. (2003). *Advance medical directives – Care in the event of incapacity.* Retrieved from www.ramq.gouv.qc.ca/en/citizens/health-insurance/advance-directives/Pages/advance-medical-directives.aspx.

Representation Agreement Act, Revised Statutes of British Columbia. (1996, c. 405). Retrieved from http://canlii.ca/t/52fhn.

Saskatchewan Association of Social Workers. (2017a). *Guidance for social workers on medical assistance in dying.* Retrieved from www.casw-acts.ca/sites/default/files/attachements/sk_paper_on_maid_for_social_workers-2017_jan_13_r1873193_0.pdf.

Saskatchewan Association of Social Workers. (2017b). *Standards of practices for registered social workers in Saskatchewan*. Retrieved from www.sasw.ca/document/4577/SASW%20Standards-of-Practice%20June%201%202017%20Approved.pdf.

Saskatchewan Health Authority. (2017). *Advance care directive (living will)*. Retrieved from www.saskatoonhealthregion.ca/patients/Pages/Advance-Care-Directive.aspx.

Seniors First BC. (2011). *Capacity continuum*. Vancouver, BC: Author. Retrieved from http://seniorsfirstbc.ca/wp-content/uploads/2011/08/capacity-continuum-e1466099198529.png.

Speak Up. (2019). *Provincial government marks national advance care planning day in Newfoundland and Labrador*. Retrieved from www.advancecareplanning.ca/acp-news/provincial-government-marks-national-advance-care-planning-day-in-newfoundland-and-labrador/.

Wahl, J., Dykeman, M. J., & Walton, T. (2016, December). *Health care consent, advance care planning, and goals of care practice tools: The challenge to get it right. Improving the last stages of life*. Commissioned by the Law Commission. Toronto, ON: Law Commission of Ontario.

Weinberg, M., & Banks, S. (2019). Practicing ethically in unethical times: Everyday resistance in Social Work. *Ethics & Social Welfare*. doi:10.1080/17496535.2019.1597141.

Chapter 6

Who cares about caregiving?

Questions to consider as you read this chapter

- Who is included in/left out from the dominant definition of "caregiver", and why is this the case?
- What discourses frame our understanding of caregivers in health and social care?
- What challenges and opportunities exist in the provision of care to caregivers?

Sachika is a 68-year-old Tamil woman who has just arrived from Sri Lanka to be reunited with her son (Arul) and her son's family, who moved to Montreal seven years ago. She speaks no English or French and knows little about the city aside from conversations she has had with her son. The apartment that her son and his family live in is quite small, so she shares a room with her youngest grandchild. Both her son and daughter-in-law (Adele) work to try to make ends meet but still struggle financially. Sachika immigrated to be close to her family and to help with her three grandchildren, all between the ages of four and 11. Sachika faces growing health concerns, but she keeps the problems to herself because she does not want to burden anyone. Her son hopes that she will be able to look after their youngest child in order to save money on daycare while both parents go out to work. Sachika is lonely and misses her friends and extended family. Her oldest grandchild seems to resent her presence and rarely acknowledges her.

One day, Sachika collapses on the kitchen floor. Her daughter-in-law arrives home to find her and calls 9-1-1. Upon evaluation, the doctors discover that she has had a stroke. Her capacity to independently take care of her activities of daily living has been affected by the stroke. She has a deficit in her left hand, which she cannot use to lift or hold objects, some loss of speech, and excessive tiredness. When Sachika is discharged, she needs to rest frequently. Adele feels that she is responsible for taking care of her mother-in-law as well as the three kids. Arul works many overtime hours to make ends meet financially and is often not available to help. Sachika tries not to be a bother, but she is feeling depressed and lonely, so Adele tries to provide emotional support and companionship. Sachika is afraid she will be abandoned by her children and put into a nursing home. Adele is afraid she will not be able to cope much longer. The social worker from the local homecare agency arrives to do a functional assessment with Sachika a few days after her discharge from hospital. Because Sachika cannot speak English or French, Adele is required to answer all the social worker's questions. This frustrates Sachika but she says nothing, only smiles. She does not want to cause a fuss. Moreover, Sachika does not trust her social worker because of the micro aggressions she experiences. For instance, Sachika observes that the social worker talks briskly without acknowledging her, sits down without asking, and rudely begins to ask Adele questions. She rarely turns to look at Sachika. Adele answers questions but says nothing about her own stress as she does not want to disrespect Sachika.

They both wait for the social worker to notice that something is wrong, but she only focusses on her forms and asks direct questions about what Sachika can and cannot do, what she needs help with, and who in the family helps her. The social worker seems pleased at how well cared for Sachika is and makes assumptions about the family's availability and well-being because she does not ask any questions about Adele or Arul, aside from those related to what they do for Sachika. Still, she hands Adele a few pamphlets on community activities available in the local area, as she departs. In the end, Sachika is not deemed eligible to receive homecare services. Her functional capacity and extensive family support are evaluated as "enough and adequate to meet current needs". "Call if anything changes, otherwise I will see you again next year", the social worker says brightly to Adele on the phone when she reports on the homecare decision to her.[1]

Sachika and Adele's story begins our chapter on caregiving (see textbox 6.1). Caregiving and aging are seen as intertwined in gerontological social work, and we know that both are highly gendered activities; thus, we pose the question "**Who cares about caregiving?**" to reflect the overall lack of recognition of caregivers within health and social care sites and sectors. Sachika and Adele's story exposes this reality in the everyday assessment process for homecare services. The older mother and daughter-in-law's case represents the complex and intersecting family and structural issues embedded within caregiving identities and relationships, as well as considerations of how migration, gender roles and expectations, family reunification, intergenerational households, reciprocity, language proficiency, economic precarity, and access to care challenge the everyday experiences of older adults and their caregivers. This chapter challenges the invisibility of caregivers in health and social care settings, contests the dominant discourse and assumptions of who counts as a caregiver, and addresses caregiving as a human rights issue.

The objectives of this chapter are to

- Introduce and define who caregivers are;
- Point to the gendered nature of caregiving;
- Extend understandings of caregiver realities to include marginalized communities;
- Contest several myths about who counts as a caregiver; and
- Provide insights and examples to foster AOP.

Directing our attention to Adele specifically, we notice how social work micro-level interventions and practices can shape how family caregivers are situated within care systems. Sachika is clearly the focus, as she is considered the "client" in this context. We believe that attention should also be given to Adele, who not only acts as the interpreter and support person for Sachika, but is also a person with her own experiences and rights. While Adele gives the social worker information on how Sachika is functioning and on her own role in providing care, there is little room to consider or respond to the stresses that Adele faces as a caregiver. This overarching identification of the caregiver as "resource" is a common assumption within health and social care services. Since the existing health and social care system is set up to respond reactively to existing problems, we as social workers often pay little attention to prevention, particularly as it relates to the caregiver. As a consequence, it is only when the caregiver has reached a point of either falling ill themselves or refusing to continue providing care that we consider their concerns and realities. Research has shown that caregivers provide care because of a strong commitment to their relationships and will continue to do so regardless of the challenges they face (Chappell, 2011). Given this, it is highly unlikely that Adele would ever refuse to care for her mother-in-law. In addition, given Adele's busy schedule and lack of access to culturally appropriate services, it is unlikely that she will find support that reflects Sachika's or her own realities within the pamphlets that were left in her home after the first visit by the social worker. We present Sachika, Adele, and Arul as an invitation for readers to consider the ways in which health and social care services currently engage with caregivers and to consider alternatives that would enhance support.

Textbox 6.1

Caregivers are those who provide unpaid care and assistance for family members or friends who are in need of support because of age, debilitating medical conditions, chronic injury, long-term illness, or disability (Carers Canada (previously the Canadian Caregiver Coalition), 2013).

Sachika and Adele's story is just one example of caregiving. More than eight million people in Canada identify as caregivers, representing approximately 30% of the entire Canadian population (Carers Canada, 2013).[2] That means there are more than eight million stories of providing care across this country. Carers Canada, a national umbrella advocacy organization, defines caregivers as those who provide care and assistance for family members or friends in need of support due to age, debilitating medical conditions, chronic injury, long-term illness, or disability (Carers Canada, 2013). We believe that this number is an under-representation of the real situation given that many people who provide unpaid care to family and friends do not identify themselves as "caregivers" but rather consider the tasks they undertake as simply part of their role (Montgomery, Rowe, & Kosloski, 2007). Caregivers care for people across the life course, but those providing care to older adults represent the majority. Caregiving accounts for approximately 80% of all unpaid community care to older adults. The economic situation is staggering; it has been estimated that caregivers contribute $25–30 billion dollars per year of unpaid labour to the Canadian economy, a figure that has tripled in only three years (Carers Canada, 2017; Fast, Keating, Lero, Eales, & Duncan, 2013). To contextualize these numbers within the entire health care system, caregiver contributions represent 11% of Canada's health care budget (Fast et al., 2013). As social workers, we must remember that caregiving is often not a choice, but rather a requirement to make up for the lack of available services. Research suggests that over 70% of caregivers feel as though they have no options, with 50% identifying a lack of available services as a contributing factor in their decision to provide care (Orzeck, 2017).

Caregiver diversity

Caregivers are diverse, representing every region and social location. The majority of caregivers in Canada and around the world are women (Calasanti & Slevin, 2001; Drummond et al., 2013; Embracing Carers, 2017; Silverman, 2013). While the proportion of men providing care has risen in the past decade (due in part to changing gender norms and women's increased workforce participation), women continue to provide most of the hands-on, personal care tasks (including bathing, dressing, cooking and cleaning) and do so for many more hours each week (Embracing Carers, 2017). Researchers have presented feminist approaches to care as seeking to understand the relationships of women who care and the context within which they care (Orzeck, 2017). Feminist approaches also identify how responsibilities for care across the lifespan shape women's autonomy and choices (Drummond et al., 2013; Hooyman & Gonyea, 1995; Orzeck, 2017) and have detrimental consequences on their financial security across the lifespan and into retirement (Calasanti & Slevin, 2001). This is a reality among both informal/ unpaid family caregivers (mostly partners/spouses and adult daughters/daughters-in- law) and among formal/paid frontline homecare workers who often work for low pay with few benefits and little security – a situation affecting mostly racialized and immigrant women (see textbox 6.2).

Textbox 6.2

Informal/unpaid versus formal/paid caregiving are terms that distinguish between those who provide care in a familial or volunteer context and those who are paid to undertake the tasks of care. Although both types of caregivers can experience emotional connection to the care receiver in the context of care, informal/unpaid caregivers are more likely to have a pre-existing personal or familial connection to the care receiver.

It has been estimated that almost 50% of caregivers to older adults are between the ages of 45 and 64 years of age, and another 24% are 65 years of age or older (Sinha, 2013). The remainder of caregivers are under the age of 45 with a growing number of youth and young adults between the ages of 15 and 24 contributing to intergenerational caregiving responsibilities within families and across generations (Charles, Stainton, & Marshall, 2012; Dellmann-Jenkins, Blan- kemeyer, & Pinkard, 2000; Stamatopoulos, 2015) (see textbox 6.3). Older adults are not only receivers of care but also givers of care within and across gener- ations. Many consequences to providing care have been documented in the litera- ture, both negative and positive. Often, caregivers experience a loss of identity and social connection because of the time and energy required to provide care (Brotman et al., 2016; Orzeck, 2016). They also face distress, depression, anxiety, chronic illness, and social isolation (Cranswick & Dosman, 2008; Pinquart & Sör- ensen, 2006). Positive aspects of care have been noted to include a deepened rela- tionship with the care receiver and an enhanced sense of personal fulfillment and purpose (Orzeck, Guberman, & Barylak, 2001).

> **Textbox 6.3**
>
> **Intergenerational care** refers to caring arrangements that take place across generations, including those in which young people provide care to older adults and those in which older adults provide care to young people, as in the case of care between grandparents and grandchildren. An example of social work intervention in the context of intergenerational care can be found within both aging and child welfare practice, for example in situations where grandparents have taken on primary care provision to grandchildren in cases of parental abuse or neglect (Hayslip, Fruhauf, & Dolbin-MacNab, 2019).

Caregiving is often a long-term commitment, lasting an average of eight to 10 years. With the majority of caregivers being middle-aged, recent attention has been placed on the problem of balancing paid work with caregiving (Brody, 2004; Lilly, 2011; Spillman & Pezzin, 2000). Those caregivers in Canada juggling work, caregiving responsibilities, and often childcare number 6.1 million (Cranswick & Dosman, 2008; Sinha, 2013). Almost one-third of caregivers say that their employment has been negatively affected by caregiving with many missing work, taking unpaid leave, experiencing reduced energy or job satisfaction, and foregoing promotion or leaving work altogether (Embracing Carers, 2017; Fast et al., 2013). Recognition and support for working caregivers through policy and program initiatives is an emerging area of advocacy.

Post-caregiving

Recently, service providers and scholars have called for the need to recognize caregiving as a life course journey, with an emphasis on the realities of post-care (Orzeck, 2016; Orzeck & Silverman, 2008). Post-care has been defined as the time between the death of the care receiver and up to two years following (see textbox 6.4). To date, there have been few services and supports targeting caregivers once the person they are caring for dies. Typically, there is an assumption made that the caregiving journey has ended, and with it the burden and stress faced by caregivers. Given that the focus of intervention in health and social care services is the "client with the health issue", namely the care receiver, there is little room to consider extending the provision of care to caregivers who are no longer actively caregiving. This means that caregivers can be left unsupported when facing the grieving process. Recent research has documented the complex experiences of grief among caregivers during the post-care period, pointing to issues including loss of role and identity, which can complicate coping with death and dying (Orzeck, 2016; Orzeck & Silverman, 2008). A focus on the death and dying process and post-care also makes room for conversations about faith and spirituality, which is otherwise an underexplored area of practice. This includes attention to the ways in which faith and spirituality are practised, its relationship to personal identity and community belonging, and the role of faith and spirituality in end-of-life decision-making and coping with grief (Lalani, Duggleby, & Olson, 2018). The potential benefits of targeting support and counselling to caregivers in the post-care period is an area worthy of consideration within health and social care services.

> **Textbox 6.4**
>
> **Post-care** is the time period in the trajectory of care immediately following the death of the care receiver. Although under-recognized in health and social care services, the post-care period has recently been identified as a significant component of the care journey in the life course of the caregiver.

Caregiving as a human rights issue

Globally, caregiving has been recognized as a significant health issue and as deserving of attention with respect to the human rights consequences of care, particularly to women across the life course (Barylak & Guberman, 2015; Embracing Carers, 2017). According to the United Nations, unpaid care represents as much as 50% of the workforce in some low-income countries (United Nations, 2009). Quoting an excerpt from a UN press release, Marilyn Waring, Professor of Public Policy at the Institute of Public Policy at AUT University in New Zealand, noted

> the invisibility of women's care work was and is not an accident. It was a strategic choice made through a series of United Nations rules imposed on countries in 1953 which described all women's unpaid work as "of little or no importance" to national accounts and excluded unpaid "household and caring work" … from economic analysis and policymaking.
>
> (United Nations, 2009, p. 2)

Advocacy efforts focussed on caregiving as a human rights issue have broadened attention to the intersectional consequences and realities of care, linking racialization, patriarchy, classism and hetero/cissexism as fundamental aspects of the caregiver experience. This supports the idea that social justice responses are required in order to increase access and equity in policy and service delivery locally and transnationally. In the context of neoliberalism and the resulting reality of resource scarcity, there has never been more pressure on family caregivers to pick up the slack of the retreating (neoliberal) welfare state (England, Earkin, Gastaldo, & McKeever, 2005). This puts caregivers, and particularly women, in a precarious position concerning their own physical, psychological, and financial well-being. This has also been contextualized to include regional variations in access and equity within and across borders (see textbox 6.5). From a national perspective, researchers and activists have, for example, pointed to the lack of available and culturally appropriate or safe health and social care services in rural and remote regions, including within Indigenous communities, as being a situation akin to a national crisis (particularly in reference to Canada's northern and remote regions). Fewer resources and long distances to urban centres in which specialized health services are more available often results in significant inequities and, as a consequence, greater responsibility for care among unpaid/informal caregivers (Crooks, Schuurman, Cinnamon, Castleden, & Johnston, 2011; Crossato & Leipert, 2006; Giesbrecht et al., 2016; Jacklin, Pace, & Warry, 2015).

Textbox 6.5

Transregional/transnational care refers to the care arrangements that exist between families and communities across borders whereby they provide and receive care transregionally (within a nation–state but across regional borders) and/or transnationally (across nation–states).

While issues regarding gender have been thoroughly explored in the research on caregiving, other aspects of identity and social location have not yet received adequate attention in the literature or in policy and practice. In practice, homogenous and restricted interpretations (heteronormative and biological) of who counts as family and which families should be prioritized for support are predominant (Neysmith, Reitsma-Street, Colins, & Porter, 2012). These interpretations significantly limit the potential of initiatives to address diversity and undermine support to the most isolated and under-served communities in contemporary society. This chapter asserts the importance of including issues of diversity as a *central feature* of analysis and understanding of caregiving. By broadening our understanding of caregiver diversity and by challenging predominant assumptions of what caregiving is and who provides care, we can both better inform the current context of informal care in Canada and reduce discrimination in service delivery responses to caregivers. The rest of the chapter is dedicated to breaking down some of the dominant myths about caregivers from marginalized communities within practice and policy settings. By doing so we hope to create opportunities for counter-discourses on caregiving and make room for AOP within health and social care services.

"They would rather take care of their own": Countering the assumption of "personal choice"

In our work with marginalized communities, we have frequently heard providers of health and social care services raise the assumption that people from these communities prefer to "take care of their own". If asked about the absence of caregivers from diverse communities on client lists, service providers suggest that the reason for this absence is that these communities prefer to provide care within the family or cultural community (Brotman, 2002). Ideas of filial piety govern perceptions about caregiving exchanges within ethno-cultural minority families (Koehn & Kobayashi, 2011) (see textbox 6.6). Filial piety is a concept drawn from Confucian philosophy and has been defined as the expression of responsibility, respect, sacrifice, and family harmony (Lai, 2010). While the concept of filial piety has been a major influence on the ways in which some families are expected to provide care for older parents, it is important to avoid reified conclusions that ethno-cultural minority communities typically adopt Confucian philosophies of care, particularly within the context of challenges to processes of acculturation and realities of living in the adopted society that have drastically shifted immigrants' perspectives on caregiving (Lai, 2010).

> **Textbox 6.6**
>
> **Filial piety** is a concept drawn from Confucian philosophy and has been defined as the expression of responsibility, respect, sacrifice, and family harmony (Lai, 2010).

Assumptions about filial piety potentially ignore the more complex realities that exist within ethno-cultural minority families. For instance, in the case of immigration, the composition of the family unit is increasingly reconstituted (and ruptured) by policies that categorize (older adult) newcomers according to their potential to contribute to the labour economy (Phillipson & Ahmed, 2004; Treas, 2008). Sponsorship in Canada, which once favoured and facilitated family reunification, is increasingly restrictive to older newcomers, with respect to accessing permanent residency status and state entitlements (Ferrer, 2015).

Life course factors contributing to cumulative disadvantage (see **Age/ism: Age as a category of difference**), such as the over-representation of ethno-cultural minority communities in the secondary labour market and higher rates of poverty, also contribute to greater strain on the availability of members to provide care (Brotman, 2002). Family members are often in the difficult position of having to work longer hours or delay retirement to make up for structural limitations on the recognition of education, access to pensions, or burdens of sponsorship. This reality was described in Sachika and Adele's story of care.

Older adults state that they would prefer to receive culturally specific services offered by and within their own communities (Brotman, 2002; Brotman, Ryan, & Cormier, 2002). However, structural limitations, including a lack of adequate funding to community groups, often make this option impossible. Mainstream services often fail to take into account the unique realities and needs of these communities, oftentimes rendering their experiences invisible (Lavoie, Guberman, & Brotman, 2010). These dynamics create realities that, on the one hand, force caregivers to protect their loved ones by not coming forward and, on the other hand, leave families isolated because there are no services to meet their needs. The result is that, as caregivers from marginalized communities are absent, they are determined by providers not to need services. Taken together, these dynamics highlight how structural inequality is at the core of "personal choice".

Incorporating intergenerational and community care into definitions of caregiving

In the current policy and practice landscape, caregivers are identified as mostly adult children and spouses, with only lip service paid to the inclusion of neighbours or friends as central and entrusted figures in the provision of care. While it is true that older adults receive most of their informal support from children and spouses (Turcotte & Schellenberg, 2007), the tendency to focus on the majority reinforces the assumption that the only caregivers who "count" are those that fit the normative model: heterosexual, Canadian-born adult children and cisgender wives/husbands. Services are targeted to offer assistance to those who fit this normative model of the traditional family. With such a narrow lens, there is limited opportunity to either offer support or include in decision-making those who are outside this norm. We would also stress that by excluding "non-normative" kinship-care, we lose sight of alternative models of caregiving that exist within and among marginalized communities. For example, Williams et al. (2015) called attention to the "ideology of community" that exists within Indigenous communities. We believe that these models can provide much-needed insight into how families and communities provide reciprocal care in contexts of adversity and scarcity and in particular when formal care provision is either not an option or is a weak one (Ferrer, Brotman, & Grenier, 2017).

Textbox 6.7

Reciprocity is the exchange of care between older adults and their chosen/families; it breaks down dominant discourses of care which assert that care is unidirectional and provided only by caregivers to care receivers.

Practices of reciprocal care, such as those within LGBTTsIQ communities, are worthy of consideration (see textbox 6.7). Although LGBTTsIQ older adults are an example of a marginalized community at risk of social isolation in later life, the extent to which this is a problem is often compounded by the fact that caregivers of LGBTTsIQ older people are often not recognized as such within the health and social care system. Existing research has documented discriminatory practices that serve as barriers to LGBTTsIQ communities' ability to access services (Brotman et al., 2007; Coon, 2007; Hash & Cramer, 2003; Moore, 2002). The importance of "chosen family networks" is especially worth highlighting, as they exist outside the recognized "traditional" family norm (Muraco & Fredriksen-Goldsen, 2011) (see textbox 6.8). When they are acknowledged, they often face exclusion, which propel some to hide their identity to protect themselves and their loved ones from the discriminatory attitudes of formal care providers (Brotman, Ferrer, Sussman, Ryan, & Richard, 2015). Same-sex partners, for instance, may not identify themselves as a spouse to service providers, opting to use terms such as "friend" to describe their long-term commitments (Brotman et al., 2015). By labelling LGBTTsIQ relationships outside the "normative" form, service providers may misinterpret what constitutes family, resulting in many lost opportunities for the inclusion of LGBTTsIQ caregivers.

Textbox 6.8

(Chosen) family are networks of people who consider themselves "family-like" and fall outside normative (nuclear) family structures. Chosen family can include extended family members and community stakeholders who are present and provide consistent care to older adults.

Within LGBTTsIQ communities, intergenerational and community caregiving practices are also common. For example, there is ample evidence of the role of lesbian community caregiver support during the early years of the HIV/AIDS pandemic (Brennan-Ing, Seidel, London, Cahill, & Karpiak, 2014). As well, the tradition of reciprocity between younger and older members of the community in terms of mentorship and role modelling related to managing stigma and discrimination and in negotiating coming out processes has been well-documented (Brotman, Ryan, & Cormier, 2003; Orel, 2004; Stein & Beckerman, 2010; Zodikoff, 2006). There has been research on the reciprocal relationship between younger members of the community who act as caregivers for older members in times of illness and disability (Brotman et al., 2007; Coon, 2007). These alternative and important contributions of intergenerational and community caregiving remain unrecognized by mainstream healthcare providers, however, both the importance of these types of caregivers in the organization of care and the capacity for these models to provide new insight for adapting healthcare initiatives are important justifications for enhancing recognition and inclusion.

In considering ethno–cultural minority communities, there continues to be little recognition of the role played by both grandchildren and community support networks within mainstream services. This shortcoming renders invisible the contributions that the intergenerational family and community members/stakeholders make to the provision of support. For example, translation and interpretation is a type of instrumental support often provided by grandchildren and community networks, who play a crucial role in serving as the intermediary between healthcare professionals and older adults (Ramnarace, 2011). This type of support also extends to navigation through the health and social care system, and state bureaucratic services where community networks take on roles of accompaniment and advocacy across sectors (i.e., immigration, retirement, and healthcare).

Conclusion

Social workers are in a unique position to bring attention to the diversity and complexity of caregiving and to the human rights of caregivers at all levels of practice and policy. We are in this unique position because of our roles in assessment, intervention, resource development, and advocacy. We will likely be the first point of contact for caregivers and key gatekeepers to services. It can take a simple act of openness to create a space for caregivers to express their own realities and concerns during assessments, but we must also create space organizationally to account for these realities more concretely (e.g., by demanding that caregivers receive their own "file" as clients eligible for services in their own right), to extend who we identify as caregivers (e.g., by broadening our definitions of caregiver to chosen family and community supports), to work more collaboratively with diverse community groups with their own expertise regarding caregiving realities within their communities (e.g., by creating partnership networks and outreach positions in conjunction with marginalized communities), and by demanding policy change and increased funding to support health promotion activities in the community to address caregiver issues (e.g., increased funding to local nonprofit, community-based culturally specific organizations and groups). Finally, existing caregiver networks must begin to take account of diversity and to create space around the table for marginalized communities to participate and make decisions. To date, caregiver networks at the local and national levels are still largely representative of mainstream people and ideas and have yet to fully acknowledge and account for the diverse range of caregivers from marginalized communities. This must change if we are to more fully capture and respond to the diversity of caregivers' realities.

We conclude this chapter by revisiting Sachika and Adele's story and by envisioning an alternative ending in which the social worker reflects AOP principles.

When the social worker calls Adele to arrange a visit, she asks Adele if Sachika can communicate in English or French. When Adele tells her no, the social worker asks if she (the social worker) can arrange for an interpreter to come with her so she can speak with Sachika directly. Adele tells her this is fine as long as she can be involved in choosing this person to make sure that she does not know them personally and that they are not in their kinship network. The social worker locates and hires a Tamil interpreter. She asks Adele if they would prefer to meet together or separately. Adele insists that she must be present at the assessment and would like her husband Arul to be present. She also would agree to a second meeting at another time so she could talk alone with the social worker. When they arrive, the social worker introduces herself and the interpreter and waits for an invitation to sit. They sit around the kitchen table. The social worker begins by asking Sachika to tell her story before asking about her functionality and supports. They engage in a more full discussion. When she meets with Adele at a later date in her office, she begins by using a care tool designed to more deeply explore Adele's unique and personal experience as a caregiver in relation to familial, social, and structural realities over time.[3] This leads to a conversation about how Adele is managing with multiple responsibilities. Adele embarrassedly admits to some of her challenges, both with respect to juggling and with respect to trying to get her husband to simply understand the weight she is under. The social worker has little to offer from within her organization, but she knows of a caregiver support group in the community and asks if Adele might be interested in attending. Adele is uncertain but says thank you, takes the phone number, and prepares to leave. The social worker, seeing the hesitation and politeness of Adele's response, offers to make inquiries to see if she can locate a more appropriate place of support and get back to Adele. She does some outreach to the Tamil community and finds a small group of retired women who are working to help other families in the community by preparing meals and providing respite. The social worker calls Adele back and Adele is pleased to have the social worker give her number to these women. The group finds Adele a babysitter and delivers dinners twice per week, which gives Adele some much needed time off. In the meantime, the social worker, with a new and relevant connection, asks her supervisor if she could start a community outreach project that would include an Advisory Committee made up of local volunteer groups to help advise them on how to better adapt services to meet the needs and desires of older people and their caregivers. She uses her intervention with Adele and Sachika to emphasize the potential usefulness and importance of this work. The social worker also joins a professional caregiver association to advocate for additional funding to help support this group of women and is successful in helping them get a small budget to cover the cost of meals and babysitting services. After five years of pushing, the agency finally agrees to create an Advisory Outreach Committee.

Exercise

*   Thinking about your practicum or work experience, consider the place of caregivers in both intervention processes and decision-making:

    a   How are caregivers perceived (as partners, resources, and/or clients)? What impact does this perception have on service options available to them?

    b   How might you advocate for the inclusion of a specific mandate within health and social care services across sites and sectors to more comprehensively include caregivers?

- Thinking about the case and counter-story presented in this chapter,

    a   Identify the main issues or problems that the older adult, family member(s), and/or social worker are facing;

    b   Highlight the potential causes/roots (personal and/or structural) of these issues or problems (historical and current);

    c   What elements would you add/change to the intervention plan proposed? How might you also include Arul and the children in such a plan?

Takeaways

- A caregiver (also known as a carer, a family caregiver, an informal caregiver or a care partner) is a person who takes on an unpaid caring role for someone who needs help because of a physical or cognitive condition, an injury, disability, or chronic life-limiting illness.
- Not all caregivers will identify themselves as such, seeing their caring work as simply part of their role as a family member or friend.
- More than three decades of research and advocacy have led to a broader understanding of the needs and realities of caregivers in society and within health and social care sites and sectors.
- The dominant discourse of caregiving in health and social care is that of "resource".
- Diversity within the caregiver population is not well accounted for in research, practice, and policy, leading to exclusion and invisibility of caregivers from marginalized communities.
- Social workers can play a key role in expanding definitions, adapting services, and advocating for change to recognize and support diverse caregivers across the life course.

Additional resources

- Carers Canada: www.carerscanada.ca/
- International Alliance of Caregiver Organizations: https://internationalcarers.org/
- Atlas of Caregiving: https://atlasofcaregiving.com/

Acknowledgement

This chapter is adapted from the original publication (Brotman, S., & Ferrer, I., 2015). Diversity within family caregiving: Extending definitions of "who counts" to include marginalized communities. *HealthcarePapers, 15*(1), 47–53, with permission from: *HealthcarePapers*: New Models for New Healthcare. Toronto, ON: Longwoods Publishing

Notes

1 Sachika's story is adapted and expanded from a brief case study (Siva) which first appeared in Grenier and Brotman (2010).

2 Canadian statistics included in this chapter are based upon findings from the 2012 Canadian Social Survey. More recent data from the Canadian Social Survey 2018 will only be made available to the public at the end of 2019. Trends are expected to be consistent with the data provided here.

3 There are many examples of caregiver-specific assessment and intervention tools that move beyond the bio-medical/functional. See The Caregiver Assessment Tool (Barylak, Guberman, Fancey, & Keefe, 2006), The Careography Tool (Orzeck, 2016), and the Atlas of Caregiving Map (atlasofcaregiving.org). These tools re-imagine genograms and ecomaps (common to social work practice) in order to more fully capture the caregiving reality and journey at personal, social and organizational/structural levels (see endnote ii in **Theorizing later life and social work praxis**).

References

Barylak, L., & Guberman, N. (2015). *Beyond recognition – Caregiving and human rights in Canada: A policy brief.* Retrieved from www.carerscanada.ca/wp-content/uploads/2016/02/CCC_Policy_brief_Human_rights_EN.pdf

Barylak, L., Guberman, N., Fancey, P., & Keefe, J. (2006). Examining the role of caregiver assessment – Barriers, outcomes, policy implications. Retrieved from www.msvu.ca/en/home/research/chairs/centresandinstitutes/centreonaging/projects/caregiverassessment/reportsandpublications.aspx

Brennan-Ing, M., Seidel, L., London, A. S., Cahill, S., & Karpiak, S. E. (2014). Service utilization among older adults with HIV: The joint association of sexual identity and gender. *Journal of Homosexuality, 61*(1), 166–196. doi:10.1080/00918369.2013.835608

Brody, E. M. (2004). *Women in the middle: Their parent care years.* New York, NY: Springer Pub.

Brotman, S. (2002). The primacy of family in elder care discourse: Home care services to older ethnic women in Canada. *Journal of Gerontological Social Work, 38*(3), 19–52.

Brotman, S., Drummond, J., Silverman, M., Sussman, T., Orzeck, P., Barylak, L., … Billette, V. (2016). Talking with spousal caregivers about sexuality and intimacy: Perspectives of service providers. *Journal of Health and Social Work, 41*(4), 263–273. doi:10.1093/hsw/hlw040

Brotman, S., Ferrer, I., Sussman, T., Ryan, B., & Richard, B. (2015). Access and equity in the design and delivery of health and social care to LGBTQ older adults: A Canadian perspective. In N. A. Orel & C. A. Fruhauf (Eds.), *Lesbian, gay, bisexual, and transgender (LGBT) older adults and their families: Current research and clinical applications* (pp. 111–140). Washington, DC: American Psychological Association.

Brotman, S., Ryan, B., Collins, S., Chamberland, L., Cormier, R., Julien, D., … Richard, B. (2007). Coming out to care: Caregivers of gay and lesbian seniors in Canada. *The Gerontologist, 47*(4), 490–503. doi:10.1093/geront/47.4.490

Brotman, S., Ryan, B., & Cormier, R. (2002). *Gay and lesbian seniors: Writings in gerontology.* Ottawa, ON: National Advisory Council on Aging.

Brotman, S., Ryan, B., & Cormier, R. (2003). The health and social service needs of gay and lesbian elders and their families in Canada. *The Gerontologist, 43*(2), 192–202. doi:10.1093/geront/43.2.192

Calasanti, T. M., & Slevin, K. F. (2001). *Gender, social inequalities and aging.* Walnut Creek, CA: AltaMira Press.

Carers Canada. (2013). Carer Facts. [Fact sheet]. Retrieved from www.carerscanada.ca/carer-facts/

Carers Canada. (2017). Advancing collective priorities: A Canadian career strategy. [Fact sheet]. Retrieved from www.carerscanada.ca/priorities/

Chappell, N. L. (2011). *Population aging and the evolving needs of older Canadians: An overview of the policy challenges.* Montreal, QC: Institute for Research on Public Policy. Retrieved from https://irpp.org/research-studies/population-aging-and-the-evolving-care-needs-of-older-canadians/

Charles, G., Stainton, T., & Marshall, S. (2012). *Young carers in Canada: The hidden costs and benefits of young caregiving*. Ottawa, ON: The Vanier Institute of the Family.

Coon, D. (2007). Exploring interventions for LGBT caregivers: Issues and examples. *Journal of Gay & Lesbian Social Services, 18*(3/4), 109–128. doi:10.1300/J041v18n03_07

Cranswick, K., & Dosman, D. (2008). Eldercare: What we know today. *Canadian Social Trends, 11*, 10. Retrieved from https://www150.statcan.gc.ca/n1/pub/11-008-x/2008002/article/10689-eng.htm

Crooks, V., Schuurman, N., Cinnamon, J., Castleden, H., & Johnston, R. (2011). Refining a location analysis model using a mixed methods approach: Community readiness as a key factor in citing rural palliative care services. *Journal of Mixed Methods Research, 5*(1), 77–95. doi:10.1177/1558689810385693

Crossato, K. E., & Leipert, B. (2006). Rural women caregivers in Canada. *Rural and Remote Health, 6*, 520. Retrieved from www.rrh.org.au/journal/article/520

Dellmann-Jenkins, M., Blankemeyer, M., & Pinkard, O. (2000). Young adult children and grandchildren in priAdele caregiver roles to older relatives and their service needs. *Family Relations, 49*(2), 177–186. doi:10.1111/j.1741-3729.2000.00177.x

Drummond, J., Brotman, S., Silverman, M., Sussman, T., Orzeck, P., Barylak, L., & Wallach, I. (2013). The impact of caregiving: Women's experiences of sexuality and intimacy. *Affilia: Journal of Women and Social Work, 28*(4), 414–427. doi:10.1177/0886109913504154

Embracing Carers. 2017. *Embracing the critical role of caregivers around the world. White paper and action plan*. Darmstadt, Germany: Merck KGaA. Retrieved from www.embracingcarers.com/content/dam/web/healthcare/corporate/embracing-carers/media/infographics/us/Merck%20KGaA%20Embracing%20Carers_White%20Paper%20Flattened.pdf

England, K., Earkin, J. M., Gastaldo, D. L., & McKeever, P. K. (2005). Neoliberalizing home care Managed competition and restructuring home care in Ontario. In K. England & K. Ward (Eds.), *Neoliberalization: Networks, states, peoples* (pp. 169–193). Oxford: Blackwell.

Fast, J., Keating, N. C., Lero, D. S., Eales, J., & Duncan, K. (2013). *The economic costs of care to family/friend caregivers: A synthesis of findings*. Edmonton, AB: University of Alberta. Retrieved from www.deslibris.ca/en-us/bookinfo.aspx?ID=245565

Ferrer, I. (2015). Examining the disjunctures between policy and care in Canada's parent and grandparent supervisa. *International Journal of Migration, Health and Social Care, 11*(4), 253–267. doi:10.1108/IJMHSC-08-2014-0030

Ferrer, I., Brotman, S., & Grenier, A. (2017). The experiences of reciprocity among Filipino older adults in Canada: Intergenerational, transnational and community considerations. *Journal of Gerontological Social Work, 60*(4), 313–327. doi:10.1080/01634372.2017.1327916

Giesbrecht, M., Crooks, V., Castleden, H., Schuurman, N., Skinner, M., & Williams, A. (2016). Palliating inside the lines: The effects of borders and boundaries on palliative care in rural Canada. *Social Science & Medicine, 168*, 273–282. doi:10.1016/j.socscimed.2016.04.037

Grenier, A., & Brotman, S. (2010). Les multiples vieillissements et leurs representations. In M. Charpentier, N. Guberman, V. Billette, J. P. Lavoie, A. Grenier, & I. Olazabal (Eds.), *Vieillir au pluriel: Perspectives sociales* (pp. 23–34). Quebec, Canada: Presses de l'Université du Québec.

Hash, K., & Cramer, E. (2003). Empowering gay and lesbian caregivers and uncovering their unique experiences through the use of qualitative methods. *Journal of Gay and Lesbian Social Services, 15*(1/2), 47–63. doi:10.1300/J041v15n01_04

Hayslip, B., Fruhauf, C., & Dolbin-MacNab, M. (2019). Grandparents raising grandchildren: What have we learned over the past decade? *The Gerontologist, 59*(3), e152–e163. doi:10.1093/geront/gnx106

Hooyman, N., & Gonyea, J. (1995). *Feminist perspectives on family care: Policies for gender justice*. Thousand Oaks, CA: Sage Publications, Inc. doi:10.4135/9781483327303

Jacklin, K., Pace, J., & Warry, W. (2015). Informal dementia caregiving among indigenous communities in Ontario, ON. *Care Management Journals, 16*(2), 106–120. doi:10.1891/1521-0987.16.2.106

Koehn, S., & Kobayashi, K. (2011). Age and ethnicity. In M. Sargeant (Ed.), *Age discrimination and diversity: Multiplied discrimination from an age perspective* (pp. 132–519). Cambridge: Cambridge University Press.

Lai, D. (2010). Filial piety, caregiving appraisal, and caregiving burden. *Research on Aging, 32*(2), 200–223. doi:10.1177/0164027509351475

Lalani, N., Duggleby, W., & Olson, J. (2018). Spirituality among family caregivers: An integrative literature review. *International Journal of Palliative Nursing, 24*(2), 80–91.

Lavoie, J. P., Guberman, N., Belleau, H., Battaglini, H., Brotman, S., & Montejo, M. E. (2007). Les limites aux solidarités familiales à l'égard des proches ayant des incapacités dans les familles d'immigration récente. *Enfances, Familles, Générations, 6.* doi:10.7202/016484ar

Lavoie, J. P., Guberman, N., & Brotman, S. (2010). Service use by immigrant families for an older relative: A question of culture or structure?. In D. Dust & M. J. MacLean (Eds.), *Diversity and aging among immigrant seniors in Canada: Changing faces and greying temples* (pp. 103–124). Calgary, AB: Detselig Enterprises.

Lilly, M. (2011). The hard work of balancing employment and caregiving: What can Canadian employers do to help? *Health Care Policy, 7*(2), 23–31.

Montgomery, R. J., Rowe, J. M., & Kosloski, K. (2007). Family caregiving. In J. A. Blackburn & C. N. Dulmus (Eds.), *Handbook of gerontology: Evidence-based approaches to theory, practice, and policy* (pp. 426–454). Hoboken: John Wiley & Sons Inc.

Moore, W. R. (2002). Lesbian and gay elders: Connecting care providers through a telephone support group. *Journal of Gay and Lesbian Social Services, 14*(3), 23–41. doi:10.1300/J041v14n03_02

Muraco, A., & Fredriksen-Goldsen, K. (2011). "That's what friends do": Informal caregiving for chronically ill midlife and older lesbian, gay, and bisexual adults. *Journal of Social and Personal Relationships, 28*(8), 1073–1092. doi:10.1177/0265407511402419

Neysmith, S., Reitsma-Street, M., Colins, S. B., & Porter, E. N. (2012). *Beyond caring labour to provisioning work.* Toronto, ON: University of Toronto Press.

Orel, N. A. (2004). Gay, lesbian, and bisexual elders: Expressed needs and concerns across focus groups. *Journal of Gerontological Social Work, 43*(2/3), 57–77. doi:10.1300/J083v43n02_05

Orzeck, P. (2016). Identities in transition: Women caregivers in bereavement. *Journal of Social Work in End-of-Life & Palliative Care, 12*(1/2), 145–161. doi:10.1080/15524256.2016.1165162

Orzeck, P. (2017). *Women's narratives of post-caregiving: A gendered lifecourse perspective.* (Doctoral dissertation). Quebec, QC: Laval University. Retrieved from https://corpus.ulaval.ca/jspui/handle/20.500.11794/28006

Orzeck, P., Guberman, N., & Barylak, L. (2001). *Responding creatively to the needs of caregivers: A resource for health care professionals.* Montreal, QC: Éditions Saint-Martin.

Orzeck, P., & Silverman, M. (2008). Recognizing post-caregiving as part of the caregiving career: Implications for practice. *Journal of Social Work Practice: Psychotherapeutic Approaches in Health, Welfare and the Community, 22*(2), 211–220. doi:10.1080/02656530802299866

Phillipson, C., & Ahmed, N. (2004). Transnational communities migration and changing identities in later life: A new research agenda. In S. O. Daatland & S. Biggs (Eds.), *Ageing and diversity: Multiple pathways and cultural migration* (pp. 157–174). Bristol: Policy Press.

Pinquart, M., & Sörensen, S. (2006). Gender differences in caregiver stressors, social resources, and health: An updated meta-analysis. *Journal of Gerontology: Psychological Sciences, 61B*(1), 33–45.

Ramnarace, C. (2011, August 11). The surprising caregiver: Your grandchild. *AARP Bulletin.* Retrieved from www.aarp.org/relationships/caregiving/info-08-2011/grandchild-as-caregiver.2.html

Silverman, M. (2013). Sighs, smiles, and worried glances: How the body reveals women caregivers' lived experiences of care to older adults. *Journal of Aging Studies, 27,* 288–297. doi:10.1016.2013.06.001

Sinha, M. (2013). *Portrait of caregivers*. Ottawa, ON: Statistics Canada. Retrieved from https://www150.statcan.gc.ca/n1/pub/89-652-x/89-652-x2013001-eng.htm

Spillman, B. C., & Pezzin, L. E. (2000). Potential and active family caregivers: Changing networks and the 'sandwich generation'. *The Milbank Quarterly*, 78(3), 347–374.

Stamatopoulos, V. (2015). One million and counting: The hidden army of young carers in Canada. *Journal of Youth Studies*, 18(6), 809–822. doi:10.1080/13676261.2014.992329

Stein, G. L., & Beckerman, N. L. (2010). Lesbian and gay elders and long-term care: Identifying the unique psychosocial perspectives and challenges. *Journal of Gerontological Social Work*, 53(5), 421–435. doi:10.1080/01634372.2010.496478

Treas, J. (2008). Transnational older adults and their families. *Family Relations*, 57(4), 468–478.

Turcotte, M., & Schellenberg, G. (2007). *A portrait of seniors in Canada*. Ottawa, ON: Statistics Canada. Retrieved from www.statcan.ca/english/freepub/89-519-XIE/89-519-XIE2006001.pdf

United Nations. (2009, March 3). *Caregiver burden must be valued shared supported by governments as crucial to sustaining society, building human capital, women's commission told*. Retrieved from www.un.org/press/en/2009/wom1715.doc.htm

Williams, A. P., Peckman, A., Kuluski, K., Lum, J., Warrick, N., Spalding, K., … Im, J. (2015). Caring for caregivers: Challenging the assumptions. *Healthcare Papers*, 15(1), 8–21.

Zodikoff, B. D. (2006). Services for lesbian, gay, bisexual and transgender older adults. In B. Berkman (Ed.), *Handbook of social work in health and aging* (pp. 569–576). New York, NY: Oxford University Press.

Chapter 7

Dementia, personhood, and citizenship as practice

Questions to consider as you read this chapter

- Do you see people with dementia as *living with* or *suffering from* dementia?
- Who is the social work client when working with older adults with cognitive impairment? Does this change based on the site and/or sector of health and social care in which you work?
- How might you facilitate voice and promote inclusion of persons with dementia as an AOP social worker?
- Does social location/ intersectionality affect dementia in any way?
- What are some ways that you can use your social work skills, knowledge, and values to support the citizenship rights of persons living with dementia and make your community more "dementia-friendly"?[1]

Harpreet is a social worker in a personal care home in Quesnel (small city in the Cariboo region of BC) where the majority of the residents have a diagnosis of dementia, often alongside other complex chronic diseases. Many of these older adults living with dementia were known to the staff from long before they started having memory problems and/or moved to the care home as they lived in Quesnel and nearby rural towns where the staff live. Harpreet herself is from Vancouver and only moved to this much smaller city when her partner got a full-time teaching position at a local high school. While she misses her family and the much larger Sikh community in Vancouver, this move was not unwelcome, as it meant leaving child protection work, which Harpreet had done for the past five years. It also gave her the chance to spend more time with her grandparents who have lived in Quesnel for over 40 years, having chosen to stay there after her grandfather's retirement from the mill. While Harpreet had never worked with older adults, she had taken a class on aging during her BSW and has always enjoyed spending time with her grandparents.

The second week at her new job, Harpreet is tasked with organizing a family meeting, as a resident named Olive has been climbing into her roommate's bed at night. Staff are concerned about how Olive's husband – who still lives at home and visits her daily – will react to this. They also worry about the safety of the other resident who has no family that they know of. Harpreet decides to meet with Olive's two daughters first to gain their support and then speak with the husband; she does not consider involving Olive as the head nurse has told her that while Olive is a lovely woman, she doesn't understand anything that's going on.

This chapter focusses on understanding dementia as a bio-psycho-social phenomenon and encouraging approaches to care/practice more consistent with AOG. We start by deconstructing the paradigms of dementia and dementia care that currently inform sites and sectors of health and social care and which often marginalize and exclude people with dementia and privilege the voices and experiences of (family) care partners and (paid) service providers. This chapter provides an in-depth and critical overview of dementia through linking the data on risk factors, types, and prevalence to social determinants of health (SDOH). We carry forward concepts discussed throughout this book including agency, equity, resilience, and resistance and situate dementia within the previous chapters on **Sites and sectors of health and social care**; **Moral, legal, and ethical issues**; and **Who cares about caregiving?** The counter-story of Harpreet and Olive is woven throughout so that readers see Harpreet's growing appreciation of Olive, first as a person and then as a citizen, and Harpreet's gradual application of AOG knowledge, skills, and values. This chapter presents a person-centred approach as a starting point before highlighting critical concepts and practice approaches that social work scholars have brought to dementia studies, including *validation therapy*, intersectionality, *cultural safety*, *citizenship as practice*, and queer theory, and address the three in italics in depth. We introduce AOG as a way to facilitate the voices, inclusion, and participation of persons living with dementia and to ensure that their needs and desires are balanced with those of their care partners through adopting a *cultural safety and citizenship as practice* approach.

The objectives of this chapter are to

- Provide an overview of dementia, including risk factors, symptoms, prevalence, and types;
- Explain the links between SDOH and dementia;
- Problematize normative understandings of dementia (what it is and how it is experienced);
- Highlight the role of social location in mediating dementia experiences; and
- Promote a cultural safety and citizenship as practice approach to social work with persons with dementia and their care partners.

Understanding dementia and dementia care

There are different ways of looking at dementia or cognitive impairment in later life, some more closely aligned to social work values and AOG than others, as we will discuss. In line with the capacity as a continuum approach introduced in **Moral, legal and ethical issues**, changes in cognitive abilities caused by biological and social determinants of health and linked to aging can be viewed as different points on a scale. Our definitions of cognitive impairment and dementia are listed in textbox 7.1 below.

Textbox 7.1

Cognitive impairment refers to diminishing thinking abilities that are usually age-associated and that may or may not develop into dementia. **Dementia** is an

> umbrella term for a range of memory loss inducing, disorienting, and judgement impairing conditions that most often occur in later life and are usually permanent (chronic).

In order to make clear the similarities and differences among the various theories of dementia, we provide brief descriptions of each, including the associated beliefs and practical applications. The six theories include: (1) dementia as a brain disease, (2) dementia as a normal part of the aging process, (3) dementia as a psycho–neurological condition, (4) dementia as a disability, (5) dementia as a social construction, and (6) dementia as a bio-psycho–social phenomenon. As you review Table 7.1 below, think about the role social work currently plays in supporting and/or challenging these approaches to dementia.

Table 7.1 Theories of dementia and their practical applications[2]

Approach	Beliefs	Practice
Bio-medical (brain disease)	Dementia is a pathological brain disease that results in particular symptoms and behavioral problems. While there are many types of dementia, none is caused by the aging process alone. The disease follows a certain course over a defined period of time.	Treatment focusses on early diagnosis, drug trials and therapies, symptom management, and individual adaptation, including preparation for the inevitable decline. Prevention focusses on reducing risk factors.
Normal aging	The brain loses strength and function over time, therefore dementia, or rather senility, is not a disease, but part of the natural aging process.	Acceptance and care in the community until institutionalization is necessary. "Warehousing" and an exclusive focus on "bed- and-body work" are the result.
Psycho-neurological condition	Dementia represents the interaction of the brain (pathology, development, and activity) and the presence of malignant social-psychology.	Person-centred care that focusses on promoting the personhood of the person living with this condition and strives to limit ill-being and maximize well-being in dementia care.
Social model of disability	Cognitive impairment is made a disabling condition by a society that is not inclusive and doesn't design dementia-friendly policies, services, and buildings.	Focus on social and environmental context and changing disabling environments; self-advocacy by persons living with dementia; alliances with other groups.
Social constructionism	Dementia is a socially constructed phenomenon whereby certain people and their actions are labelled as deviant and thereby socially excluded. Its meaning varies across time and space.	Efforts at reducing the stigma associated with dementia, promoting citizenship rights of those affected, and challenging societal definitions of "normalcy".
Bio-psycho-social phenomenon	Dementia is a syndrome caused by biological and social determinants of health, and its expression and recognition are mediated by the socio-cultural and political-economic context.	Seek to understand the embodied illness experience from the perspectives of persons living with dementia and adopt a cultural safety and citizenship as practice approach.

In reviewing Table 7.1, can you identify which of these approaches are the most dominant in sites and sectors of health and social care today? Which resonate the most with social work values and AOG?

An overview of symptoms, prevalence, risk factors, and costs

If people are familiar with the word dementia, they usually associate it with memory loss in later life, particularly if the type of dementia is Alzheimer's Disease (AD). Other symptoms are less familiar (see Table 7.2), including impaired judgement, disorientation (to time, place, and person), and language difficulties. While "dementia can also affect mood and behaviour" (Public Health Agency of Canada (PHAC), 2019, p. 82), not everyone living with dementia is affected in this way. These changes are often a sign that the illness is progressing. You may hear the behaviours listed in Table 7.2 referred to as symptoms, as in "behavioural and psychological symptoms of dementia"; however, these are not signs that someone has dementia. Further, while you may hear complaints of "challenging behaviours," we would prefer you to say "behaviours that challenge" as this slight shift indicates that it is the care/service provider's job to determine the needs and wishes of a person whose ability to communicate is compromised and that the system is challenged or ill-equipped to support persons with dementia. This is in line with the social model of disability introduced in **Theorizing later life and social work praxis**.

> *As Harpreet learns more about dementia through her work at the care home, she begins to recognize the signs of disorientation. For example, Jimmy will get restless at the end of the day and search for his hat, coat, and briefcase. He believes that it is time for him to leave work and go home for dinner, and Harpreet understands this to mean that he is disoriented to time and place. This occurs a few hours after Clara begins to ask when her mother is picking her up from school. Harpreet witnesses the staff reorienting both of these residents to the present and wonders if this is the best approach, as Clara is distressed to learn that her mother has died and Jimmy worries that he has lost or will lose his job given that it is not the place he has spent the day. Harpreet starts to think it might be better to "jump into their realities".[3]*

While dementia is the most feared disease of later life (George & Whitehouse, 2014; Whitehouse & George, 2008), the majority of those over the age of 65 do not have any form of cognitive impairment. Early research indicated 16% of those over the age

Table 7.2 Symptoms of dementia and associated behaviours

Common symptoms of dementia	Associated behaviours (that challenge)
Memory loss	Aggressiveness
Disorientation (time, place, person)	Disinhibition – sexual and other types
Impaired judgement	Wandering, restlessness
Language difficulties	Hoarding

of 65 have cognitive impairment and another 8% are diagnosed with AD or another dementia (Canadian Institutes of Health Research (CIHR), 2007, p. 6). Canada's National Dementia strategy, which was released on June 17, 2019, states that 6.9% of those aged 65 or older are living with diagnosed dementia, 63% of whom are women (PHAC, 2019). This figure is 1% lower than the 2007 CIHR estimate and includes neither those living with early onset AD (under the age of 65) nor those who have not been diagnosed. Rates of dementia are increasing for First Nations people in Canada (Walker & Jacklin, 2019) and for Indigenous populations in other countries (Warren, Shi, Young, Borenstein, & Martinuik, 2015). The onset tends to be earlier for both Indigenous people and people with Down Syndrome; these two groups are at higher risk for dementia, as are women, older adults, and those with previous health conditions such as hypertension (PHAC, 2019).

As dementia is associated with aging, the percentage of older adults who have dementia is higher amongst the "oldest-old" or those in "the fourth age" (the 85+ age group). Early research determined that two-thirds of people over age 85 have cognitive impairment (CIHR, 2002, p. 1) and 35% have dementia (Canadian Study of Health and Aging Working Group (CSHA), 1994). Given the aging of the population – with the current 15.3% of the Canadian population aged 65 and older in 2013 expected to become 22.2–23.6% by 2030 (Statistics Canada, 2014) – and the age association of dementia, epidemiologists (those who study the spread of disease) have expected that this figure will rise; however, this appears not to be the case. Recent evidence indicates that while incidence rates are increasing in low- and middle-income countries, they are coming down in high-income countries (Patterson, 2018). Population aging is a global phenomenon as is the increase of persons living with dementia; currently 50 million people around the world are living with dementia, and this number is expected to rise to 152 million by 2050 (Patterson, 2018, pp. 6–7); however, the global distribution is changing.

Canada currently has approximately 419,000 people living with diagnosed dementia (PHAC, 2019), down from 500,000 10 years ago (Alzheimer Society of Canada (ASC), 2010), despite the projected doubling of this figure from 2010–2040. These earlier demographic data along with advocacy from family care partners, health care professionals, the Alzheimer Society of Canada, and persons living with dementia led to Canada's becoming the 30th country to have a national dementia strategy. Bill C-233 *An Act respecting a national strategy for Alzheimer's disease and other dementias* was passed in June 2017 (ASC, 2017) and *A Dementia Strategy for Canada: Together We Aspire* (PHAC, 2019) was released two years later by Minister Petipas-Taylor, a former social worker and daughter of a woman living with dementia.

In line with apocalyptic demography (see textbox 1.1), there has been much emphasis on the costs of caring for persons with dementia. For example, the BC Medical Association (2004) estimated this to be $22,727 per person per year; however, this calculation did not include the significant amount of care provided by family members and friends (informal care partners/providers), most of whom are women, as this work is not often seen to have economic value (see **Who cares about caregiving?**). However, when out-of-pocket caregiver expenses were added to total health care costs, the annual cost of dementia in 2011 rose to $8.3 billion and is projected to reach $16.6 billion by 2031 (PHAC, 2019, p. 3). Economic analyses such as these undoubtedly informed Bill C-233, along with pressure from groups like the Canadian Medical Association (CMA), which "along with many other medical and health organizations, ha[d] been calling for a national dementia plan given the impact dementia will continue to have on health and social systems as well as on families and caregivers" (CMA, 2016, p. 11).

Another problem with these cost calculations is that caring is not seen to be reciprocal in the sense that there is an exchange of care or other positive emotions; rather, the relationship is characterized as "burdensome" and unidirectional. As AOP social workers, we are concerned with the focus on costs especially as it accompanies the dominant discourse on dementia, one that is overwhelmingly negative and portrays dementia as "a loss of self" and "hellish experience" and objectifies or depersonalizes those living with dementia (Beard, 2016; Hulko, 2009). At the same time, it is important that a role for social workers is implicitly recognized in some of these economic calculations, particularly when it is noted that "system navigators" could reduce the economic burden of dementia by delaying admissions to residential care and by reducing informal caregiver burden (Risk Analytica, 2009). It is also essential to reflect upon the ways in which calculations of the cost or "burden" of dementia might differ if we viewed caring as reciprocal rather than one-directional and valued interdependence over independence in our consideration of these calculations.

The risk factors for dementia are varied, with age and genetic factors (i.e., presence of the apoE4 gene) being the major ones. As you review Table 7.3 on risk factors for dementia, think about what you know about the SDOH (see endnote 2 in the **Introduction**) and consider how particular risk factors may be more significant for the older adults, their families, and communities with which you work or will be working. For example, while diabetes has been a major health concern for Indigenous peoples for some time now, it is only recently that it has been added to the list of risk factors for dementia (see Hulko, Wilson, & Balestrery, 2019 for more on Indigenous people and dementia). At the same time, there is now a belief among many dementia researchers that "it is all vascular", particularly as one-third of all cases of AD are said to be preventable (Norton, Mathews, Barnes, Jaffe & Brayne, 2014). Doctors have been advising "what is good for the heart, is good for the head" (e.g., exercise regularly, refrain from smoking, limit alcohol) for a long time, and Indigenous people similarly stress the importance of "connecting the head and the heart" in line with a holistic approach to health (Hulko, Camille, Antifeau, Arnouse, Bachynski & Taylor, 2010; Hulko et al. 2019).

Table 7.3 Risk factors for dementia

Diabetes	Mild cognitive impairment	Family history
Post-menopausal state in women	Down Syndrome	Chronic inflammatory conditions
Head injury (traumatic brain injury)	History of episodes of clinical depression	Strokes or mini-strokes
High cholesterol levels	High blood pressure	Inadequate exercising of the brain
Lack of physical exercise	Low socio-economic status	Obesity
"Unhealthy" eating habits	Stress	Low levels of formal education

In their analysis of the evolving classification of dementia before the 2013 release of the 5th edition of the *Diagnostic and Statistical Manual* (DSM), critical dementia scholars George, Whitehouse, and Ballenger (2011) stated that "like autism and Asperger's [other forms of neuro-diversity], a case can be made on evidentiary grounds for viewing AD as the latter stage of a spectrum of cognitive changes associated with normal aging" (p. 429). In fact, dementia was reclassified as a neurocognitive disorder in the DSM-5 (Sachdev et al., 2014). This is reflected in part in the definition of dementia in Canada's new strategy where

> dementia is an umbrella term used to describe a set of symptoms affecting brain function that are caused by *neurodegenerative* [our emphasis] and vascular diseases or injuries. It is characterized by a decline in cognitive abilities such as memory; awareness of person, place, and time; language, basic math skills; judgement; and planning.
>
> (PHAC, 2019, p. 82)

Before the family meeting, Harpreet learns more about Olive from reading the chart notes, which depict Olive as frequently disoriented, unable to form complete sentences, and restless. The notes also query whether climbing into her neighbour's bed is a sign of sexual disinhibition. Harpreet asks the head nurse whether the previous social worker had completed a social history with Olive and/or her family and wonders if this might help the team better understand Olive's current behaviour and provide more person-centred care. Learning that the previous social worker felt Olive was too cognitively impaired to be a reliable informant, Harpreet feels reassured that her plan to meet with the daughters makes sense.

*   When she meets with the daughters and apprises them of Olive's nocturnal activities, they do not seem concerned about this and report that their mother has always been an adventurous person. They ask if the neighbour and/or her family are upset at all, and Harpreet says the team's concern has been Olive's husband, rather than the neighbour as the latter appears comfortable with this arrangement. The daughters suggest they allow this to continue but ask that Harpreet continue to withhold this information from their father so as not to upset him.*

As mentioned in Table 7.1, there are many types of dementia, the main ones being AD at 63% and vascular or multi-infarct dementia at up to 20% (Risk Analytica, 2009; see also www.alzheimer.ca). Lewy body dementia, which represents 5 to 15% of all dementias, can occur with AD, with Parkinson's disease, or on its own. Dementia is connected to anxiety, depression, and psychotic symptoms (MacCourt, 2005) and is one of several chronic conditions with which anxiety is often associated (Gellis & McCracken, 2008). Depression is both a risk factor for dementia (Diniz, Butters, Albert, & Dew, 2013) and common amongst those with dementia (Snowden, Atkins, Steinman, Bell, Bryant, Copeland, & Fitzpatrick, 2015).

Putting yourself in the shoes of persons with dementia and their care partners

A few days after meeting with Olive's daughters, Harpreet happens upon Olive's husband Milton in the dining room and introduces herself as the new social worker. Milton seems keen to talk with her and tells her that the couple met at university when they were both graduate students and student activists who crossed paths frequently at protests and demonstrations, as well as social gatherings. Harpreet enjoys listening to his tales of being on the frontlines of civil rights and anti-war protests, as it reminds her of why she wanted to be a social worker in the first place and also why she left child protection work. Milton describes Olive as a "real fire-cracker" who always made life interesting, smiling in fondness at his wife's antics in their younger years. He talks of Olive's involvement in the women's movement and her anger over the ousting of lesbian women – "the lavender menace" in the 1970s – and the couple's support of gay rights. Milton then leans towards her and says quietly, "Olive was in a relationship with a woman before we met and she still likes women, you know". Harpreet thanks Milton for sharing this with her and invites him to stop by her office and chat the next time he comes to visit Olive. As she walks away, she smiles to herself, thinking about Olive and her roommate and wondering if Olive is "in the closet" or if her daughters have put her in there. Harpreet is intrigued by this image of Olive that Milton conjures for her and wonders if she might get to know this person. She decides the starting point has to be seeing Olive as a person living with dementia – as she was taught in her BSW program – rather than suffering from it – as the media and so many health professionals depict it. She decides to try to speak directly with Olive and brings along some images of older adults so that she can try photo elicitation and third-party questioning, a technique she recalls reading about in the BCASW newsletter and her AOP social work textbook.

If we believe in the social work mantra "start where the client is at", then it should be obvious that we approach persons with dementia before their care partners and try to find ways to listen to their voices or at least include them in our assessments and interventions, as Harpreet attempts to do with Olive after learning about 'the person behind the disease'. Olive's story reflects the reality that dementia is a "women's issue". The reasons for this are varied, but speak to the fact that, on average, women still live longer than men and so there are more women living with dementia. As well, more women are represented as caregivers. See Table 7.4 for information on dementia as a "women's issue" and the significance of the ratio 2/3.

Table 7.4 2/3: Why dementia is a "women's issue"?

More women than men have dementia. 72% of Canadians living with dementia are women (Alzheimer Society of Canada, 2018). This is connected to the *feminization of aging* in that women live longer than men, and age is the biggest risk factor for dementia.
More women than men care for persons living with dementia whether they are paid for this or not. Two-thirds of the primary (informal) care partners are women and the majority of the paid dementia care workforce is made up of women. Globally, this figure is now 71% (Patterson, 2018).
At the same time, there has been little research explicitly focussed on gender and dementia (Errol, Brooker, & Peel, 2015), and those studies that do exist focus almost exclusively on caregiving (Bartlett, Gjernes, Lotherington, & Obstefelder, 2018).
The dominant discourse on dementia as resulting in a loss of self effectively de-genders persons with dementia, while person-centred approaches serve to re-gender persons with dementia so that they fall (back) in line with the sex/gender system (Sandberg, 2018).

According to research with social workers in Ireland, persons with dementia are excluded from decision-making processes for the following reasons: assumptions that they lack capacity; family member preference that the person not be involved; communication difficulties; time constraints; little or no opportunity given; and, the person delegated decision-making to others (Donnelly, Begley, & O'Brien, 2018). Thus, the story of Olive in this chapter is sadly typical. What is rare – though increasing – is the approach that Harpreet adopts after learning more about Olive as a person, an approach more aligned with the strength's perspective and the capabilities approach (see **Theorizing later life and social work praxis**). For example, McCormick, Becker, and Grabowski (2018) adopted a strengths-based approach to their patient handbook project, collaborating with 24 persons with memory loss as well as 37 professionals, care partners, and community members; they concluded that the strengths perspective "underscores that people have a right to participate in the development of the care they are going to receive [and that] memory loss alone does not prevent people from participating in decisions that affect their life" (p. 362; McGovern, 2015).

Social work approaches to working with persons with dementia and their care partners

While the strengths perspective is increasingly adopted in dementia care, often paired with a personhood approach, social work has not always been so progressive in working with persons with dementia. For example, a social work practitioner-researcher in England in the 1940s–1950s called those with whom she worked "the dements" and saw her primary role as supporting families and ensuring continuity of care (Manthorpe, 2016). This neglect of the person with dementia persisted, with the common belief being *"you can't talk to people with dementia"*, as a social work academic that I (Wendy) admired very much said in 2000 upon hearing my plans to explore the experiences of persons living with dementia for my PhD research.

More recently, albeit to a limited extent, social work in the context of dementia has begun to discard the belief that "persons with dementia are incapable of communicating and lacking in insight", and shift its gaze from families/care partners to persons with dementia who are increasingly seen as clients in their own right. Dementia is now a growing area of specialty with attention placed not only on caregiver-centred work (which is still the main focus of the field) but also on reciprocity. In addition, greater attention is being paid to culturally and linguistically diverse (CALD) older adults. It has been found, for example, that language reversion amongst CALD older adults with dementia (learned another language before English or the contextually appropriate language and reverted to first language with dementia) is compounded by social isolation (Tipping & Whiteside, 2015). Taking a strengths perspective, we can see this language reversal as representing a possibility to renew languages, especially Indigenous languages that are in danger of becoming extinct; this is due mainly to the removal of children from their families and communities and placement in state care, which started with residential schools and continues to this day through child welfare/ protection. In other words, settler colonialism continues, and hence culturally safe practice is critical, not only for Indigenous people, but for all older adults from equity-seeking groups.

Validation therapy

Perhaps one of social work's most innovative and overlooked contributions to dementia care and practice is validation therapy, which was developed by Naomi Feil (2002). The video of Naomi Feil practicing this therapy with Gladys Wilson, a severely cognitively impaired woman living in a care home, is illuminating (Memorybridge, 2009). Gladys is largely non-responsive when Naomi first approaches her. However, as she experiences Naomi's use of validation therapy's techniques, including maintaining genuine, close eye contact; using a clear, low, loving tone of voice; mirroring (the actions of the other person); touching; and, music (Feil, 2002), Gladys gradually begins to tap along to the music and then to sing a song with Naomi. Gently and purposively, Naomi discovered Gladys Wilson's preferred sense and made use of it to draw her out. This video alone is testament to the potential and ongoing relevance of validation therapy, a social work innovation that builds on our focus on strengths. The "retained abilities" of persons with dementia enumerated by occupational therapist Jitka Zgola (1999) can also help social workers shift our focus away from deficits or "challenging behaviours" and towards the strengths of persons with dementia and thereby discover possibilities for engagement. A few of these retained abilities are remembering things from the distant past; holding an opinion or offering advice; performing habitual, overlearned patterns of behavior; and responding to and expressing emotion (Zgola, 1999). Consider how, by adopting the strengths perspective or capabilities approach and/or drawing on retained abilities such as these, you could facilitate the voice and inclusion of persons living with dementia as an AOP social worker.

Building on the pioneering work of Naomi Feil (2002), social work scholars in dementia studies have championed the application of a social model of disability to understand and respond to dementia (Marshall & Tibbs, 2006); analyzing views and experiences of dementia through the lens of intersectionality and interlocking oppressions (Hulko, 2002, 2016; O'Connor, Phinney, & Hulko, 2010); taking a culturally safe approach to care and practice with Indigenous Elders and/or Jewish older adults (Hulko & Stern, 2009; Hulko et al., 2010, 2019; Stern, 2012); adopting a citizenship as practice approach (Bartlett, 2016; Bartlett & O'Connor, 2010); taking a human rights approach (Cahill, 2018); and making use of queer theory (Ward & Price, 2016). For example, through her grounded theory research on dementia and intersectionality, Hulko (2009, 2011) found that social location affects experiencing, othering, and theorizing dementia with those participants who were multiply privileged (white, majority ethnic, wealthy, mostly male) viewing dementia as a hellish experience, being 'othered' (ignored/dismissed/silenced) frequently, and espousing the brain disease theory of dementia. This was in sharp contrast to those who were multiply marginalized (racialized and/or minority ethnic, poor, mostly women) who saw dementia as not a big deal, retained their social relationships, and (strategically) made use of normal aging theory. This research showed not only that persons with dementia have much to say, but also that social location affects their experiences, i.e. diversity makes a difference.

Culturally safe dementia care/practice

As you learned in **Sites and sectors of health and social care** and **Theorizing later life and social work praxis**, cultural safety moves beyond cultural sensitivity, cultural competence, and cultural appropriateness to consider power in our interactions with service users and stresses the need to transfer (more) power to the service user so that the outcome of our intervention is one they consider to be culturally safe. Based on her critical ethnography of intercultural care in a Jewish long-term care facility, Stern (2012) calls for a culturally safe approach to dementia care, recognizing that

> current models of cultural competency tend to focus on education that examines the relationships between static and defined cultural groups that do not take into account the wide range of cultural identities that individuals can construct. It fails to make the next step that recognizes the diversity of both the people receiving care and those providing it.
>
> (p. 9)

Further, researchers recommend

> consulting with Elders or other community members to learn cultural and health status information [as this] can shift the power differential from one in which the health care provider is the 'expert' to one in which the Elder teaches or guides the provider about the cultural aspects of their memory loss and care needs.
>
> (Hulko et al., 2010, p. 375)

As Harpreet gains more experience being a member of the inter-professional health care team, gets to know Olive as a person, and meets other residents in the care home, she wonders if social histories might be of benefit. After listening to Olive talk about both her past and present, Harpreet is particularly interested in applying an intersectional life course approach to make evident the diversity of the residents' lives and the ways in which they have shown resilience and resistance in the face of interlocking oppressions, much like her own grandparents. She decides to try constructing a social history for a newly admitted First Nation man who has dementia as there are no other Indigenous residents in the home and staff have not yet taken the provincial Indigenous cultural competency training.[4] Below is the first social history Harpreet writes:

Michael is a 76-year old Dene man who has lived away from his home community in the Northwest Territories since he was 6. He and his siblings were taken away to a residential school down South where Michael spent eight painful years before he ran away from it with his older brother Stan. They made their way to the Prince George area where they found work in a mill and relied on one another for support as they had in the residential school. Stan returned to their home community in the North five years later, seeking reconnection with his culture, family, and community, and healing from his residential school experiences. Michael stayed as he had met and fallen for a local white woman named June who he married the following year after which they moved to a small town outside Prince George. June's family never fully accepted him and that was one of the reasons the couple decided not to have children. Michael had good friends at the mill with whom he enjoyed fishing and hunting on the weekends. He was forced to retire eight years ago when he was diagnosed with dementia and three years later June died suddenly, leaving him on his own to take care of himself and their small house. For a long time, Michael managed on his own, but with his increasing cognitive and physical challenges and having few supports due to Stan and the rest of his Dene family and community being far away and his friends still working full-time, it became unsafe for him to live alone. As a result, he has been 'placed' in this care home in Prince George. It is an hour's drive from the small town where Michael lived for over 60 years and he is the only Indigenous resident. Michael was sent to residential school at the age of 6. During that time, he lost both of his parents. Not all of his siblings survived residential school and Michael has tried to forget the abuse they all suffered there, yet the memories remain.

After spending time with Michael to write his social history, Harpreet speaks to the Head Nurse about making both trauma-informed practice and ICC training a priority for all staff. She offers to facilitate a discussion at the next staff meeting and/or host an in-service on ways they can all make the care home more culturally safe, not only for Michael, but also for the staff. This includes the two Carrier (a First Nation in Northern BC) nurses and the Métis cook with whom she has spoken about their inter-actions with the white residents, as well as the few racialized staff, including herself and two South Asian care aides who are casual employees. Knowing that dementia rates are increasing for Indigenous people and having seen how the first available bed policy plays out, Harpreet expects there to be more Indigenous residents in the future, as well as more Sikh residents until her community is able to build its own care home. She has invited a few of her colleagues to the Gurdwara (Sikh temple) she visits every weekend with her grandparents to enjoy a meal with the community and attend the service. Har-preet believes that if more people understand that her religion is a peaceful and loving one and that the Gurdwara is open to all, then they will be better able to provide cul-turally appropriate or safe care to the Sikh residents. Harpreet would like to have a dialogue about racism in the workplace as well; however, she thinks it might be safer to start with the residents and is hopeful that her white colleagues who claim to be allies will broaden the discussion to include racism experienced by both residents and staff. In constructing Michael's social history, she has enjoyed the opportunity to expand her knowledge and skills beyond strengths and person-centred approaches and looks forward to learning more about cultural safety and other approaches more aligned with AOP social work.

A social history such as the one Harpreet constructed has the potential to sensitize care staff to the losses and trauma that residents have endured throughout their life course as well as their resilience in the face of settler-colonialism and other forms of structural violence (see **Mapping trauma across the life course** and **Addressing mistreat-ment and violence**).

Citizenship as practice

The movement from personhood to citizenship has been led by social work scholars Ruth Bartlett in the UK and Deborah O'Connor in Canada, and it is within social work that this approach has really taken hold (see Figure 7.1). Bartlett and O'Connor (2010) describe this approach as the "fourth moment" in the development of our understanding of dementia: the first being dementia as *a natural part of aging* (senility); second, as *a bio-medical condition*; and third, a *relational* understanding (personhood) that "sees" the person behind the diagnosis. A shift to citizenship de-centres dementia as an "individual experi-ence" and focusses instead on how people with dementia are shaped by socio-cultural practices and discourses. For example, Olive may not be the only resident who was a feminist and civil rights activist and has been in a relationship with a woman, as the

Personhood is "a standing or status bestowed on one human being, by others, in the context of relationship and social well-being" (Kitwood, 1997, p.8)

Personhood resides at the interface of subjective experiences, interpersonal relationships and the socio-cultural context (O'Connor, Phinney, Smith, Small, Purves, Perry et al., 2007)

Embodied selfhood (Kontos, 2003) highlights the ways in which personhood is enacted through the body and observable in habitual bodily movements in particular

Citizenship indicates a focus on rights and entitlements and a recognition that socio-cultural practices and discourses shape experiences (Bartlett & O'Conner, 2010)

Relational citizenship integrates the central tenets of relationship-centred care and embodied selfhood theory into citizenship (Kontos, Miller & Kontos, 2017)

Figure 7.1 From personhood to relational citizenship

majority of those living in residential care are women and many of them are baby boomers like Olive. Also, Michael may not be the only Indigenous person in the home; there may be Métis residents or others with Indigenous ancestry who are perceived to be white by the staff or are passing as white like they did when they were younger when it was not as safe to identify as Indigenous as it is now.

If we don't create space and time for people to talk about their multiple and complex identities and affirm their marginalized social statuses when they disclose them to us, then we miss the opportunity to see how socio-cultural practices and discourses have shaped their lives and be able to engage in citizenship as practice. Bartlett and O'Connor (2010) note that citizenship can be enacted in the following ways:

1.   As an opportunity for growth;
2.   To be recognized holistically, beyond the diagnosis;
3.   To retain purpose in one's life;
4.   To participate as an active agent;
5.   To create a sense of solidarity and belonging with others; and
6.   To have the right to live free from discrimination.

Applying this conceptualization to their research on social work assessments, Österholm and Hydén (2016) determined several ways that social workers support citizenship as practice when persons with dementia run into communication problems. These include allowing time for the person with dementia to "self-repair", rather than jumping in to help or correct, acknowledging that communication is a challenge and expressing appreciation for their contributions, and making use of forced response (yes/no) questions when input cannot be elicited otherwise. We add to this list techniques associated with validation therapy and the use of photo elicitation and third-party questioning.

Supporting self-advocacy and making communities more inclusive

Peer support and self-advocacy is vibrantly alive in the dementia community and AOG social workers are well poised to support this work. This includes the work of the Dementia Advocacy and Support Network International (DASNI), which was formed on-line in 2000 and had the involvement of two British Columbia residents (Lynn Jackson and Jim Mann), both of whom are affiliated with the Centre for Research on Personhood in Dementia Care (CRPD) at the University of British Columbia. At the same time, it took until 2003 for the first person with dementia to be appointed to the board of Alzheimer's Disease International. The slow progress in ensuring persons living with dementia are included in Alzheimer associations and invited to speak at scientific gatherings (Bartlett, 2014; Beard, 2004) led activists to form Dementia Alliance International (DAI). DAI incorporated as a non-profit, and it restricts membership to persons with dementia, adopting the disability rights mantra "nothing about us, without us".

Based on her diary interview and participant observation research with 16 dementia activists, social work scholar Ruth Bartlett (2014) determined there are three modes of dementia activism: "protecting-self against decline", "(re) gaining respect", and "creating connections with other people with dementia". Unsurprisingly, time was found to play a significant role in participants' activism, and Bartlett (2014) further suggests that engaging in activism can prevent decline. Cultural relevance or safety is an important consideration in determining what approaches will work in particular communities and contexts. For example, amongst Indigenous Elders healing ceremonies can lead to "re-mentia". As one Secwepemc Elder offers in a teaching story, "if the emotional bruises are healed – through sweats, smudging, love, and the Creator – then the dementia can be healed or the impact of living with it lessened" (Elder et al., 2019, p. 21).

Groups such as DASNI and DAI and individuals living with dementia are also very active on social media, including Twitter. For example, Tommy Dunne (@Tommy-Tommytee18) tweets regularly, does public speaking, and opened a dementia-friendly checkout lane at the Chester Tesco [grocery] store in the UK in May 2015 and then reported on it for Dementia Diaries (www.onourradar.org/dementia/2015/05/19/theyve-opened-a-dementia-friendly-check-out). Social workers can follow these accounts to learn more about life with dementia and support the self-advocacy work of persons living with dementia. They could also start their own campaigns, as Andy Tsoe, a dementia nurse, did with #DementiaDo and Dementia Advocacy Canada has done with #makedementiamatter. The first of these two Twitter threads stresses what persons with dementia can do and challenges negative media portrayals, while the second is used to advocate for the implementation of Canada's national dementia strategy. Table 7.5 below gives examples of the contrasting media messages about dementia one can hear on the radio and read on Twitter.

Another community-building initiative is Dementia Friends Canada (www.dementiafriends.ca), a joint initiative of the Alzheimer Society of Canada and the

Table 7.5 Contrasting media messages about dementia

B100 Radio on March 7, 2016	#DementiaDo on Twitter
The scourge of dementia	#DementiaDo something about the distress, misery, and false hope generated by these headlines
Wrestling with Alzheimer's disease	#DementiaDo to treat each person as a person not a sufferer

Government of Canada to raise awareness and engage the public. It was inspired by the UK Dementia Friends program, which was based on Japan's Dementia Supporters. There are three simple steps to take to be a Dementia Friend – watch the video, register, and commit to action – and over a million Canadians had already done this by June 2018. As you read **Building inclusive communities**, consider other ways that you – as an AOG social worker – could support persons living with dementia to create more inclusive communities in rural towns, small cities, and large urban centres throughout Canada. Envision how to shift your practice and that of others to reflect that persons with dementia are still citizens with rights and responsibilities and that their social locations not only vary, but also mediate their experiences of dementia.

Conclusion

People living with dementia are increasing in both numbers and influence. There has been a gradual shift from viewing persons with dementia as incapable and sub-human to recognizing them as citizens with lives left to be lived. This is occurring as persons with dementia author their own stories, engage in self-advocacy on Twitter, create and exhibit art, and speak at conferences. The experiences of persons with dementia are as varied as those who live with cognitive impairment in later life. There is no master narrative about dementia, nor are persons with dementia a homogenous group; rather, their views on and experiences of dementia are profoundly shaped by socio-cultural and political-economic contexts, as are ours as social workers. Social workers can assist persons with dementia by "jumping into their reality" (Vittoria, 1998), ensuring voice and inclusion, and building inclusive communities.

Exercise

Discuss these questions in small groups, drawing on your personal and practice experiences.

- What can we do as social workers to promote voice and facilitate inclusion/interaction of persons living with dementia like Olive and Michael? Consider individual, family, community, and societal levels.
- Continue the story of Harpreet and Olive by explaining how Harpreet could adopt a citizenship-as-practice approach in addressing the initial concern (about

Olive climbing into her roommate's bed at night) after she has gotten to know Olive as a person and spent time with her family members.

- How do we get there (dementia-friendly communities) from here ("diagnosis, drugs and decay")? Can we apply our AOG principles to dementia care? Why? Why not?
- What do we need to know more about as social workers, care partners, and/or citizens in order to improve the lives of persons living with dementia?

Takeaways

- There are many ways of viewing dementia; some are more consistent with AOP social work than others, including dementia as a psycho-neurological condition, dementia as a disability, dementia as a social construction, and dementia as a biopsychosocial phenomenon.
- While basic knowledge of the biological and psychological aspects of dementia is helpful, it is more important for gerontological social workers to ascertain how our clients make sense of their illness experience and determine the influence of their social location.
- It is possible to communicate with persons living with dementia throughout their illness experience if we consider dementia to be a disability and use patience, creativity, and skill.
- Social workers have been leaders in moving dementia studies forward and ensuring that persons living with dementia are not only included, but also supported to participate as citizens with voice and authority and to have their intersecting identities affirmed.

Additional resources

- Alzheimer Society of Canada: www.alzheimer.ca.
- Brain X Change (formerly Canadian Dementia Knowledge Translation Network): http://brainxchange.ca/Public/Home.aspx
- Dementia Advocacy and Support Network International (DASNI): www.dasninternational.org/.
- Dementia Advocacy Canada: https://dementiacanada.com/events
- Dementia Diaries: https://dementiadiaries.org/.

Notes

1 "Dementia-friendly" generates much discussion amongst persons with dementia on Twitter, as do dementia villages, with not all seeing dementia-friendly community (DFC) initiatives as progressive or enabling inclusion of persons with dementia (Swaffer, 2014). However, inclusion was the original intent of the DFC movement (Marshall, 1999). See Lin (2017) for more on DFCs and see Lin and Lewis (2015) for the distinction between "capable", "friendly", and "positive" in relation to dementia.

2 This is an updated version of a chart developed by W. Hulko for a 2003 guest lecture at the McMaster Summer Institute on Gerontology and shared with participants in an effort to change practice. Bio-medical is listed first as it represents the dominant discourse, and the last

row (bio-psycho-social) is one we have added for this chapter and represents another counter-narrative.

3 "Jump into their realities" is a phrase/directive from Anne Vittoria's 1998 article on identity work in dementia care settings.

4 ICC is an on-line training program for health care providers in BC developed by the Provincial Health Services Authority to educate health care practitioners on the impacts of colonization and residential schools on Indigenous peoples and prepare them to work in a more respectful (culturally safe) way. It takes 8–12 hours to complete the program.

References

Alzheimer Society of Canada (ASC). (2010). *A rising tide: The impact of dementia on Canadian society*. Toronto: Author.

Alzheimer Society of Canada (ASC). (2017, June 22). *Canada to become 30th country with national dementia strategy*. Toronto: Author. Retrieved from https://alzheimer.ca/sites/default/files/national/media-centre

Alzheimer Society of Canada (ASC). (2018, January 2). Alzheimer awareness month. Spreading awareness about the 72%. Retrieved from www.alzheimer.ca/en/the72percent

Baines, D. (2017). *Doing anti-oppressive practice: Social justice social work* (3rd ed.). Halifax, NS: Fernwood Publishing.

Bartlett, R. (2014). The emergent modes of dementia activism. *Ageing & Society*, *34*(4), 623–644. doi:10.1017/S0144686X12001158

Bartlett, R. (2016). Scanning the conceptual horizons of citizenship. *Dementia*, *15*(30), 453–461. doi:10.117/1471 301-216-644114

Bartlett, R., Gjernes, T., Lotherington, T. A., & Obstefelder, A. (2018). Gender, citizenship and dementia care: A scoping review of studies to inform policy and future research. *Health and Social Care in the Community*, *26*(1), 14–26. doi:10.1111/hsc.12340

Bartlett, R., & O'Connor, D. (2010). *Broadening the dementia debate: Toward social citizenship*. Bristol: Policy Press.

Beard, R. (2004). Advocating voice: Organisational, historical and social milieu of the Alzheimer's disease movement. *Sociology of Health and Illness*, *27*(6), 797–819. doi:10.1111/j.0141-9889.200.00419.x

Beard, R. L. (2016). *Living with Alzheimer's: Managing memory loss, identity and illness*. New York: New York University Press.

British Columbia Medical Association (BCMA). (2004, April). *Building bridges: A call for a coordinated dementia strategy in British Columbia*. Vancouver, BC: BCMA.

Cahill, S. (2018). *Dementia and human rights*. London: Policy Press.

Canadian Institutes of Health Research (CIHR). (2002). Cognitive impairment in aging strategy and partnership. Retrieved from www.cihr-ihsc.gc.ca/cgibin/print-imprimer.pl.

Canadian Institutes of Health Research (CIHR). (2007). The future is aging: The CIHR institute of aging strategic plan 2007-2012. Retrieved from www.cihr-irsc.gc.ca/cgi-bin/print-imprimer.pl.

Canadian Medical Association (CMA). (2016, September). *The state of seniors' health care in Canada*. Ottawa: CMA.

Canadian Study of Health and Aging Working Group. (1994). Canadian study of health and aging: Study methods and prevalence of dementia. *Canadian Medical Association Journal*, *150*(60), 899–913. Retrieved from www.ncbi.nlm.nih.gov/pmc/articles/PMC1486712/

Diniz, B., Butters, M., Albert, S. & Dew, M.A. (2013). Late life depression and risk of vascular dementia and Alzheimer's disease: Systematic review and meta-analysis of community-based cohort studies. *The British Journal of Psychiatry*, *202*(5), 329–335. doi:10.1192/bjp.bp.112.118307

Donnelly, S., Begley, E., & O'Brien, M. (2018). How are people with dementia involved in care-planning and decision-making? An Irish social work perspective. *Dementia*, *0*(0), 1–19. doi:10.1177/1471301218763180

Elder, S., Hulko, W., Wilson, D., Mahara, S., Campbell McArthur, G., William, J., … Moller, E. P. (2019). We call it healing. In W. Hulko, D. Wilson, & J. Balestrery (Eds.), *Indigenous peoples and dementia: New understandings of memory loss and memory care* (pp. 19–22). Vancouver, BC: UBC Press.

Errol, R., Brooker, D., & Peel, E. (2015, June). *Women and dementia: A global research review*. London: Alzheimer Disease International.

Feil, N. (2002). *The validation breakthrough: Simple techniques for communicating with people with "Alzheimer's-type dementia"* (2nd ed.). Baltimore, MD: Health Professions Press.

Gellis, Z. & McCracken, S. (2008). Mental health and aging. *Aging Times- the CSWE Gero-Ed Center*, *4*(3). Retrieved from https://www.cswe.org/Centers-Initiatives/Centers/Gero-Ed-Center/News-and-Media/Aging-Times-Archive/2008.aspx#ZviGellis

George, D. R., & Whitehouse, P. J. (2014). The war (on terror) on Alzheimer's. *Dementia*, *13*(1), 120–130. doi:10.1177/1471301212451382

George, D. R., Whitehouse, P. J., & Ballenger, J. (2011). The evolving classification of dementia: Placing the DSM-V in a meaningful historical and cultural context and pondering the future of "Alzheimer's". *Culture, Medicine & Psychiatry*, *35*, 417–435. doi:10.1007/s11013-011-9219-x

Hulko, W. (2002). Making the links: Social theories, experiences of people with dementia, and intersectionality. In A. Leibing & L. Scheinkman (Eds.), *The diversity of Alzheimer's disease: Different approaches and contexts* (pp. 231–264). Rio de Janeiro: CUCA-IPUB.

Hulko, W. (2009). From 'not a big deal' to 'hellish': Experiences of older people with dementia. *Journal of Aging Studies*, *23*(3), 131–144. doi:10.1016/j.jaging.2007.11.002

Hulko, W. (2011). Intersectionality in the context of later life experiences of dementia. In O. Hankivsky (Ed.), *Health inequities in Canada: Intersectional frameworks and practices* (pp. 198–220). Vancouver, BC: UBC Press.

Hulko, W. (2016). LGBT* individuals and dementia: An intersectional approach. In S. Westwood & L. Price (Eds.), *Lesbian, Gay, bisexual and trans* individuals living with dementia: Concepts, practice, and rights* (pp. 35–50). Abingdon: Routledge.

Hulko, W., & Stern, L. (2009). Cultural safety, decision-making, and dementia: Troubling notions of autonomy and personhood. In D. O'Connor & B. Purves (Eds.), *Decision-making, personhood and dementia: Exploring the interface* (pp. 70–87). London: Jessica Kingsley.

Hulko, W., Camille, E., Antifeau, E., Arnouse, M., Bachinski, N., & Taylor, D. (2010). Views of First Nation Elders on memory loss and memory care in later life. *Journal of Cross-Cultural Gerontology*, *25*, 317–342.

Hulko, W., Brotman, S., & Ferrer, I. (2017). Counter-storytelling: Anti-oppressive social work with older adults. In D. Baines (Ed.), *Doing anti-oppressive practice: Social justice social work* (3rd ed., pp. 193–211). Halifax, NS: Fernwood Publishing.

Hulko, W., Wilson, D., & Balestrery, J. (Eds.). (2019). *Indigenous peoples and dementia: New understandings of memory loss and memory care*. Vancouver, BC: UBC Press.

Kitwood, T. (1997). *Dementia reconsidered: The person comes first*. Buckingham: Open University Press.

Kontos, P., Miller, K.-L., & Kontos, A. (2017). Relational citizenship: Supporting embodied selfhood and relationality in dementia care. *Sociology of Health and Illness*, *39*(2), 182–198. doi:10.1111/1467-9566.12453

Lin, S.-Y. (2017). 'Dementia-friendly communities' and being dementia-friendly in healthcare settings. *Current Opinion Psychiatry*, *30*(2), 145–150. doi:10.1097/YCO.0000000000000304

Lin, S.-Y., & Lewis, F. M. (2015). Dementia friendly, dementia capable, and dementia positive: Concepts to prepare for the future. *The Gerontologist*, *55*(2), 237–244. doi:10.1093/geront/gnu122

MacCourt, P. (2005, June 8). *Presentation to standing senate committee on social affairs, science and technology's study on mental health issues round table meeting on senior's mental health.* Vancouver, BC. Retrieved from https://ccsmh.ca/wp-content/uploads/2016/03/KIRBY_writtenSubmission FinalOct31_2005.pdf

Manthorpe, J. (2016). The dement in the community: Social work practice with people with dementia revisited. *Dementia, 15*(5), 1100–1111. doi:10.1177/1471301214554810

Marshall, M. (1999). What do service planners and policy-makers need from research? *International Journal of Geriatric Psychiatry, 14*(2), 86–96. doi:10.1002/(SICI)1099-1166(1999902)

Marshall, M., & Tibbs, M. A. (2006). *Social work and people with dementia: Partnerships, practice and persistence* (Revised 2nd ed.). Bristol: The Policy Press.

McCormick, A. J., Becker, M. J., & Grabowski, T. J. (2018). Involving people with memory loss in the development of a patient handbook: A strengths-based approach. *Social Work, 63*(4), 357–364. doi:10.1093/sw/swy043

McGovern, J. (2015). Living better with dementia: Strengths-based social work practice and dementia care. *Social Work in Health Care, 54*(5), 408–421. doi:10.1080/00981389.2015.1029661

Memorybridge. (2009, May 26). Gladys Wilson and Naomi Feil. [Video file]. Retrieved from www.youtube.com/watch?v=CrZXz10FcVM

Norton, S., Mathews, F. E., Barnes, D. E., Yaffe, K., & Brayne, C. (2014). Potential for primary prevention of Alzheimer's disease: An analysis of population-based data. *The Lancet, 13*(8), 788–794. doi:10.1016/S14744422(14)70136-X

O'Connor, D., Phinney, A., & Hulko, W. (2010). Dementia at the intersections: A unique case study exploring social location. *Journal of Aging Studies, 24*, 30–39. doi:10.1016/j.jaging.2008.08.001

O'Connor, D., Phinney, A., Smith, A., Small, J., Purves, B., Perry, J., & Beattie, L. (2007). Personhood in dementia care: Developing a research agenda for broadening the vision. *Dementia, 6*(1), 121–142. doi:10.1177/1471301207075648

Österholm, J. H., & Hydén, L.-C. (2016). Citizenship as practice: Handling communication problems in encounters between persons with dementia and social workers. *Dementia, 15*(6), 1457–1473. doi:10.1177/1471301214563959

Patterson, C. (2018). *World Alzheimer report 2018. The state of the art of dementia research: New frontiers.* London: Alzheimer Disease International. Retrieved from www.alz.co.uk/research/world-report-2018

Public Health Agency of Canada (PHAC). (2019). *A dementia strategy for Canada: Together we aspire.* Ottawa: Author. Retrieved from www.canada.ca/en/public-health/serices/publications/dieases-conditions/dementia-strategy.html

Risk Analytica. (2009). *Rising tide: The impact of dementia in British Columbia 2008–2038.* Vancouver, BC: Alzheimer Society of BC. Retrieved from https://alzheimer.ca/en/bc

Sachdev, P. S., Blacker, D., Blazer, D. G., Ganguli, M., Jeste, D. V., Paulsen, J. S., & Petersen, R. C. (2014). Classifying neurocognitive disorders: The DSM-5 approach. *Nature Reviews Neurology, 10*, 642–643. doi:10.1038/nrneurol.2014.181

Sandberg, L. (2018). Dementia and the gender trouble? Theorising dementia, gendered subjectivity and embodiment. *Journal of Aging Studies, 45*, 25–31. doi:10.1016/j.jaging.2018.01.004

Snowden, M., Atkins, D., Steinman, L., Bell, J., Bryant, L., Copeland, C., & Fitzpatrick, A. (2015). Longitudinal Association of dementia and depression. *American Journal of Geriatric Psychiatry, 23*(9), 897–905. doi:10.1016/j.jagp.2014.09.002

Statistics Canada. (2014, September 26). *Canada's population estimates: Age and sex, 2014.* Retrieved from www.150.statcan.gc.ca/n1/daily-quotidien/140926/dq140926b-eng.htm

Stern, L. A. (2012). *The cultural whisper in our ear: Intercultural dementia care in a Jewish long-term care facility.* Vancouver, BC: University of British Columbia (doctoral thesis).

Swaffer, K. (2014). Dementia: Stigma, language, and dementia-friendly. *Dementia, 13*(6), 709–716. doi:10.1177/1471301214548143

Tipping, S. A., & Whiteside, M. (2015). Language reversion among people with dementia from culturally and linguistically diverse backgrounds: The family experience. *Australian Social Work*, *68*(2), 184–197. doi:10.1080/0312407X.2014.953187

Vittoria, A. (1998). Preserving selves: Identity work and dementia. *Research in Aging*, *20*(1), 91–136. Retrieved September 20, 2019, from https://journals-sagepub-com.proxy3.library.mcgill.ca/doi/pdf/10.1177/0164027598201006

Walker, J., & Jacklin, K. (2019). Dementia prevalence. In W. Hulko, D. Wilson, & J. Balestrery (Eds.), *Indigenous peoples and dementia: New understandings of memory loss and memory care* (pp. 24–40). Vancouver, BC: UBC Press.

Ward, R., & Price, E. (2016). Reconceptualising dementia: Towards a politics of senility. In S. Westwood & E. Price (Eds.), *Lesbian, gay, bisexual and trans** individuals living with dementia: Concepts, practice and rights (pp. 65–78). London: Routledge Press.

Warren, L. A., Shi, Q., Young, K., Borenstein, A., & Martinuik, A. (2015). Prevalence and incidence of dementia among Indigenous populations: A systematic review. *International Psychogeriatrics*, *27*(12), 1959–1970. doi:10.1017/S1041610215000861

Whitehouse, P., with D. George. (2008). *The myth of Alzheimer's: What you aren't being told about today's most dreaded diagnosis*. New York: St. Martin's Press.

Zgola, J. (1999). *Care that works: A relationship approach to persons with dementia*. Baltimore, MD: John Hopkins University Press.

Chapter 8

Mapping trauma across the life course

Questions to consider as you read this chapter

- How do you think trauma comes to be hidden in the lives of older adults?
- What are some underlying assumptions you have about the experience of those with trauma and how people recover? How will this influence your practice with older adults?
- What particular responses or behaviours of those you are assisting might trigger you? How do you know when this is happening? How will you respond?
- How prepared are you to work with older adults and their families to address trauma and to make your workplace more trauma-informed?
- What social work skills and values fit into a trauma-informed approach?

Gerontological social workers will, at times, witness the outcomes and expressions of different forms of trauma older adults may have experienced across their life course – everything from intimate partner violence, genocide, colonization, child abuse and neglect, and natural disasters. Regardless of what the trauma was, when it was experienced, and past coping mechanisms and strategies, the potential stresses of aging (such as experiences of loss, transitions, cognitive and physiological changes, requiring support) can result in unique experiences of trauma. While the relationship between trauma and aging has not been well studied, there is enough evidence to suggest that their interaction differs significantly from the experiences of trauma among other age-based cohorts, specifically as it relates to cognitive, biological, and psycho-social processes common to aging (Lapp, Agbokou, & Ferreri, 2011). Trauma is often the "hidden variable" in older adults' lives (Cook & O'Donnell, 2005), not disclosed by them or their families, buried in the past, and overlooked or misunderstood. Like other health and social care practitioners, social workers often have limited education and training regarding trauma and are, in turn, unprepared to recognize it in older adults and work within a framework that can support survivors of trauma (Giberovitch & Berry, 2013; Graziano, 2004).

The way in which trauma is examined and understood in much of the practice and research literature is as something that happens to, and affects only, the individual – as in psychological trauma. However, trauma can also be historical, collective, and inter-generational in nature, with impacts resonating across families, groups, communities, and generations. Trauma can be the outcome of membership in groups and communities who have experienced and are currently experiencing violence, discrimination, displacement, and mistreatment. The risk for exposure to trauma and adverse trauma responses can be linked to cumulative inequality, disadvantage, and oppression throughout the life course that may be due to gender, socio-economic status, race, ability, gender identity and expression, and sexual orientation (Ferraro & Shippee, 2009). Effects therefore are not just experienced or embedded in the individual, but also in the very socio-cultural fabric in which they live. This can be problematic and/ or it can be the source of resilience, resistance, and healing.

Trauma (and the potential to re-traumatize) can also be embedded in systems, institutions, and structures. The sites and sectors of health and social care that older adults must access can reinforce oppression, create greater harm through re-traumatization, and result in a lack of safety and control for those who have been impacted by trauma. This is especially true for those individuals and groups who have a mistrust of traditional health and social care services because of historical oppression and exclusion within these systems. Sites of care such as hospitals and long-term care facilities are structured in ways that privilege the treatment of medical and physical issues, often to the exclusion of the psycho-social. A lack of knowledge and attention to older adults' trauma histories has been shown to have a negative impact on care relationships and outcomes, especially in institutional settings (Anderson, Fields, & Dobb, 2011; Teshuva, Borowski, & Wells, 2016), where the potential to misdiagnose, re-trigger, or exacerbate symptoms is high (David & Pelly, 2003). This includes, for example, continually having to re-tell one's story, being treated as a diagnostic label, having a lack of choice or involvement in care planning, and being subject to care practices that require physical and emotional vulnerability without safety (undressing and dressing, personal care, body care).

This chapter connects individual and psychological trauma with an understanding of the socio-cultural context in which it occurred (and continues to occur) as it relates to the lived experiences of older adults. It uses an intersectional life course perspective (see **Age/ism: age as a category of difference**) to understand the relationship between trauma and aging with a particular focus on context and meaning. For example, we consider how the events throughout a person's life, both individually and structurally, may have contributed to, exacerbated, re-triggered, and protected older adults. Finally, we explore and integrate how social workers can adopt trauma-informed approaches to care into their practice with older adults, their families, their workplaces, and the broader sites and sectors of care.

The objectives of this chapter are to

- Define trauma and describe how it interacts with aging;
- Explore the experiences of trauma and aging with an individual and collective lens; and
- Understand how trauma-informed care can be integrated into AOP.

A reflection on trauma

The impacts of trauma and the importance of enacting a trauma-informed practice (TIP) approach in the work we do as social workers has recently emerged in the practice and research literature, but very little of it relates to working with older adults. In reflecting on this, I (Louise) thought back to my own practice and where a lack of knowledge and insight about trauma may have been detrimental. I thought back to my work as the coordinator of a day program for people living with dementia over 20 years ago and wondered "*How can I imagine it differently*"?

> *One of my favourite clients was BB. He was adored by staff and the other participants at the program because he was a gentle soul with a beautiful smile. He was always wanting hugs – always telling us how much he loved us all. He had a very poor memory, and he really did not speak much, but he was an important presence in our group.*
>
> *I often saw dark clouds behind his kind eyes. He would repeat a number – especially when he was stressed or anxious or when he was overstimulated by the noise and the environment. When we would ask him about what the number meant, he would tear up and cry. One day, on the way to the washroom, he got lost and ended up in the furnace room. I found him clinging desperately to a pole and crying while reciting the number.*
>
> *We asked his family about the meaning behind the number and they told us his story. He had a terrible childhood experience. He was an orphan – a child who was a survivor of the Armenian genocide of the 1920s – who was brought to Canada with other child survivors as refugees and ended up in an institution that raised him to be a farm labourer. He lost most of his language and culture (although because of his dementia, his language was coming back). He had a hard-working life, grew up, and had a family; they were all thriving and well. The number was the individual identification number he was given, as were all children who were transported to Canada; it was used throughout his childhood here. It was a piece of his identity left over from a past trauma.*

As a fairly new social worker at the time, and with very limited information on trauma available 20 years ago, I did not have the language or knowledge to put a name to what I was seeing and what BB was experiencing. All I knew is that what worked with him was to create a space where he felt safe and cared for; for us to understand what his "triggers" were and how they might be exacerbated by his dementia; and when to create these safe spaces for him so he was not overly stimulated. We did not pathologize or problematize his "behaviours". On reflection, this was because of a number of factors. First, his behaviours had a context for us. His past experiences appeared to be real for him in the present; and because we had a strong biography of his life (through assessment), we were able to make those links. Second, we had created an environment where relationship was central to the work we did, both with BB and his family. The longer we worked with him, the more we understood his reactions and triggers. We asked the family to provide us with some Armenian words to use to calm him down, and we were able to identify when he might be responding negatively to stress. Finally, BB was easy to care for and engage with, even when agitated. If he hadn't been a person who was easy to care for and if his behaviours had been considered antagonistic, aggressive, or irritating to others around him, we might not have been so inclined to make those links between his past and his present. We might have just attributed them to the symptoms of his dementia.

What this reflection made evident to me some 20 years later (and now armed with the language and knowledge about trauma) is that there is an imperative for social workers to be better informed about and engaged with trauma and aging and their relationship with one another. Trauma should not just be understood as something that happens in the "present", but something that may have taken place in the past, with the potential to re-emerge at any time. In fact, trauma and TIP are applicable to nearly all of the chapters and topics addressed in this book, particularly those that focus on practice – specifically **Mental health, mental wellness, and substance mis/use** and **Addressing mistreatment and violence**. TIP needs to become an everyday fixture in our practice toolboxes. Moving forward, social workers must become more aware of what trauma is, how it is experienced and known, and how it impacts or is impacted by the aging process.

Trauma

Trauma is the term used to describe *what happens* when an *individual* has an adverse internal *response* to external events (or their exposure to them) as indicated below in textbox 8.1.

Textbox 8.1

Trauma results from an event, series of events, or set of circumstances that is experienced by an individual as physically or emotionally harmful or life threatening and that has lasting adverse effects on the individual's functioning and mental, physical, social, emotional, or spiritual well-being (SAMHSA, 2014a, p. 7).

Not everyone reacts to traumatic events and experiences or develops symptoms in ways that could be considered problematic or that interfere with their quality of life and their functioning. In fact, *the event itself does not cause the trauma; rather, trauma is caused by how it is experienced and the meaning attributed to it*. This means that a combination of factors can impact (negatively and positively) how a traumatic event is experienced by individuals. These include

- the age of the person and the stage of development in which it is experienced;
- the frequency, duration, and intensity of the event(s);
- whether it originates from interpersonal or external sources; and
- the socio-cultural context in which it is experienced.

In general, practice and research literature examining trauma has been more focussed on the first three factors, with less emphasis placed on understanding the socio-cultural context in which it is experienced.

Traumatic events are differentiated based on how many times and at what point in the life course the trauma occurs and by how many people or generations are affected/ harmed by it (see Table 8.1)

Individuals have the potential to have been exposed to numerous (including collective and historical) traumatic events across their lives that could contribute to the complex and problematic nature of their current experiences. This is particularly relevant to the lived experiences of older adults for whom cumulative trauma may be present. A number of different responses (or symptoms) to trauma are illustrated in Table 8.2. As noted, not every person will respond in the same way or exhibit the same

Table 8.1 Types of trauma

Single Incident	One-time unexpected and overwhelming event or situation. *Example*: car accident, witnessing violence, sudden loss, assault (physical or sexual)
Complex, Repetitive	Ongoing abuse *Example*: intimate partner violence, being trapped emotionally and physically in a relationship
Developmental	Early exposure (infancy and childhood) to ongoing and repetitive trauma within caring context. Outcomes interfere with healthy development and attachment *Example*: neglect, physical, sexual and emotional abuse, abandonment
Intergenerational	Effects of those living with trauma (coping and adaptation) are transmitted interpersonally, within family, socio-culturally, and biologically
Historical Trauma	Cumulative trauma and wounding over lifespan and across generations as a result of mass group trauma (linked to intergenerational) Example: genocide, colonization, slavery

symptomology, but an awareness of potential expressions of trauma is important for social work practitioners in order to better integrate a trauma–informed approach to practice. As you read these, you may notice overlap with some conditions that may be related to aging – especially in the physical and cognitive responses sections. This is one reason trauma is often undetected or misdiagnosed in older adults; the untangling of these responses from co-occurring conditions can be challenging.

Individual (psychological) trauma and aging

Research suggests that 70 to 90% of older adults (over the age of 65) have been exposed to at least one traumatic event in their lifetime (Ogle, Rubin, & Siegler, 2013). This seems accurate when we consider how broad the category of "traumatic events" is (see Table 8.1). However, older adults (specifically the current cohort) are less likely to identify their problems from a psychological perspective or make the link to past traumatic events; they exhibit these effects in other behaviours such as mental illness, substance (mis)use, and somatic complaints and are reluctant to disclose information because of dominant societal discourses of stigma and shame (Hiskey & McPherson, 2013; Ogle et al., 2013). The current cohort of older adults may have grown up in a time when, because of social and political discrimination, disclosure of experiences, such as intimate partner violence or sexual orientation, would not have been considered an option.

Older adults can be affected by trauma in the following ways, specific to different ages and stages of their lives: **early in life** and with a later re-emergence as they age (such as child abuse, neglect, and abandonment); **throughout the life span** (such as abusive relationships, incarceration, discrimination, and oppression); **later in life** (such as losses, institutionalization, and disability); or through **historical and collective experiences** (such as genocide, colonialism, and racism). It can be attributed to a **single event** such as an accident or loss or to complex forms of

Table 8.2 Trauma responses and symptoms

1. Emotional Responses
- Difficulty with self-regulation
- Difficulty labelling or expressing feelings
- Difficulty communicating wishes and needs
- Internalizing symptoms such as anxiety and depression

2. Physical Responses (Body and Brain)
- Analgesia (inability to feel pain)
- Coordination, balance, and tone
- Somatization
- Increased medical problems
- Developmental delays/regressive behaviours

3. Relationships and Attachments
- Relationship problems with family and peers
- Attachment and separation anxiety and fears
- Problems with boundaries
- Distrust and suspicion
- Social and emotional isolation
- Difficulty attuning to and relating to other people's perspectives

4. Behaviour
- Impulse control
- Risk taking (self-destructive, aggression)
- Externalizing behaviours
- Sleep disturbance
- Eating disturbance
- Substance misuse
- Oppositional behavior

5. Cognitive Responses
- Difficulties with executive functioning
- Lack of curiosity
- Problems with information processing
- Lack of ability to focus and complete tasks
- Language
- Learning difficulties

6. Disassociation
- Disconnect between thoughts, emotions, and perceptions
- Amnesia/loss of memory of events
- Depersonalization (detachment)
- Experiences alterations or shifts in consciousness

ongoing and repetitive trauma, such as neglect and abuse, intimate partner violence, and war.

What is known about trauma and aging is limited, especially when compared to what is known about trauma in children, youth, and adults (Cook & Simiola, 2018; Maschi, Baer, Morrissey, & Moreno, 2013). The Adverse Childhood Experiences Study (Felitti et al., 1998) brought attention to the prevalence of childhood traumatic experiences and made significant links between traumatic experiences and poor health and social outcomes across the life course. The premise is that exposure to traumatic events (especially accumulated exposure) leads to impacts that resonate across time. The impacts of childhood trauma on individuals as they enter "old age" have not been well examined, but initial findings show that childhood trauma is significantly associated with poor mental health outcomes (including dementia and PTSD), substance mis/use, violence, re-victimization, and chronic health conditions among older adults (Bachner, Carmel, & O'Rourke, 2017; Burri, Maerker, Krammer, & Simmon-Janevska, 2013; Cook, McCarthy, & Thorp, 2016; Maschi et al., 2013).

Ogle et al. (2013) found that older adults who experienced trauma earlier in life had more severe symptoms of PTSD and lower levels of happiness than those who experienced trauma later in life. The authors see this as a cumulative effect, in that the impacts, such as dysregulation and disturbances across different areas of functioning, increase susceptibility to other negative outcomes through their lives, including problematic coping strategies and limited social supports. Findings from the Jerusalem Longitudinal Study, which looked at effects of Holocaust exposure during adulthood, showed that while there was evidence of psycho-social and functional impairments for survivors, there were no real differences in health outcomes. Because the trauma exposure happened during adulthood, rather than in childhood, survivors appeared less susceptible to certain physiological and neurological impacts (Stessman et al., 2008). These findings point to the potentially enduring nature of trauma across one's life course and the importance of age and stage of exposure.

There is evidence that the emergence of trauma responses can happen later in life, even when individuals have not shown prior evidence, and long after the events may have occurred (Hiskey, Luckie, Davies, & Brewin, 2008). There are a number of explanations for this including the onset of new life events associated with aging (such as social and interpersonal losses), changes to roles and status, and the experience of cognitive and neuro-biological changes (such as cognitive impairment or dementia) that may trigger a past memory and/or create conditions whereby the older adult is more vulnerable to experiencing negative consequences from that memory. The onset of dementia and related cognitive changes can exacerbate trauma symptomology such as agitation, aggression, and the reliving of hidden memories (Mittal, Torres, Abashidze, & Jimerson, 2001). Finally, the presence of trauma outcomes such as PTSD has been shown to increase the incidence and prevalence of dementia (Qureshi et al., 2010).

Less examined is trauma exposure that happens later in life. Research that compared the impacts of early and late life trauma in centenarians (people 100 years and older) showed that trauma experienced later in life was more associated with health problems and depression than earlier experiences (Oseland, Bishop, Gallus, & Randall, 2016). The authors posit that the responses of "the old-old" to trauma are possibly shaped by their cohort membership, which has allowed them to develop collective hardiness and resilience (i.e., the Great Depression of the 1930s) that mitigated the long-term effects of earlier trauma; and that proximity to events may impact perceived severity. This has been more challenging to explore in the context of aging and dementia, because dementia symptoms appear to mimic those associated with trauma, including PTSD (Lapp et al., 2011); people with dementia may not be able to "report" the trauma. An example is the case presentation of a woman with dementia who had been sexually assaulted in a long-term care facility. While the woman was unable to narrate her experience, she had an "emotional and embodied memory" of the trauma that was expressed through symptoms that were described as "inconsolable agitation ... a tendency to bolt ... pac[ing] relentlessly ... and avoidance of male staff" (McCartney & Severson, 1997, p. 76). All of this provides evidence that trauma can occur at different times across the life course and impact older adults differentially.

While there is a relationship between trauma and poor outcomes later in life, there is also evidence of resilience and resistance to pathology in other life domains that continues even in the context of aging and adversity. As people age, and with an emerging awareness of trauma and its impacts across the life course, a focus on how trauma manifests itself in older adults provides an opportunity to examine both vulnerability and resilience.

Collective/historical trauma and aging

As evidenced in the previous section, the understanding of trauma, its causes, symptoms, and outcomes are primarily focussed on individual responses and experiences and neglect collective responses and experiences. These collective responses and experiences are encapsulated in the definition of historical and collective trauma (see textbox 8.2).

Textbox 8.2

Historical and collective trauma is defined as the cumulative emotional and psychological wounding from massive group trauma across generations, including the lifespan (Braveheart, 1998).

Collective and historical trauma may directly affect individuals (such as attendance at residential schools or being direct survivors of the Rwandan genocide) and/or impact through familial and cultural proximity (intergenerational transmission, racism, institutional, and structural forms of oppression). While not every member of a collective will manifest psychological trauma, latent symptomology may be evident in high rates of substance mis/use or mental health challenges, changes to community and family cohesion, and health disparities, for example. These stressors then become normalized, incorporated into culture, and passed down inter-generationally (Wesley-Esquimaux & Smolewski, 2004).

> Within an Indigenous context, the intergenerational transmission of trauma may occur at many levels, including: *interpersonally*, through altered parenting; within *families*, which may be disrupted by loss of members or exposure to stressors like domestic violence; at the level of the *community*, when many individuals and families are impacted by disturbances of social networks and experiences of safety and solidarity that affect health; and at the level of *nation*, where the suppression of culture and the disruption of family and community threaten the continuity of whole peoples.
>
> (Kirmayer, Gone, and Moses, 2014, pp. 308–309)

This means that many older adults who have lived and are living within cultural communities in which trauma is deeply embedded and transmitted through bio-psycho -social and spiritual processes may still be dealing with structural impacts of historical trauma.

Older adults who have experienced ongoing and sustained historical traumas stemming from genocide and colonization and/or structural discrimination and oppression including racism, homophobia, and transphobia may be more susceptible to the emergence of adverse trauma outcomes as they age. Research on older trans adults, for example, demonstrates that trauma effects can re-emerge in later life and that post-trauma symptoms can worsen as people age often because of ongoing small-t (micro-aggressions) and large-t (sexual assault and hate crimes) traumas they continue to experience (Munson, 2016).

Rather than just focussing on psychological forms of trauma – and interventions that look primarily at individual needs – there must also be consideration of the collective context of trauma when working with older adults, especially those from groups who dealt with or still are dealing with different forms of oppression. Interestingly, research in the area of collective and historical forms of trauma has shifted away from pathology and "vulnerability", to "resilience". Research focussing on Indigenous Elders and Holocaust survivors has provided a model for how to integrate a framework of resilience and has consistently noted how vulnerability to poor trauma outcomes often co-exists with resilience (Hatala, Desjardins, & Bombay, 2016; Shmotkin, Shrira, Goldberg, & Palvi, 2011). In this context, resilience is not conceptualized as just "individual traits or characteristics", but rather something that also has collective and communal dimensions (Kirmayer, Dandenau, Marshall, Phillips, & Williamson, 2011). Collective forms of resilience are made up of protective factors situated in a specific socio-cultural context – such as family and social supports, spirituality/religion, customs of grieving, and ways of meaning-making and transmitting memory about collective traumas as a form of social justice education.

The medicalization of trauma

As noted earlier, the socio-cultural context of the experience of trauma (and aging) has not been well examined or explored. An awareness of trauma and its integration into AOP social work (through trauma-informed approaches) is needed and warranted. This includes the need to be aware of the hazards of adopting new approaches without first engaging in a critical analysis of the prevailing assumptions and discourses that inform and construct these approaches. For example, the use of a "trauma discourse" model within mental health services (Suarez, 2016) has emerged within the context of the increasing medicalization of human responses to adversity, suffering, and distress (Conrad, 2007) (as outlined in **Mental health, mental wellness, and substance mis/use**). The medicalization of these responses as "disordered" is reflected in the inclusion of post-traumatic stress disorder (PTSD) as a diagnostic category in the DSM 5.[1]

PTSD (as defined in the DSM-5) is seen as the gold standard measure for understanding trauma outcomes, but this is problematic for a number of reasons. For one, it is a Western psychiatric construct that is applied universally and globally, ignoring how culture shapes psycho-social aspects of responses to traumatic events and how local communities draw on their own methods of meaning making, remembrance, coping strategies, and resources (Marsella, 2010; Suarez, 2016). The DSM categorizes trauma responses as universal in nature, ignoring the fact that these responses are culture-bound – varying across time and place – and therefore cannot be standardized (Summerfield, 2004).

Second, PTSD does not capture how trauma remains deeply rooted in structural problems such as racism, poverty, and sexism, nor is it able to capture these types of trauma in the assessment process. For example, racism is often subtle, ambiguous, and insidious in nature – rather than an overt event – so that the distress that emerges from it will produce different "symptoms" that are not easily categorized (Miller, 2009). Lastly, PTSD has been critiqued as being "pathologically" focussed, which may negate the resilience and resistance inherent in the lived experiences of older survivors and from within specific socio-cultural contexts.

Trauma-informed practice

The medicalization of trauma has implications for the approaches used to provide care and support. As Summerfield (2004) notes, practitioners have a duty to recognize distress but also to attend to what people carrying the distress want to signal by it. Social workers need to be aware of these implications when working with older adults, who are already subject to the medicalization of many of their problems (see textbox 3.4). In this section, we look at what AOG social workers can do to address trauma and work with older adults through the application of a TIP approach, a strengths-based framework and set of principles that take into account the presence of trauma in all aspects of service delivery and care (Trauma-Informed Practice Guide (TIP), 2013). It starts from the premise that an individual's current difficulties may be experienced within the context of past traumas (Knight, 2015, p. 25). The traumatic event does not have to be disclosed, acknowledged, or even experienced directly by the individual because they can be traumatized through the witnessing of events or through the inter-generational transmission of trauma. The *presumption* of its potential presence can provide practitioners with a context for understanding the problem, treatment, and care of older adults regardless of setting or care needs. Unlike trauma-specific services that attempt to directly address the need for healing from traumatic life experiences, trauma-informed approaches do not intentionally treat the trauma directly, but rather consider how trauma is expressed, how it is manifested in lived experience, and how the organizations and institutions that care and support individuals, groups, and communities may be complicit in re-traumatizing and re-triggering. While not explicitly labelled as trauma-informed, you will see how some of the principles of TIP were actually drawn on and integrated into the story of BB.

TIP is useful for AOP social work, but there are cautions to adopting this approach, including its emphasis on the needs of individuals over the collective and its neglect of how trauma is rooted in structural problems of oppression. There is a concern that TIP reinforces the medicalization of trauma in a more "appealing" package. Even with this caution, the principles underpinning this approach do fit with the social work values of empowerment, advocacy, collaboration, and self-determination. Because it does not require disclosure or memory of events, or even for the person to have directly experienced the traumatic event(s), it can be useful for work with people who have cognitive (memory) challenges, fears of disclosure, or disassociation with past traumatic events. Social workers must look to biographical/narrative and socio-cultural context to make potential links to the presence of trauma and to the larger structural impacts on the experiences of older adults across the life course, including oppression and discrimination.

Trauma-informed approaches to practice are concerned with application at the personal, professional, and organizational levels. We would expand this to take into account the structural:

- **PERSONAL**: how self-aware we are as practitioners of the impacts of trauma in our own lived experiences, including our social locations and how they may influence our work with others. This includes recognition of the potential for vicarious and secondary trauma in our work.
- **PROFESSIONAL**: how we recognize trauma in our work with individuals, groups, and communities and how we integrate trauma-informed principles through all phases of social work practice.
- **ORGANIZATIONAL**: how we work to create organizational and system practices and environments (including policies and procedures) that are trauma-informed.

A number of useful resources and manuals focus in depth on understanding and integrating trauma-informed approaches to practice (see additional resources at the end of this chapter). None of these is specific to older adults, but all of the principles espoused by them can be used and adapted to AOG social work practice. This section will also be useful when you are reading **Mental health, mental wellness, and substance mis/use** and **Addressing mistreatment and violence**, where this approach is also addressed and applied. A number of different configurations and iterations of these principles appear in the literature, but here we will use a distillation of those we feel are the most pertinent and relevant to an AOG framework:

- Trauma awareness;
- Safety and trustworthiness;
- Choice, collaboration, and control;
- Strengths-based approach;
- Cultural, historical, and gender issues.

To illustrate and illuminate these principles, we introduce the following case study. The goal of this is for you to consider what how you would re-vision Amina's story of care.

Amina

Amina is a 64-year-old woman who was recently admitted to the rehab unit of a regional hospital after suffering a stroke. The stroke has left her with right-sided weakness, some short-term memory loss, and the need for assistance with walking and personal care.

The staff are struggling with both her behaviour and care needs. The focus is to get her up and mobilizing independently and performing her own activities of daily living so that she can return to some form of independent living. She is often angry and refuses to work with the physiotherapist. She often breaks down and cries when the staff "make demands of her".

The staff are aware she is "not from Canada", but they really do not have an understanding of her past and how this may be impacting her current status and the ability to move forward.

Amina is a Sudanese, Muslim woman who came to Canada 15 years ago as a political refugee. She was a social justice activist and one evening was arrested and separated from her partner and small child. She was jailed and experienced sexual, physical, and psychological torture while in jail. After five years, she was released, but her partner had also been jailed. She reconnected with her daughter (Hiba); out of fear and to ensure a better life for Hiba, she applied for and was granted refugee status in Canada.

Once in Canada, Amina continued her equity work and found employment as a support worker for political refugees as they resettled. She continued to be what she described as a "social justice warrior", "fiercely independent" and "tough as nails". Hiba is involved with her mother, but feels powerless in her limited ability to influence her mother.

The first principle is **trauma awareness,** which requires an understanding of the high prevalence of all forms of trauma and the wide range of responses, effects, and adaptations among individuals, groups, and communities. Social workers need to bring this awareness of the impacts of trauma to all aspects of the social work process, including assessment, intervention, evaluation, and termination. AOG social workers need to develop knowledge about:

- what trauma may look like in older adults (as opposed to younger adults);
- how it can be manifested over the life course (both as vulnerabilities and strengths);
- forms of resilience and resistance;
- how individuals who have experienced different forms of oppression across their lives may be exposed to unique and interrelated forms of traumatic events and experiences;
- how it may present later in life, especially as it intersects with physical and cognitive changes that can be associated with aging; and
- how it is often ignored, misdiagnosed, or misinterpreted in the care of older adults.

Finally, social workers need to be critically reflective of their own relationship to trauma and to protect themselves from the potential of vicarious and secondary traumatization.[2]

The second principle is **safety and trustworthiness,** which is the provision of physical, spiritual, emotional, and cultural safety. Safety is a central principle of trauma-informed practice because trauma survivors often feel unsafe, are likely to have experienced abuse of power in important relationships, and may currently be in unsafe relationships or living situations (TIP Guide, 2013, p. 13). The provision of multiple forms of safety allows the social worker to address the oppressive dynamics of authority and power that have been evident in the lives of clients and the communities in which clients reside. The challenge with creating safety is that it needs to be integrated and enacted at the organizational level, as well as the professional level. While the social worker can integrate safety into their individual work with older adult clients, creating environmental and cultural safety can be more challenging, especially in institutional care settings.

The third principle is *choice, collaboration, and control*, which is the encouragement and facilitation of environments that create opportunities for inclusion in care planning and support and self-efficacy, self-determination, dignity, and personal control. As noted throughout this book, ageism creates conditions in which older adults are excluded from decision-making and planning in their care, especially when cognitive and behavioural challenges are perceived to be present. A lack of awareness of the presence of trauma and misdiagnosis can pathologize these behaviours and cause further exclusion. Connected to this is the fourth principle, *strengths-based approach*, which is the examination of resiliency/resistance, coping skills, and strategies used by the individual throughout the life span to protect and thrive even through extreme adversity.

The fifth principle is an acknowledgement of *cultural, historical, and gender issues* which recognizes and addresses the impacts of historical and collective forms of trauma on individuals and communities. This is an understanding that individuals may be part of cultural groups that are particularly vulnerable to trauma, less willing to engage with traditional care systems because of past traumas, and concerned they will be treated in culturally insensitive and unsafe ways, particularly within mainstream health and social care sites and sectors. Social workers must recognize that culture influences the following:

- the ways in which some individuals, groups, and cultural communities become more susceptible and vulnerable to experiencing trauma events because of historic and/or systemic abuses;
- whether or not events are labelled as traumatic and how the individual ascribes meaning to them;
- the range of "acceptable" responses to trauma and how it is expressed;
- whether or not individuals seek out support and treatment;
- the provision of a sense of strength, support, and strategies for healing (SAMHSA, 2014b, p. 27).

Final reflections

Amina's and BB's stories illustrate the extent to which many different types of trauma can be hidden in the lives of older adults and how it may deeply impact their care. The first step to "pulling back the curtains" on trauma is *awareness* at the personal, professional, and organizational levels. Without awareness, Amina's and BB's behaviours may continue to be "problematized", primarily attributed to symptoms of their "dementia" or "stroke", or simply deemed to be the result of a challenging personality. Without awareness, health and social service providers would likely continue to ask, *"What is wrong with them?"* rather than *"What happened to them?"* and miss important contextual and biographical clues. Without adapted interventions, Amina and BB may continue to be re-triggered or re-traumatized and become more resistant to care and less amenable to rehab or participating in the day program. Their trauma responses may be heightened, which in turn may exacerbate symptoms of their dementia (memory loss, confusion) or their stroke (memory loss, emotional lability). Both stories demonstrate that there is a long list of *"clues"* regarding how and why trauma can remain unexplored, especially when trauma is not the primary reason for intervention. We need to be attentive to trauma across the life course. Finally, interventions need to be undertaken in ways that do not perpetuate the medicalization or "disordering" of older adults' responses, behaviours, or experiences and that consider them in a wider socio-cultural context.

AOG social workers have an important role to play in that they can act as the starting point for "awareness" at all three levels. This includes becoming knowledgeable about *all types* of trauma across the life course, trauma's intersection with the processes of aging, how some individuals and groups may be more susceptible to traumatic responses (and triggers), and the extent to which institutions and structures can themselves traumatize or exacerbate problematic responses. Most importantly, social workers can advocate for the inclusion of trauma-informed approaches to care in the sites and sectors in which they work. Going back to BB's story, I (Louise) do not think *I could have imagined it differently*. The principles and values underpinning a trauma-informed approach to practice were evident despite not having originally labelled them as such because what we did as service providers fit with social work values and the client-focussed and relational nature of the day program. The stories presented in this chapter demonstrate that a trauma-informed approach is possible if one is equipped with the knowledge and skills required to identify it and to adapt interventions that address the multiple forms of trauma that are experienced by older adults across the life course.

Exercise

- We would like you to consider how we could re-vision Amina's care with the application and integration of the five trauma-informed principles at the personal, professional, and organizational levels. As you take on this task, reflect on some of the challenges and barriers that you may face in implementing these principles. How would you address them? We have provided you with a chart (Table 8.3) to help you to complete this task.

Takeaways

- Social workers do not routinely take into account trauma in their work with older adults, yet trauma has been a routine part of the life course of older adults.
- Trauma is mostly understood as a psychological/individual experience, with little focus on collective/historical impacts of trauma with older adults, the socio-cultural context in which it is experienced, and the meaning derived from it.
- Environmental and socio-cultural contexts can impact trauma responses either by minimizing or exacerbating them.
- Trauma-informed approaches to practice with older adults need to be implemented at personal, professional, and organizational levels.
- The impacts of oppression, marginalization, and discrimination across the life course can affect older adults in traumatic ways.
- Traumatic responses intersect and interact with processes of aging including age-related health conditions such as dementia.

Table 8.3 Application of a trauma-informed approach to Amina's care

Personal Level	Practicing self-awareness and reflection	Awareness:
	Awareness of potential for vicarious and secondary trauma	Safety and Trustworthiness:
	Social location	Choice, Collaboration, and Control:
		Strengths-based:
		Cultural, Historical, and Gender Issues Awareness:
Professional Level	Integration into social work practice	
	Skills, ethics, processes	Safety and Trustworthiness:
		Choice, Collaboration, and Control:
		Strengths-based:
		Cultural, Historical, and Gender Issues:
Organizational Level	Environment	Trauma Awareness:
	Policies and procedures of the organization	Safety and Trustworthiness:
		Choice, Collaboration, and Control:
		Strengths-based:
		Cultural, Historical, and Gender Issues:

Additional resources

- Trauma Informed Practice Guide (2013, May): http://bccewh.bc.ca/wp-content/uploads/2012/05/2013_TIP-Guide.pdf
- Klinic Community Health Centre (2013) The Trauma Toolkit (2nd Ed.): https://trauma-informed.ca/wp-content/uploads/2013/10/Trauma-informed_Toolkit.pdf
- Substance Abuse and Mental Health Services Administration (2014a) SAMHSA's Concept of Trauma and Guidance for a Trauma-Informed Approach: https://store.samhsa.gov/system/files/sma14-4884.pdf
- Substance Abuse and Mental Health Services Administration SAMHSA (2014b) Trauma-Informed Care in Behavioral Health Services: https://store.samhsa.gov/system/files/sma14-4816.pdf
- Canadian Centre on Substance Abuse (2014) The Essentials of Trauma-Informed Care: www.ccsa.ca/Resource%20Library/CCSA-Trauma-informed-Care-Toolkit-2014-en.pdf
- University at Buffalo School of Social Work Self-Care Resources: http://socialwork.buffalo.edu/resources/self-care-starter-kit/how-to-flourish-in-social-work/self-care-nasw.html

Notes

1 PTSD was first included in the DSM III in 1980 as a co-creation between psychiatry and veterans' advocacy groups (primarily from the Vietnam War) as an official recognition of the trauma and impacts of war and combat.
2 People working with people who have been traumatized are also at risk for traumatization and re-traumatization. **Vicarious trauma** is a permanent change in the practitioner resulting from empathetic engagement with multiple clients' situations and trauma or trauma background. The practitioner may have triggers related to this work. Symptoms are more pervasive than burnout because it impacts all facets of life – body, mind, character, and belief system. Vicarious trauma develops over a period of time. **Secondary trauma** occurs when a practitioner relates to a specific client's situation. The practitioner begins to mirror or exhibit similar symptoms to the client. This can happen suddenly in one interaction. Prevention strategies include self-care plans, self-reflection, supervision, peer support, and the opportunity to debrief. See the Additional resources at the end of the chapter for resources specific to self-care (UB School of Social Work). All the TIP resources listed also include information on vicarious and secondary trauma.

References

Anderson, K. A., Fields, N. L., & Dobb, L. A. (2011). Understanding the impact of early-life trauma in nursing home residents. *Journal of Gerontological Social Work*, *54*(8), 755–767. doi:10.1080/01634372.2011.596917.

Bachner, Y. G., Carmel, S., & O'Rourke, N. (2017). The paradox of well-being and Holocaust survivors. *Journal of American Psychiatric Nurses Association*. doi:10.1177/1078390317705450.

Braveheart, M. Y. H. (1998). The return to the sacred path: Healing the historic trauma response among the Lakota. *Smith College Studies in Social Work*, *68*(3), 287–305. doi:10.3138/ijih.v5i2.28981.

Burri, A., Maerker, A., Krammer, S., & Simmon-Janevska, K. (2013). Childhood trauma and PTSD symptoms increase the risk of cognitive impairment in a sample of former indentured child labourers in old age. *PLoS One*, *8*(2), 1–8. doi:10.1371/journal.pone.0057826.

Conrad, P. (2007). *The medicalization of society: On the transformation of human conditions into treatable disorders*. Baltimore, MD: Johns Hopkins University Press.

Cook, J. M. & O'Donnell, C. (2005). Assessment and psychological treatment of PTSD in older adults. *Journal of Geriatric Psychiatry and Neurology, 18*(2), 61–71.

Cook, J. M., McCarthy, E., & Thorp, S. R. (2016). Older adults with PTSD: Brief state of research and evidence-based psychotherapy case illustration. *The American Journal of Geriatric Psychiatry, 25*(5), 522–530. doi:10.1016/j.jagp.2016.12.016.

Cook, J. M., & Simiola, V. (2018). Trauma and aging. *Current Psychiatric Reports, 20*(10), 93. doi:10.1007/s/11920-018-0943-6.

David, P., & Pelly, S. (Eds.). (2003). *Caring for aging Holocaust survivors: A practice manual*. Toronto, Ontario, Canada: Baycrest Centre for Geriatric Care.

Felitti, V. J., Anda, R. F., Nordenberg, D., Williamson, D. F., Spitz, A. M., Edwards, V., … Marks, J. S. (1998). Relationship of childhood abuse and household dysfunction to many of the learning causes of death in adults: The adverse childhood experiences (ACE) study. *American Journal of Preventive Medicine, 14*(4), 245–258.

Ferraro, K. F., & Shippee, T. P. (2009). Aging and cumulative inequality: How does inequality get under the skin? *Gerontologist, 49*(3), 333–343. doi:10.1093/geront/gnp034.

Giberovitch, M., & Berry, R. G. (2013). *Recovery from genocidal trauma: An information and practice guide to working with Holocaust survivors*. Toronto, Ontario, Canada: University of Toronto Press.

Graziano, R. (2004). Trauma and aging. *Journal of Gerontological Social Work, 40*(4), 3–21. doi:10.1300/J083v40n04_02.

Hatala, A. R., Desjardins, M., & Bombay, A. (2016). Reframing narratives of aboriginal health inequality: Exploring Cree elder resilience and well-being in contexts of historical trauma. *Qualitative Health Research, 26*(14), 1911–1927. doi:10.1177/1049732315609569.

Hiskey, S., Luckie, M., Davies, S., & Brewin, C. R. (2008). The emergence of PTSD in later life: A review. *Journal of Geriatric Psychiatry and Neurology, 21*(4), 232–241. doi:10.1177/0891988708324937.

Hiskey, S., & McPherson, S. (2013). That's just life: Older adult constructs of trauma. *Aging and Mental Health, 17*(6), 689–696. doi:10.1080/13607863.2013.765832.

Kirmayer, L. J., Dandenau, S., Marshall, E., Phillips, M. K., & Williamson, K. J. (2011). Rethinking resilience from Indigenous perspectives. *Canadian Journal of Psychiatry, 56*(2), 84–91. doi:10.1177/07064371105600203.

Kirmayer, L. J., Gone, J. P., & Moses, J. (2014). Rethinking historical trauma. *Transcultural Psychiatry, 51*(3), 299–319. doi:10.1177/1363461514536358.

Knight, C. (2015). Trauma informed social work practice: Practice considerations and challenges. *Clinical Social Work Journal, 43*(1), 25–37. doi:10.1007/s10615-014-0481-6.

Lapp, K. L., Agbokou, C., & Ferreri, F. (2011). PTSD in the elderly: The interaction between trauma and aging. *International Psychogeriatrics, 23*(6), 858–868. doi:10.1017/S1041610211000366.

Marsella, A. J. (2010). Ethno-cultural aspects of PTSD: An overview of concepts, issues, and treatments. *Traumatology, 16*(4), 17–26. doi:10.1177/1534765610388062d.

Maschi, T., Baer, J., Morrissey, M. B., & Moreno, C. (2013). The aftermath of childhood trauma on late life mental and physical health: A review of the literature. *Traumatology, 19*(1), 49–64. doi:10.1177/1534765612437377.

McCartney, J. R., & Severson, K. (1997). Sexual violence, post-traumatic stress disorder and dementia. *Journal of the American Geriatrics Society, 45*(1), 76–78. doi:10.1111/j.1532-5415.1997.tb00982.x.

Miller, G. H. (2009). The trauma of insidious racism. *The Journal of the American Academy of Psychiatry and the Law, 41*(4), 37–41.

Mittal, D., Torres, R., Abashidze, A., & Jimerson, N. (2001). Worsening of PTSD symptoms with cognitive decline. *Journal of Geriatric Psychiatry and Neurology, 14*(1), 17–20. doi:10.1177/089198870101400105.

Munson, M. (2016). FORGE's trauma-informed trans aging work. *Generations, 40*(2), 71–72.

Ogle, C. M., Rubin, D. C., & Siegler, I. C. (2013). The impact of the developmental timing of trauma exposure on PTSD symptoms and psychosocial functioning among older adults. *Developmental Psychology, 49*(11), 2191–2200. doi:10.1037/a0031985dot.

Oseland, L. M., Bishop, A. J., Gallus, K. L., & Randall, G. K. (2016). Early and late life exposure to trauma and biopsychosocial well-being in centenarians. *Journal of Loss and Trauma, 21*(5), 433–443. doi:10.1080/15325024.2015.1117927.

Qureshi, S. U., Kimbrell, T., Pyne, J. M., Magruder, K. M., Hudson, T. J., Peterson, N. J., … Kunik, M. E. (2010). Greater prevalence and incidence in dementia in older veterans with PTSD. *Journal of American Geriatrics Society, 58*(9), 1627–1633. doi:10.1111/j.1532-5415.2010.02977.x.

Shmotkin, D., Shrira, A., Goldberg, S. C., & Palvi, Y. (2011). Resilience and vulnerability among aging holocaust survivors and their families: An intergenerational overview. *Journal of Intergenerational Relationships, 9*(1), 7–21. doi:10.1080/15350770.2011.544202.

Stein, G. L., Beckerman, N. L., & Sherman, P. A. (2010). Lesbian and gay elders and long-term care: Identifying the unique psychosocial perspectives and challenges. *Journal of Gerontological Social Work, 53*(5), 421–435. doi:10.1080/01634372.2010.496478.

Stern, L. (2012). *The cultural whisper in our ear: Intercultural dementia care in a Jewish long-term care facility* (Unpublished doctoral dissertation). Vancouver, BC: University of British Columbia.

Stessman, J., Cohen, A., Hammerman-Rozenburg, R., Bursztyn, M., Azoulay, D., Maaravi, Y., & Jacobs, J. M. (2008). Holocaust survivors in old age: The Jerusalem longitudinal study. *Journal of the American Geriatrics Society, 56*(3), 470–477. doi:10.1111/j.1532-5415.2007.01575.x.

Suarez, E. B. (2016). Trauma in global contexts: Integrating local practices and socio-cultural meanings into new explanatory frameworks of trauma. *International Social Work, 59*(1), 141–153. doi:10.1177/0020872813503859.

Summerfield, D. (2004). Cross-cultural perspectives on the medicalization of human suffering. In G. M. Rosen (Ed.), *Posttraumatic stress disorder: Issues and controversies* (pp. 233–245). New York, NY: John Wiley & Sons Ltd. doi:10.1002/9780470713570.ch12.

Teshuva, K., Borowski, A., & Wells, Y. (2016). The lived experience of providing care and support services for holocaust survivors in Australia. *Qualitative Health Research*. Advace online publication. doi:10.1177/1049732316667702.

Teshuva, K., & Wells, Y. (2014). Experiences of ageing and aged care in Australia of older survivors of genocide. *Ageing & Society, 34*, 518–537. doi:10.1017/S0144686X12001109.

Trauma informed practice guide. (2013, May). Vancouver, BC: British Columbia Mental Health and Substance Use Planning Council. doi: 10.13140/RG.2.1.5116.

Wesley-Esquimaux, C. C., & Smolewski, M. (2004). *Historic trauma and aboriginal healing.* Ottawa, ON: The Aboriginal Healing Foundation.

Chapter 9

Mental health, mental wellness, and substance mis/use

Questions to consider as you read this chapter

- What do you know about mental health issues and older adults?
- What are some "myths" that you can identify related to aging and mental illness?
- Do we have to work differently with older adults in this area of practice than we would with younger adults? Why? Why not?
- What are your own personal beliefs and values relating to mental health and wellness? How do personal beliefs and values potentially impact practice?

Penny is a 79-year-old woman who is living with a diagnosis of bi-polar disorder. Penny's history with the mental health system has been troubling. As a young woman, her parents took her to a psychiatrist to "cure her of the homosexuality", which at the time was considered a "disorder".[1] During this time, she became deeply depressed and attempted suicide. She was then hospitalized for six months during which she was diagnosed with bi-polar disorder.

After her discharge, Penny left home and moved to Winnipeg where she began a career as a community organizer. She managed her mental health through exercise, counselling, and involvement with a group of survivors who became strong advocates for system change in the Manitoba mental health care system.

During her 60s, Penny was again hospitalized after a severe bout of depression and was given electroconvulsive therapy treatment. After this, she noted a change in her short-term memory. Since this last treatment, Penny has remained actively involved in the consumer movement, becoming a peer mentor and educator about mental health issues within both seniors and LGBTTsIQ communities in Manitoba.

She is the caregiver for her partner Susan who was diagnosed with Multiple Sclerosis five years ago. They have been together for 32 years. Though she has been living well with her diagnosis, she is fearful of her mental health and wellness being affected by the stresses of caregiving and what the future may hold as she struggles to keep Susan at home.

We use Penny's story to illustrate a number of different themes this chapter will address. It illustrates an older adult's mental health and well-being as it is shaped by earlier experiences, the historical period in which they live, and socio-cultural context (Mechanic & McAlpine, 2011). It is an example of how individuals, especially those occupying marginalized social identities, live with "stigmatizing", "discriminatory", and "oppressive" practices situated inside and outside mental health systems. Systems are able to label and disorder identities and everyday responses to distress (including stigma) as pathology. As people age, they may meet with new challenges (as Penny did) that could exacerbate pre-existing challenges. They could also experience the onset of mental health challenges for the first time or experience behavioral and psychological symptoms that are related to conditions such as dementia or Parkinson's (MacCourt, Wilson, & Tourigny-Rivard, 2011). Their interactions with mental health systems will undoubtedly be shaped by the fact that these systems are not prepared and/or cognizant of the diversity of needs and experiences that older adults may have compared to younger adults. As a result, they will face both sanism (see textbox 9.1) and ageism.

Textbox 9.1

Sanism

Sanism is systematized discrimination, antagonism, or exclusion directed against neuro-divergent people based on the belief that neuro-typical cognition is superior. Divergence from normal ways of thinking and behaving is seen as pathology.

(From: Simmons University Library LibGuides https://simmons.libguides.com/anti-oppression/anti-sanism)

Social workers' exposure to information and knowledge about mental health (and substance mis/use) within the older adult population is limited. And yet, social workers will find themselves working in mental health and substance use facilities and institutions (psychiatric units, mental health teams, treatment facilities, shelters) where they will work with older adults and will work in settings specific to older adults (long term care, community health, day programs), where they will address mental health and substance use challenges. Much of the training and knowledge they receive about these issues do not necessarily come from academic environments, where they may have one course on mental health and/or substance mis/use and possibly aging. Instead, it is derived from the sites and sectors where they practice. While there has recently been a re-visioning of the Canadian mental health system to adopt a recovery approach to prevention, treatment and care and address the unique and diverse needs of older adults (MHCC, 2011, 2015), this change has been slow. Treatment and care continue to be dominated by a bio-medical discourse of mental illness, even within the mental heath recovery movement itself (Poole, 2011). This results in a considerable lack of resources, knowledge, and support for the development of relevant critical and anti-oppressive practice for social workers.

As part of AOP, social workers need to "trouble" and challenge oppressive forms of practice that perpetuate power imbalances and disempower the people, groups, and communities with whom they work. Unfortunately, in the mental health field, social work has largely been complicit with bio-medical discourses and systems of care. Morley (2003) asserts that the current role of social work is a "support to psychiatric and medical treatment" in which we use "an uncritical embrace of the tenets of the bio-medical model" (p. 66). Larson (2008) concurs and states, there is a "lack of fit between general anti-oppressive, structural and feminist frameworks taught in social work education and the literature and practice used in mental health settings" (p. 40).

Larson goes on to add that while social workers in mental health may focus their individual practice around social-environmental factors, the "basis of care in mental health organizations, and the interventions and the organizational structures typically emanate from a medical model" (p. 42).

This infers that because social work has mostly aligned itself with a psychiatric medical model, it often acts against anti-oppressive and critical social work values. For example, current social work education and practice models have been critiqued for ignoring the impacts of "sanism" – the systematic subjugation of people who have received a mental health diagnosis or treatment (Poole et al., 2012, p. 20) – and doing little to address the impacts of mental health stigma and discrimination at both the micro (personal), meso (community/social-relational), and macro (structural) levels (Gormley & Quinn, 2009; Scheyett, 2005).

The objectives of this chapter are to

*   Make evident how mental health practice is situated in systems informed by bio-medical discourse of mental illness (medicalization);
*   Examine how ageism and sanism intersect with other forms of oppression and the impact on older adults; and
*   Examine and apply anti-oppressive approaches to the care and support of older adults that take into account diverse lived experiences across the life course, and within a broader socio-cultural, historical, and political context as they navigate mental wellness.

Definitions

As in the other practice chapters, having a definition of the concepts that are being addressed is an important place to start analysis. This is done with the understanding that these definitions are socially constructed, reflecting dominant discourses of what are considered normal behaviours, feelings, and (re)actions to the distresses of everyday life (Tew, 2005). As you read the definitions in Table 9.1, note the differences between the first two (mental health and mental wellness) and the last two (mental illness and mental disorder).

This chapter does not address substance mis/use as thoroughly as it does mental health and wellness, though the two are inextricably linked. This connection between mental illness and substance mis/use is encapsulated in bio-medical terms such as 'dual diagnoses', 'concurrent disorders' and 'multi-morbidity', as a common occurrence. Figure 9.1 depicts substance mis/use as existing on a continuum and Table 9.2 is a short overview of substance mis/use specific to older adults. We provide this content early in the chapter so that you will consider substance mis/use in relation to mental health and mental wellness. Substance mis/use is specifically addressed again in the case example used in the chapter and in the resources list provided for your reference.

The medicalization of mental health and illness

Conrad (2007) describes medicalization as "the process by which non-medical problems become defined and treated as medical problems, usually in terms of illnesses or disorders" (p. 4). Aspects of this process include

Table 9.1 Definitions of health, wellness, disorder, illness

Mental Health	Defined as "a state of well-being" in which every individual realizes their own potential, can cope with the normal stresses of life, can work productively and fruitfully, and is able to make a contribution to [their] community (WHO, 2014).
Mental Wellness	Based on an Indigenous worldview, mental wellness is a holistic strengths-based understanding built on the integration of the physical, mental, emotional, and spiritual at the individual, family, and community levels. Mental wellness happens along a continuum and is supported by culture, language, Elders, families, and creation (First Nations Mental Wellness Continuum Framework, 2015).
Mental Disorder	A *clinically* significant behavioural or psychological syndrome or pattern that occurs in an individual and is associated with present distress (e.g., a painful symptom) or disability (i.e., impairment in one or more important areas of functioning) or with a significantly increased risk of suffering death, pain, disability, or an important loss of freedom.
Mental Illness	Mental illness is a collection of disorders such as depression, bipolar disorder, schizophrenia, and anxiety. The symptoms can range from loss of motivation and energy, changed sleep patterns, extreme mood swings, disturbances in thought or perception, or overwhelming obsessions or fears. It can be episodic or persistent in nature. Mental illness can interfere with relationships and affects a person's ability to function on a day-to-day basis, often leading to social isolation.

Not all individuals who use prescription or non-prescription substances will encounter problems with its use. Substance use occurs across a continuum:

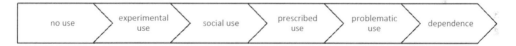

Figure 9.1 The continuum of substance mis/use

- Defining normal or acceptable behaviours, actions, and experiences as abnormal;
- Situating the source of the problem in the individual (rather than the environment or social world);
- Prioritizing individual medical interventions, rather than collective or social ones; and
- Increasing levels of medical social control of human behaviours and actions.

There has been a long history of asserting that the challenges related to mental health and wellness should be recognized and understood as "diseases" or "disorders". Even the terms used to describe these experiences such as "mental illness", "mental disorder", and "disease" infer a specific way of thinking about mental health challenges: as pathology or deficit. In this context, mental illness is conceived of as an "objective bio-physical phenomenon that is characterized by a change in the functioning of the

Table 9.2 Older adults and substance mis/use (based on Flint, Merali & Vaacarino, 2018; National Initiative for the Care of the Elderly, n.d.)

Age and Substance Mis/use	Services and Supports
Seen as an issue only relevant to younger adults (not recognized or addressed)	No consensus on appropriate screening and assessment tools specific to age and stage; diagnostic criteria is not applicable to older adults
Stigma and reluctance to address by both practitioners and older adults	Limited age-specific care and treatment options
Symptoms often misdiagnosed or misattributed to "getting older" or age-related problems (dementia)	Treatment can be complex because of societal stigmas and barriers and the unique complexities of physical and mental health
Age related factors can result in different impacts and outcomes (interaction with medications, changing physiology changes how substances effect person)	Age-specific approaches should not just focus on abstinence; the use of harm reduction approaches should take into account quality of life
Risk factors:	
• social isolation and exclusion • personal, social, and functional losses • mental health challenges • presence of chronic medical conditions	

biological organism of the body" (Chappell, 2008, p. 128). The bio-medical framing of mental illness emphasizes that the pathology or the location of the "problem" is in the individual, specifically their brain (biology and chemistry). It can be known (and diagnosed) through the clinical assessment and evaluation of specific and observable categorical symptoms, using the Diagnostic and Statistical Manual (DSM-5). With each revision of the DSM, new "disorders" are created or expanded upon – and sometimes, as with homosexuality and masturbation – are de-medicalized and removed. Treatment is focussed on cure, primarily through the use of medications and the alleviation and/or elimination of symptoms. Social control is exerted through the role of "experts" and "systems" (psychiatrists, scientists, drug companies) and their *authority and power* to define and label people, behaviours, and things (Conrad, 2007, p. 8). Social control is also exerted in the legislation and laws that are used to "protect" individuals diagnosed with mental illness for "their own good" or "to protect others and society at large" (Spencer, 2009).

The process of medicalization infiltrates all aspects of people's lives, specifically the ways social problems are understood and managed (Suissa, 2009). Individuals and groups who are the most socially excluded and marginalized in society are more likely to be subject to the medicalization of their behaviours. While Suissa (2009) uses the example of the medicalization of people with addictions to emphasize this point, in general, the assertion that the medicalization of any behaviour should be understood as a form of social control can be applied to many marginalized communities (p. 44). Older adults are particularly susceptible to the medicalization of their symptoms and behaviours, which are often attributed or mislabelled as being outcomes or responses to the aging process. Magoteaux and Bonniver (2009), for example, assert that the accuracy of assessing personality disorders in older adults is often distorted by ageist stereotypes and a lack of understanding of cultural and cohort-based contexts (p. 19). The diagnostic categorization of the *"eccentric and crazy old lady"* who is *"resistant to care"* as "disordered" is problematic. Based on this, any ensuing interventions can unintentionally be disempowering, paternalistic, and discriminatory. Yet, whether intentional or not, mental health (and addictions), systems of treatment, and care are currently built around this biased understanding of mental illness. Many older adults will find themselves, voluntarily or involuntarily, seeking and getting help within this context, as will social workers find themselves working.

Challenges to medicalization

Social models of mental health were conceptualized in resistance to its medicalization. Influenced by the disability movement, these models reject the stigmatizing reductionism of identities and experiences to diagnostic labels (Tew, 2005). In Table 9.3, we have outlined the differences between the two models and how they influence treatment.

In the definitions provided in Table 9.1, you will note the inclusion of the term "mental wellness", which presents an alternative worldview or understanding of mental health challenges. Although the bio-medical worldview of mental illness dominates, many culturally specific frameworks or perspectives challenge this discourse and resist narrow definitions of the etiology of mental health. Attitudes and beliefs about mental health are culturally situated and constructed. They are shaped by personal knowledge and experiences, cultural stereotypes and beliefs, the media, stigma, and institutional practices (Choudhry, Mani, Mong, & Khan, 2016). For example, Indigenous perspectives on mental health challenge the individualist dualism inherent in a deficits and pathology model that permeates Eurocentric or Western thought. In many instances, diagnostic labels used in Western frameworks do not even exist or translate into Indigenous languages or contexts. Instead of "mentally healthy" or

Table 9.3 Bio-medical vs. social model of mental illness

Bio-medical Model	Social Model
Mental illness is an individual brain disease or disorder	Mental illness is greatly influenced by, and a product of, an unaccommodating and oppressive society, and it is not simply a medical problem.
	Mental illness as a label pathologizes problems of daily living through processes of stigma and discrimination.
Medical intervention = limit or cure of the brain disorder through medical intervention (i.e., medication/ECT)	Societal and political change required; address discrimination and accommodation
	Medical/psychosocial intervention in conjunction with structural change

"mentally ill", the term "mental wellness" is more commonly used in Indigenous contexts with a focus on holism and strengths. According to a mental wellness perspective, wellness occurs across a continuum from minimal to optimal. A person's place on the continuum at any given time is the result of internal and or external factors, with a balance of mind, body, and spirit being optimal. Most importantly, this conceptualization of wellness presumes that the well-being of the individual cannot be separate from the social collective and whole of creation (Mussell, 2014).

Stigma, discrimination, and ageism in mental health

The social model described in Table 9.2 notes the importance of identifying and addressing socio-cultural context when considering mental health. The goal is to make visible the prevalence of stigma and discrimination in the lives of individuals living with mental health challenges. Stigma and discrimination can be present at different levels simultaneously: from the interpersonal (such as through micro-aggressions) to the structural (discrimination through policies, laws, and systems). Textbox 9.2 below defines stigma and distinguishes between three types of stigma.

Textbox 9.2

Stigma and mental illness

Stigma is a "complex social process which works together to marginalize and disenfranchise people diagnosed with mental illness". The MHCC (2013) defines three types of stigma:

Self-stigma: when people with a mental health diagnosis accept and agree with negative stereotypes.
Public stigma: prejudicial attitudes and discriminatory behaviours expressed to people with a mental health diagnosis by members of the public.
Structural stigma: at levels of institutions, policies and laws people may be denied their human rights or their mental health issues are not given priority.
Discrimination is an action or behaviour that treats individuals or groups differently because of their mental health diagnosis.

Regarding micro-aggressions (see textbox 9.3), Gonzales, Davidoff, Nadal, and Yanos (2015) explored examples of micro-aggressions that people living with mental illness experience. These include one's experiences with mental illness being minimized; seeing all feelings and behaviours as potentially problematic; the denial of individual agency; assuming lower intelligence and abilities; a fear of contamination; and shaming. Familiarity with micro-aggressions which can be verbal or non-verbal and include actions such as eye-rolling, ignoring, turning away, and silencing, is critical knowledge for AOP social workers to have in their work with older adults from equity-seeking groups.

Textbox 9.3

Micro-aggressions

Micro-aggressions are the "everyday verbal, nonverbal, and environmental slights, snubs, or insults, whether intentional or unintentional, that communicate hostile, derogatory, or negative messages to target persons based solely upon their marginalized group membership" (Sue, 2010, p. 3).

Stigma and discrimination can prevent individuals with a mental health diagnosis from accessing basic economic and social resources, including employment and education; prevent them from accessing treatment and care because of fear and shame; or exclude them from services that are specific to their culture, age, gender, and/or other aspects of their identity. Systems do not just discriminate against people with a mental health diagnosis; they may also exclude certain categories of people within this group, including older adults and/or other equity- seeking groups. Older adults experience unique forms of oppression in the mental health system when taking into account ageism and other forms of oppression.

Mental health practice, policy, and research have historically tended to exclude older adults (MacCourt, 2008). This trickles down into the mental health care systems that older adults need to access. Though not well studied, ageism is present in these systems through the ageist attitudes of practitioners and clinicians, their training and education, assessment and diagnostic tools,[2] and the availability and sites of treatment and care. Mental health practitioners have shown age-related bias and discrimination in both their perceptions of the relationship between mental health and older adults, and the ways they treat them (Bodner, Palgi, & Wyman, 2018). For example, the perception that poor mental health, including depression or low mood is considered a natural and normal consequence of aging is quite common. This incorrect perception illustrates how bias and stigma can lead to discriminatory practices. For example, in long-term care facilities in Canada, over 44% of older adults were diagnosed as or showed symptoms of being depressed. Of this number, only 18% were actively being treated for their depression, with the assumption being that depression was a normal part of aging in long-term care (CIHI, 2010).

The belief that mental health challenges are simply a part of aging results in the inequitable allocation of mental health resources for older adults. Older adults are less frequently referred and assessed, most likely to be given medications to treat symptoms, and less likely to receive psycho-social and alternative supports to treatment (MacCourt, 2008). Misidentification and under-reporting of mental health and substance mis/use issues for older adults naturally follow this. Like mental health, substance mis/use has been misperceived as a younger person's problem, so older adults are under-represented in the research and practice literature that informs systems of care and treatment (Koechl, Unger, & Fischer, 2012, p. 543). Because of this, substance mis/use is often missed or misdiagnosed in older adults, and its signs and symptoms are often attributed to "getting older" (mobility, dementia, memory loss, social isolation). In general, the use of mental health services among older adults is lower than any other age cohort (Quinn, Laidlaw, & Murray, 2009). The most frequently identified barriers include personal beliefs (*I don't need help*); mistrust and negative attitudes of care providers; not believing treatment would work; and not wanting to talk with strangers about private affairs (Brenes, Danhauer, Lyles, Hogan, & Miller, 2015).

From a legal perspective, Spencer (2009) notes that guardianship legislation addressing mental capacity and decision-making are predisposed to being both ageist and sanist, thereby acting as tools of social control for the old. Older adults are most likely to have their mental capacity called into question – especially those who are very old and/or those diagnosed with dementia. Spencer further states that, relating to mental capacity and mental health, older adults are commonly not consulted or are circumvented in regards to decision-making (see **Deconstructing risk and frailty**).

Tools used to assess and diagnose mental illness in older adults have also been noted as problematic. Generally, the DSM has been critiqued for its lack of attention to the socio-political and cultural context of emotional distress; using an ethnocentric, racially biased framework; and facilitating the widening of diagnostic boundaries that have the potential to pathologize natural reactions and expressions of feelings (Burstow, 2005). These are all relevant to aging, and there are also specific issues related to their use with older adults. The tools such as the DSM-5 and ICD-11[3] inadequately discern between age-related problems and mental illness and age differences in symptom presentation (Bodner et al., 2018). Pertaining to the diagnostic criteria linked to mental disorders and aging, research shows that distress is expressed as physical (somatic) rather than psychological complaints more commonly amongst older adults, when compared to younger adults (Mechanic & McAlpine, 2011, p. 487). Despite this, the DSM remains the gold standard for diagnosis and treatment in the mental health system. Social workers may find it challenging to resist the medical categorization of highly complex life events in the sites and sectors of care where they are working.

The role of ageism and the intersectional nature of oppression that many older adults face has not been well understood. Older lesbian, gay, bisexual, and trans adults, for example, are at higher risk of disability and poorer mental health outcomes than their heterosexual counterparts because of the multiple forms of discrimination and stigma they experience across the life course, as well as the lack of culturally safe services that address their specific needs and realities (Hoy-Ellis, Ator, Kerr, & Milford, 2016). For Indigenous Elders, mental wellness challenges can be linked to colonial oppression across the life course, including but not limited to experiences in residential schools and the persistence of social and political inequities (Mussell, 2014). There is an assertion that the history of mental illness and of racism are closely intertwined, yet there is limited research on what that looks like in the context of older adults in Canada. Both bio-medical psychiatry and racism rely on interlocking forms of oppression, which make possible the denial of personhood, potential, and rights that occurs in the interaction between marginalized people and formal mental health systems and institutions (Mad in America, 2013).

Application to practice

This section will focus on exploring how AOG social workers can introduce and apply three models/approaches to support older adults who are dealing with mental health challenges (and substance mis/use or a combination). These include **recovery, harm reduction,** and **trauma-informed**. We centre this discussion on the case of Estella in order to ground the information in practice.

Estella

Estella is a 78-year-old Jamaican-Canadian woman who has recently moved into supportive housing. Previously, she experienced insecure housing, and she had been moving between boarding homes and homeless shelters. Much of this appears to be linked to her long history of mental health challenges and substance misuse. The psychiatrist on the mental health team has diagnosed her as having Borderline Personality Disorder. Her admission chart notes the following symptoms: inflexibility and resistance to care, anti-social behaviour, emotional instability, Type 1 Diabetes, poor personal hygiene, short-term memory loss and poor recall, and hypertension.

Estella emigrated with her mother from Jamaica when she was eight years old. Her mother died when she was 10 years old. She lived with her aunt until she began to show signs of "problem behaviours" and was taken into care at age 13 when her aunt said, "she couldn't take it anymore" and Estella was placed in a group home. Estella was married at age 18 and had two daughters by the age of 21. She described her marriage as "volatile". She separated from her husband 20 years ago and was able to work part time in retail until 10 years ago when her daughters noted a decline in her functional and cognitive abilities. She lost her employment and then her apartment. Her daughters tried to intervene and support her, but she was resistant and has a distant relationship with them. A combination of housing and financial insecurity has resulted in some untreated medical challenges. Estella describes her placement in the supportive housing building as "the last straw" and is resistant to accepting care and support from the staff and the mental health team. She is adamant that she wants to leave.

The psychiatrist on the mental health team has confirmed the diagnosis of Borderline Personality disorder. This diagnosis relates to pervasive disturbance, including impulsivity and emotional distress within an individual's personality and behaviour that often has a negative effect on social functioning and relationships.

Central to Estella's treatment and care from the team and the supportive housing staff is the consistent administration of medication; management of "problematic" behaviours or symptoms; and ensuring compliance to the regulation of abstinence from alcohol use.

Estella is skeptical of her diagnosis and the intervention of the mental health team. She is resistant to the use of the medications, explaining that "they make me feel not normal" and "like I am not living in reality". She denies drinking excessively and states, "I just like a nip to keep me on the straight and narrow". She feels that the other residents and staff at the site are the problem – she says they are racist and treat her as if she is a child. They are always trying to tell her what to do and all she wants is "peace and quiet". The staff complain of her "manipulative" and "overly dramatic" behaviours and her resistance to taking her medications.

Recovery model

Mainstream bio-medical models of mental health treatment tend to view recovery as a linear process consisting of the expert driven identification of clinical symptoms, leading to diagnosis and then to a specific treatment protocol. In reaction to this and conceived as an alternative to an emphasis on clinical symptomatology, the recovery model was introduced to situate recovery as a process that provides a holistic view of people with mental illness, one that focusses on the person, not just their symptoms. Recovery practice does not necessarily mean returning back to "life before" symptoms, but instead focusses on learning to *live a new life with* the condition (Jacob, 2015,

p. 119). The central tenet of the recovery model is that people who are living with mental illness can and do recover, not as a result of the elimination of symptoms or behaviours, but rather because they are living a *satisfying life beyond their psychiatric diagnosis* (Carpenter, 2002, p. 88). The principles and values informing the recovery model (see Figure 9.2) fit well with social work values and address many of the challenges social workers may have working in mainstream mental health systems.

Though there is limited application of recovery to older adults, it could be useful in treatment and care because it emphasizes autonomy and agency in goal setting and treatment. Daley, Newton, Slade, Murray, and Banerjee (2012) caution that there is a difference in "recovery" goals for older adults than for younger and middle-age adults, especially as it relates to aging outcomes such as physical and cognitive changes and stigma. Koder (2018) concurs and highlights that the difference in a recovery model for older adults is centred on adapting concepts to better represent the needs and realities of aging. This includes, for example, exploring and responding to the personal narratives of older adults and considering ways to facilitate agency even when there may be cognitive or physical challenges. This can be difficult in institutional or residential care settings where the incidence of mental health problems is high, yet services and supports may be minimal and most often addressed through pharmacological treatment. This requires us to reconsider non–pharmacological forms of support that could enhance a sense of agency and be open to the reduction or removal of pharmacological treatment as a baseline requirement for participation.

Recovery is an individual journey and process – and it is ultimately up to the individual to define the illness and the meaning it has in their lives (Carpenter, 2002). The social

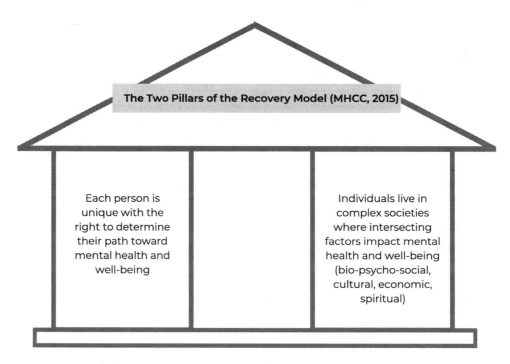

Figure 9.2 The two pillars of the recovery model (MHCC, 2015)

worker's role in working with Estella using the recovery model then would entail addressing how she understands her condition (*starting where the client is at*); identifying strengths and resiliencies she can draw on; allowing for voice and choice in relation to care planning, goal setting, and medication use; and making visible the presence and power of stigma and marginalization in her life. People who are socially isolated and who live on the margins, especially those who are older and racialized like Estella, are more likely to lose control of their ability to make decisions about their own lives. As such, the social worker may want to explore the process and specific incident(s) that brought Estella to the facility in the first place. Why was she placed? Were other options explored? What are her wishes?

While recovery is central to the most recent Canadian Mental Health Strategy (MHCC, 2015), there has been resistance to its implementation, especially in the context of medicalized settings that tend to be hierarchical and expert driven. On the other hand, recovery has been critiqued for not being anti-oppressive because it still situates the "problem" in the individual, rather than the environment or social world; it may not appeal to people from more collectivist cultures; and it ignores how social, economic and political processes may cause someone to be unable to recover (Poole, 2011). Poole (2011) suggests a focus on *critical recovery* – derived from narrative deconstruction or counter-stories – and alternative understandings of what living with a mental health diagnosis may look like and choices made related to "getting better". This critical approach also takes into account the impacts of oppression (such as the naming of racism, ageism, poverty) and working to address them. This means working to ensure access to rights, funding, services, housing, and other material supports that many people living with mental health diagnoses may be excluded from, including Estella.

A trauma-informed approach to mental health practice

As was noted in **Mapping trauma across the life course**, trauma-informed practice operates from the acknowledgement and awareness of the potential impacts of past traumas on current situations. The relationship between trauma, mental health, and substance mis/use are significant and well documented (SAMHSA, 2004). Despite this, trauma often goes unexplored and acknowledged in the lives of older adults within sites and sectors of care. In exploring mental health services, Harris and Fallot (2001) described "being trauma informed" as two different things:

> First to be trauma informed means to know the history of past and current abuse in the life of the consumer with whom one is working. Such information allows for more holistic and integrated treatment planning. But, second … to be trauma informed means to understand the role that violence and victimization plays in the life of most consumers of mental health services and substance abuse services and to use that understanding to design service systems that accommodate the vulnerabilities of trauma survivors.
>
> (p. 4)

Using a trauma-informed analysis, several issues across Estella's life course are foregrounded. These include the impact of immigration as a racialized woman at a young age; the loss of her mother and placement in a residential care setting at the age of 13; and the reality of precarious housing and homelessness. Childhood trauma (or adverse childhood experiences) has been linked to increased risk for mental health, substance mis/use, breakdowns in social relationships and poor health outcomes as people age. Contextual factors informed by the "intersection of race, class, gender ... add to the complex and disproportionate exposure to trauma" of individuals and groups who experience historical trauma, marginalization, and oppression (CSWE, 2012, p. 2; see also CSWE, 2015). Relating to Estella's housing insecurity and homelessness, there is a relationship between childhood trauma and risk of homelessness in adulthood and between mental illness, substance mis/use, and homelessness (Gulliver & Campney, 2015). For others, the trauma occurs because of being homeless. Often, a history of trauma makes it difficult for individuals to leave the streets because of long-standing coping mechanisms and life choices. Solutions will not be simple for someone like Estella who has a history of housing insecurity and street entrenchment, and who has faced multiple forms of oppression, especially marginalization, violence, and powerlessness, based on her race, gender, age, and mental health status.

Using a trauma-informed approach with Estella, the social worker would attempt to reframe "problem behaviours" as attempts to deal with past traumas and experiences. As noted by Haskell (2003), within this context, "disorders" that are seen as "responses" and "symptoms" become instead "adaptations". The question a social worker would want to focus on with the team is "What has happened to Estella?" rather than "What is wrong with Estella?" and subsequently attempt to make links to current issues and concerns. Intervention would focus on upholding trauma-informed principles of safety (personal/emotional, physical and cultural), preventing re-traumatization, working collaboratively and providing choice in care and treatment, and focussing on strengths rather than pathologies. All of these approaches are often antithetical to current bio-medical practices. For example, placement in structured, institutional settings is significantly problematic for people like Estella because staff are often not aware of traumas that many of their residents have experienced and their impacts. In turn, older adults may be placed in settings where the highly regulated environment and the procedural nature of care can re-trigger and exacerbate emotional and behavioural responses that are then understood as being related to their mental health diagnosis. The social worker should consider how Estella's resistance to care could be linked to her childhood placement, and/or to her experience of systemic racism and cultural isolation within the institutional care setting (Mullings, 2006). Making this link explicit to the care team would be useful in helping to identify ways in which their interventions may re-trigger or re-traumatize her.

Harm reduction

> From the mental health team's perspective, Estella is at risk for a number of social and health based harms: potential exacerbation of symptoms due to the interaction of medications and alcohol; risk of falling and physical outcomes; risk of being evicted from assisted living facility; risk of social isolation.

Eliminating risk from older adult's lives can result in a significant loss of self-determination and autonomy in the decision-making process (see **Deconstructing risk and frailty**). Harm reduction is an approach that social workers can adopt in order to address the reality of "risk" in their client's lives. It reflects many of the fundamental values of social work, including the inherent worth and dignity of individuals, collaboration, and client self-determination. Harm reduction has traditionally been applied to the treatment of substance mis/use and is also compatible when applied to managing mental illness, especially when there is evidence of concurrent disorders. Harm reduction is considered Best Practice and should be applied to the lives of older adults *broadly* as it relates to their quality of life (Health Canada, 2004).

Harm reduction can be defined as "policies, programs and practices that aim to reduce the negative health and social consequences that ensue from the use of (legal and illegal) substances without necessarily reducing the use of them" (Anbar, Buckland, Hope, Layland, & Peckham, 2012, p. i). The focus of harm reduction then is not to eliminate the use of substances or behaviours, but to improve quality of life as defined by the older person. Mancini and Wyrick-Waugh (2013) describe three harm-reduction practices specific to mental health and substance mis/use:

1.   Low threshold access to supports and service: Clients should be able to access support regardless of whether they are "actively using" or are resistant to prescribed treatment including medication and/or therapy;
2.   Unconditional support and motivational strategies to engage and assist in a move to healthy behaviours; and
3.   Education and practical guidance to reduce harm and enhance recovery (p. 14).

A harm-reduction approach for Estella would focus not on "compliance" behaviours, but rather on the mitigation of harms that come from her choices or that facilitate these choices. For example, addressing factors like poverty, social isolation, racism, and sanism that have influenced and still impact her current situation would also explicitly become part of the intervention plan. For many older adults who have been dealing with mental illness and substance mis/use over a long period of time, the goal of abstinence or "cure" is not necessary or realistic (Health Canada, 2004). A harm reduction approach would better acknowledge the complexities of Estella's life situation both past and present. This includes recognition of the cumulative nature of social determinants of health like poverty, gender, race, social isolation, and lack of housing (MHCC, 2011, p. 30) that are prominent in Estella's case and undoubtedly impact her functioning .

A harm reduction approach allows social workers and other mental health professionals to more comprehensively focus on non-stigmatizing, non-judgmental approaches that minimize risks and their consequences and that are inclusive of the older adult's voice and wishes. Using this approach with Estella as the team social worker, your role would be to inform and educate team members about the ways in which labelling behaviours as "non-compliant" increases experiences of stigma. Behaviours can then be reframed from "deliberate individual choices" to "ways of coping and managing adverse events across her life". Educating other team members can be a challenging task as many practitioners in the field of mental health operate using a bio-medical lens. As such, de-centring mental health professionals from being experts who need to "fix" the person to a support role in which the older adult is positioned as the expert in their own life takes time and a commitment (Lago, Peter, & Bogus, 2017).

Another important social work role is related to reducing the potential impacts and harms that substance mis/use can have on intervention outcomes. Estella frames her alcohol use as a way to "keep her on the straight and narrow". This could be understood as a form of self-medication or a way in which to maintain her social functioning. Social workers should be careful not to pathologize the use of substances in older adult's lives, without understanding both history and context. It would be useful to explore Estella's relationship to alcohol and to negotiate potential ways in which to manage use without asking her to give it up completely. This could be done collaboratively with the care team to ensure that she is safe and that use is managed, especially in recognition of how alcohol interacts with her other medications. For those wanting to use, regardless of where they are living and under what constraints they are under, they are most likely to find ways to access their substance of choice. Acknowledging and negotiating use will help to control negative outcomes and to make Estella feel as if she has some control in what would otherwise be a disempowering situation.

Conclusion

To conclude this chapter, we return to Penny's narrative of recovery and wellness, which provides a useful counter-story with its focus on ageism, pathology, and sanism. Mental wellness supports for older adults need to move beyond individualized, deficit-oriented treatment models to embrace approaches that take into account the social and political impacts of living with a diagnosis of mental illness. It also requires the use of a life course perspective that makes evident how mental illness can be both the consequence and the cause of inequalities and exclusion in older adult's lives (MacCourt et al., 2011, p. 31).

Exercise

Imagine that you are the social worker assisting Penny:

- Consider what you would want to focus on to support her mental well-being.
- What would be some challenges that both you and Penny would want to address?
- What are some of Penny's strengths and resources that you could draw on to support her?
- How does her role as caregiver fit into this plan?

Takeaways

- Mental distress is often manifested differently in older adults (expressed as physical/somatic rather than psychological) and can be linked to changes in physical and cognitive functioning, social and relational losses, co-morbid conditions, and increased use of medications.
- Ageism and sanism (and other forms of oppression) intersect to create unique forms of stigma and discrimination in the care and support of older adults with mental health challenges, including attitudes and actions of care providers, tools used to assess and diagnose, and treatment options and accessibility.
- Older adults would benefit from aging specific mental health services and supports that attend to a holistic view of mental health and well-being and that use a life course perspective to make links between micro and macro barriers and strengths.

Additional resources

- Health Canada (2015). *First Nations Continuum Wellness Framework*. Ottawa: ON. https://thunderbirdpf.org/wp-content/uploads/2015/01/24-14-1273-FN-Mental-Wellness-Framework-EN05_low.pdf
- Canadian Centre on Substance Abuse. (2009*). Substance Abuse in Canada: Concurrent Disorders*. Ottawa, ON: Canadian Centre on Substance Abuse. www.ccsa.ca/sites/default/files/2019-04/ccsa-011811-2010.pdf
- CAMH Health Aging Project (2006). *Responding to older adults with substance use, mental health and gambling challenges: A guide for workers and volunteers.* www.camh.ca/-/media/files/guides-and-publications/responding-to-older-adults-en.pdf
- Canadian Mental Health Association: https://cmha.ca/
- Canadian Coalition for Seniors Mental Health: https://ccsmh.ca/

Notes

1 Homosexuality was first identified in 1952 as a mental disorder in the *Diagnostic and Statistical Manual* (DSM) and was not removed until 1973.
2 Examples of these screening and assessment tools (other than the DSM 5):
   - Geriatric Depression Scale (GDS): https://web.stanford.edu/~yesavage/GDS.html
   - SIGECAPS: http://webmedia.unmc.edu/intmed/geriatrics/reynolds/pearlcards/depression/sigecaps.htm
   - Cornell Scale for Depression in Dementia: www.scalesandmeasures.net/files/files/The%20Cornell%20Scale%20for%20Depression%20in%20Dementia.pdf
   - Centre for Epidemiological Studies Depression Scale (CES-D): www.chcr.brown.edu/pcoc/cesdscale.pdf
   - SMAST – Geriatric Version (alcohol use in older adults): www.healthvermont.gov/sites/default/files/documents/pdf/ADAP_SMAST-G.pdf

   While not specific to older adults, examples of screening and assessment tools for substance mis/use:
   - CAGE-AID: www.integration.samhsa.gov/images/res/CAGEAID.pdf
   - Drug Abuse Screen Test (DAST): www.sbirtoregon.org/wp-content/uploads/DAST-English-pdf.pdf

3 ICD – International Classification of Diseases (11th edition) World Health Organization

References

Anbar, M., Buckland, D., Hope, S., Layland, L., & Peckham, M. (2012, December). *Harm reduction policy for social work practice: Policy considerations for the Ontario College of Social Workers and Social Service Workers*. Toronto, ON: Canadian Harm Reduction Network. Retrieved from http://fileserver.idpc.net/library/Harm_reduction_policy_for_social_work_practice.pdf.

Bodner, E., Palgi, Y., & Wyman, M. F. (2018). Ageism in mental health assessment and treatment of older adults. In L. Ayalon & C. Tesch-Römer (Eds.), *Contemporary perspectives on ageism: International perspectives on aging* (Vol. 19, pp. 241–262). Cham: Springer.

Brenes, G. A., Danhauer, S. C., Lyles, M. F., Hogan, P. E., & Miller, M. E. (2015). Barriers to mental health treatment in rural older adults. *American Journal of Geriatric Psychiatry*, *23*(11), 1172–1178. doi:10.1016/j.jagp.2015.06.002.

Burstow, B. (2005). A critique of PTSD and the DSM. *Journal of Humanistic Psychology*, *45*(4), 429–445. doi:10.1177/0022167805280265.

Canadian Institute for Health Information (CIHI) (2010). Depression among seniors in residential care: Analysis in brief. Retrieved from https://secure.cihi.ca/free_products/ccrs_depression_among_se niors_e.pdf.

Carpenter, J. (2002). Mental health recovery paradigm: Implications for social work. *Health and Social Work*, 2(1), 86–94. doi:10.1093/hsw/27.2.86.

Chappell, N. (2008). Aging and mental health. *Social Work in Mental Health*, 7(1–3), 122–138. doi:10.1080/15332980802072454.

Choudhry, F. R., Mani, V., Ming, L. C., & Khan, T. M. (2016). Beliefs and perception about mental health issues: A meta-synthesis. *Neuropsychiatric Disease and Treatment*, 31. doi:10.2147/NDT.S111543.

Conrad, P. (2007). *The medicalization of society: On the transformation of human conditions into treatable disorders*. Baltimore, MD: John Hopkins University Press.

Council on Social Work Education (CSWE). (2012). *Advanced social work practice in trauma*. Retrieved from https://www.cswe.org/getattachment/Accreditation/Other/EPAS-Implemen tation/TraumabrochurefinalforWeb.pdf.aspx.

Council on Social Work Education (CSWE). (2015). Specialized practice curricular guide for trauma-informed social work practice. Retrieved from www.cswe.org/getattachment/Education-Resources/2015-Curricular-Guides/2015EPAS_TraumaInformedSW_Final-WEB.pdf.

Daley, S., Newton, D., Slade, M., Murray, J., & Banerjee, S. (2013). Development of a framework for recovery in older people with mental disorder. *International Journal of Geriatric Psychiatry*, 28(5), 522–529. doi: 10.1002/gps.3855.

Flint, A., Merali, Z., & Vaccarino, F. (Eds.). (2018). *Substance use in Canada: Improving quality of life: Substance use and aging*. Ottawa, ON: Canadian Centre on Substance Use and Addiction. Retrieved from www.ccsa.ca/sites/default/files/2019-04/CCSA-Substance-Use-and-Aging-Report-2018-en.pdf.

Gonzales, L., Davidoff, K. C., Nadal, K. L., & Yanos, P. T. (2015). Micro-aggressions experienced by persons with mental illnesses: An exploratory study. *Psychiatric Rehabilitation Journal*, 38(3), 234–241. doi:10.1037%2Fprj0000096.

Gormley, D., & Quinn, N. (2009). Mental health stigma and discrimination: The experience within social work. *Practice: Social Work in Action*, 21(4), 259–272. doi:10.1080/09503150902993621.

Gulliver, T., & Campney, A. (2012). Healing the pain and hurt: Dealing with the trauma of homelessness. In Inclusion Working Group, Canadian Observatory on Homelessness (Eds.), *Homelessness is only one piece of the puzzle: Implications for policy and practice* (pp. 136–151). Toronto, ON: Canadian Observatory on Homelessness. Retrieved from https://homelesshub.ca/sites/default/files/23%20-%20Trauma%20Informed%20Services.pdf.

Harris, M., & Fallot, R. D. (Eds.). (2001). *New directions for mental health services: Using trauma theory to design service systems*. San Francisco, CA: Jossey-Bass.

Health Canada. (2004). Best practices: Using harm reduction. Aging in Canada Best Practices Information Sheets #3. Retrieved from www.agingincanada.ca/Best_3.pdf.

Haskell, L. (2003). *First stage trauma treatment: A guide for mental health professionals working with women*. Toronto, ON: Centre for Addiction and Mental Health.

Hoy-Ellis, C. P., Ator, M., Kerr, C., & Milford, J. (2016). Innovative approaches addressing aging and mental health needs in LGBTQ communities. *Generations*, 40(2), 56–62. Retrieved from www.ncbi.nlm.nih.gov/pmc/articles/PMC5375170/.

Jacob, K. S. (2015). Recovery model of mental illness: A complementary approach to psychiatric care. *Indian Journal of Psychological Medicine*, 37(2), 117–119.

Koder, D. (2018). Recovery oriented care for older people: Staff attitudes and practices. *International Journal of Psycho-social Rehabilitation*, 22(2), 46–54. Retrieved from www.psychosocial.com/IJPR_22/Recovery_Koder.html.

Koechl, B., Unger, A., & Fischer, G. (2012). Age-related aspects of addictions. *Gerontology*, 58(6), 540–544. doi:10.1159/000339095.

Lago, R. R., Peter, E., & Bogus, C. M. (2017). Harm reduction and tensions in trust and distrust in a mental health service a qualitative approach. *Substance Abuse, Treatment, Prevention, and Policy, 12*(12), 1–9. doi:10.1186/s13011-017-0098-1.

Larson, G. (2008). Anti-oppressive practice in mental health. *Journal of Progressive Human Services, 19*(1), 39–54. doi:10.1080/10428230802070223.

MacCourt, P. (2008). Promoting senior's well-being: The senior's mental health policy lens toolkit. BC Psychogeriatric Association. Retrieved from www.mentalhealthcommission.ca/sites/default/files/Seniors_Seniors_Mental_Health_Policy_Lens_Toolkit_ENG_0_1.pdf.

MacCourt, P., Wilson, K., & Tourigny-Rivard, M.-F. (2011). *Guidelines for comprehensive mental health services for older adults in Canada.* Seniors Advisory Committee, Mental Health Commission of Canada. Retrieved from www.mentalhealthcommission.ca/sites/default/files/2017-09/mhcc_seniors_guidelines_0.pdf.

Mad in America (2013). The intersection between race and mental illness. Retrieved from www.madinamerica.com/2013/01/the-intersection-between-race-and-mental-illness/.

Magoteaux, A. L., & Bonniver, J. H. (2009). Distinguishing between personality disorders, stereotypes, and eccentricities in older adults. *Journal of Psychosocial Nursing and Mental Health Services, 47*(7), 19–24.

Mancini, M. A., & Wyrick-Waugh, W. (2013). Consumer and practitioner perceptions of the harm reduction approach in a community mental health setting. *Community Mental Health Journal, 49*(1), 14–24. doi:10.1007/s10597-011-9451-4.

Mechanic, D., & McAlpine, D. D. (2011). Mental health and aging: A life-course perspective. In R. A. Settersten, Jr. & J. L. Angel (Eds.), *Handbook of sociology of aging, handbooks of sociology and social research* (pp. 477–493). Springer. doi:10.1007/978-1-4419-7374-0_30.

Mental Health Commission of Canada. (2011). Guidelines for comprehensive mental health services for older adults in canada: Executive summary. Retrieved from www.mentalhealthcommission.ca/sites/default/files/Seniors_MHCC_Seniors_Guidelines_ExecutiveSummary_ENG_0_1.pdf.

Mental Health Commission of Canada. (2013). *Opening Minds: Interim Report.* Retrieved from www.mentalhealthcommission.ca/sites/default/files/opening_minds_interim_report_0.pdf.

Mental Health Commission of Canada (2015). *Guidelines for recovery-oriented practice.* Retrieved from www.mentalhealthcommission.ca/sites/default/files/2016-07/MHCC_Recovery_Guidelines_2016_ENG.PDF.

Morley, C. (2003). Towards critical social work practice in mental health. *Journal of Progressive Social Services, 14*(1), 61–84. doi:10.1300/J059v14n01_05.

Mullings, D. V. (2006). Policy needs of older Caribbean Canadian women: A long term care discussion. *Caribbean Journal of Social Work, 5*, 143–158. Retrieved from: https://www.researchgate.net/publication/264416446.

Mussell, B. (2014). Mental health from an indigenous perspective. In P. Menzies & L. F. Lavalee (Eds.), *Journey to Healing: Aboriginal Perspectives with Addiction and Mental Health* (pp. 187–199). Toronto, ON: CAMH.

National Initiative for the Care of the Elderly (NICE). (n.d.). *Introduction to older adults and substance use.* Retrieved from www.nicenet.ca/tools-introduction-to-older-adults-and-substance-use.

Poole, J. (2011). *Behind the rhetoric: Mental health recovery in Ontario.* Halifax, NS: Fernwood Publishing.

Poole, J., Jivraj, T., Arslanian, A., Bellows, K., Chiasson, S., Hakimy, H., … Reid, J. (2012). Sanism, 'mental health' and social work education: A review and call to action. *Intersectionalities, 1*, 20–36. Retrieved from www.researchgate.net/publication/262374063_Sanism_'mental_health'_and_social_workeducation_A_review_and_call_to_action.

Quinn, K. M., Laidlaw, K., & Murray, L. K. (2009). Older people's attitudes to mental illness. *Clinical Psychology and Psychotherapy, 16*(1), 33–45. doi:10.1002/cpp.598.

Scheyett, A. (2005). The mark of madness: Stigma, serious mental illnesses, and social work. *Social Work in Mental Health: The Journal of Behavioral and Psychiatric Social Work, 3*(4), 79–97. doi:10.1300/J200v03n04_05.

Spencer, C. (2009). Ageism and the law: Emerging concepts and practices in housing and health. Law Commission of Ontario. Retrieved from www.lco-cdo.org/wp-content/uploads/2014/01/older-adults-commissioned-paper-spencer.pdf.

Substance Abuse and Mental Health Services Administration (SAMHSA). (2014). *SAMHSA's concept of trauma and guidance for a trauma-informed approach.* Retrieved from https://store.samhsa.gov/system/files/sma14-4884.pdf.

Sue, D. W. (2010). *Microaggressions and marginality: Manifestation, dynamics and impact.* Hoboken, NJ: John Wiley and Sons, Inc.

Suissa, A. J. (2009). Medicalization and addictions: Markers and psycho-social issues. *Canadian Social Work Review, 26*(1), 43–58. Retrieved from www.jstor.org/stable/41669901.

Tew, J. (2005). *Social perspectives in mental health: Developing social models to understand and work with mental distress.* London: Jessica Kingsley Publishing.

World Health Organization. (2014). *Mental health: A state of well-being.* Retrieved from www.who.int/features/factfiles/mental_health/en/.

Chapter 10

Addressing mistreatment and violence

Questions to consider as you read this chapter

- Why do you think older adults show reluctance to self-disclose and seek support in relation to mistreatment and violence in their lives?
- To what degree should we "protect" older adults?
- What ethical challenges can you identify in addressing mistreatment and violence in the lives of older adults?
- What anti-oppressive knowledge and skills can be used when addressing and investigating mistreatment and violence in the lives of older adults?

Here are some common images of older adult mistreatment represented in the media and within society more generally:

- A "little old lady" who has been scammed by telemarketers;
- Nursing home residents confined to their wheelchairs or their beds and not provided proper care;
- An 'elderly' widower who has been targeted by an online dating site "catfish-er";
- Family members who have taken financial advantage of their "elderly" parents;
- "Elderly" hoarders who live in homes filled to the ceiling with "garbage".

In these scenarios, the older adults are portrayed as being frail, vulnerable, victimized, and in need of protection. While these are common representations, the mistreatment and violence against older adults is much more complex than the sensationalized and de-contextualized way it is often portrayed. The representations above only show one component of violence and mistreatment. They exclude other "faces" and "experiences" or types of violence that older adults may face – especially those whose stories are often hidden and marginalized in the discourse of outrage that we often see in the mainstream media. Consider these:

- An older lesbian woman moving into a care setting who feels she must hide her identity out of fear of being "outed" or "mistreated";
- Living in a rural community and the only care facility is 50 kilometres away, meaning older adults who need long-term support (i.e. residential care) will be placed far away from family and community supports;
- Living in a long-term, violent intimate partner relationship and feeling obligated to act as a caregiver to the perpetrator;

- Older adult immigrants who are sponsored by their families and who feel they are isolated in the home and "forced" to spend many hours cleaning, cooking, and providing care;
- Indigenous Elders who are still "waiting" for residential school compensation from the federal government;
- Incarcerated older adults who have no access to adequate care or treatment as they age.

These examples are thought provoking and potentially challenging. In this book, we discuss the impacts of ageism and other forms of oppression on the life course experiences of older adults. However, this chapter really speaks to and illustrates their "extreme" outcomes. Exposure to violence and mistreatment can elicit a number of different feelings and reactions on the part of social workers and other professionals. As a social worker, you may feel triggered, angry, scared, sad, vulnerable, powerless, and ethically compromised. You may assume that mistreatment and violence is overt and easily identifiable, but it is not. You will struggle to find appropriate practice frameworks or "best practices" outside of the legal and criminal justice systems from which to draw to guide your interventions. It can be difficult work.

Like many of the topics covered in this book, the realities of mistreatment and violence among older adults are not well explored in the research and practice literature; when they are, the exploration tends to focus on the more common experiences we noted at the beginning. The ways we think about the relationship between mistreatment and violence and older adults is centred on the concept of "*elder abuse and neglect*", which is understood as something that happens *to* (individual) older adults because of their old age, and almost always in an interpersonal context where they are particularly vulnerable (families, relationships, and strangers). A singular individualistic (age-based) and/or relational focus neglects the exploration of structural and socio-cultural factors that create and facilitate the conditions for mistreatment and violence as a person ages, or as it carries on from the past.

In this chapter, we explore violence and mistreatment in the lives of older adults by de-centring the personal (individual) in order to render the structural more apparent. This means critically examining the systems, practices, and processes that create, support, and facilitate violence and mistreatment in older adults' lives. What is it about aging and being a woman and/or a member of a marginalized community that potentially exposes someone to violence and mistreatment from others? How are mistreatment and violence supported and reinforced in specific socio-cultural and geo-political contexts? How, as AOG social workers, do we make these experiences more visible in our practice? Finally, how do we intervene in ways that respect an older adult's right to make decisions even when we may not necessarily agree with them?

The objectives of this chapter are to

- develop a critical understanding of how mistreatment and violence are conceptualized in the lives of older adults;
- explore the different ways that older adults experience mistreatment and violence, including across the life course; and
- understand the work (and interventions) that social workers can draw upon in their practice that are based upon AOP.

Elder abuse and neglect

"*Elder abuse and neglect*" (see textbox 10.1) is the common terminology used to describe and understand the mistreatment and violence that older adults experience.

Textbox 10.1

Elder abuse is "a single, or repeated act, or lack of appropriate action, occurring within any relationship where there is an expectation of trust which causes harm or distress to an older person". Elder abuse can take various forms such as financial, physical, psychological, and sexual. It can also be the result of intentional or unintentional neglect (WHO, 2002).

Access any website, textbook, research study, or resource specific to this topic and you will find a definition of types of elder abuse and descriptions of what these actions/events look like. This "list" is useful for social work practitioners, because it can help provide an indication of what to look for in practice. Figure 10.1 provides an example of this for your reference.

The term elder abuse is problematic, conceptualized as a social problem informed by ageist social discourse (Jackson, 2016; Podnieks, 2008). As you may notice from the chart in Figure 10.1, "elder abuse and neglect" is constructed as a wide-ranging social phenomenon and problem that occurs across different sites and sectors of care and types of relationships. The challenge is that there is no *one* definition or explanation of this "phenomenon" – it is rather, a group of phenomena – the only common denominator being the specifics of a person's age (Harbison et al., 2012). The difficulty with using one term to describe a multitude of experiences is that "elder abuse and neglect" mirrors dominant biomedical discourses of decline, frailty, and vulnerability in relation to older adults.

The current conceptualization of elder abuse and neglect is primarily informed by expert knowledge (research, legal, legislative, and practice). Privileging these definitions tends to discount the perspectives of older adults, both in how the problem is identified and how it is addressed. Also, expert-based definitions of abuse and mistreatment are often different from those of older adults. Research demonstrates that there are gaps between theoretical, legal, and clinical definitions of mistreatment used by professionals in legal, health, and social care, and the ways in which older adults themselves experience it (NICE, 2015). For example, older adults do not readily associate abusive behaviours that have occurred within their own lives as actual "elder abuse", or if they do, some types are considered more problematic than others. Older adults also have broader views about mistreatment, including the role of wider society and institutions in the facilitation and sanctioning of mistreatment (Naughton, Drennan, Lyons, & Lafferty, 2013, p. 1258). Older adults also have difficulty when experts use stigmatizing language to describe their experiences and note that "abuse" is something that "did not happen to them" while "mistreatment" represented something "they admit happens" (WHO/IPNEA, 2002, p. 9).

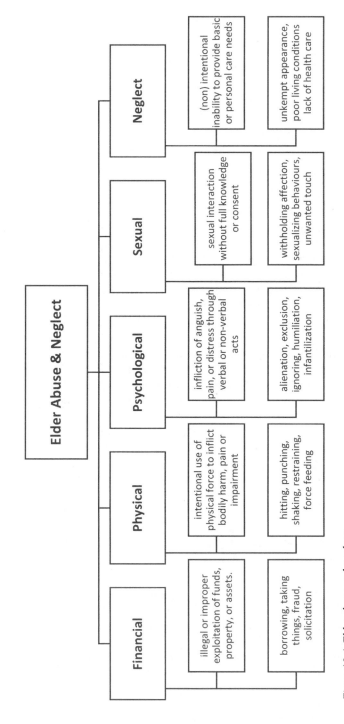

Figure 10.1 Elder abuse and neglect

To address these concerns, in this chapter we do not use the term "elder abuse and neglect" unless describing the concept, preferring instead to label these experiences as "elder mistreatment" and/or "violence". We believe that this terminology is more inclusive and reflective of the diverse types of experiences older adults have across the life course (not just when they are old) and is less stigmatizing. Still, it is important to understand that both current scholarship and resources specific to this topic will, more likely than not, use the term "elder abuse and neglect".

Current conceptualizations of elder mistreatment locate the problem in two distinct ways. First, it is interpreted as an individual problem, something that happens to an older person *because of their age* and the resulting physical and cognitive vulnerabilities that emerge as a result of aging. Second, it is primarily viewed as a "family" or relational (care) problem, something that happens in the context of a relationship with a family member or care provider, or even with strangers. The recognition and examination of structural and systemic forms of mistreatment and violence are often not included as part of this definition. For older adults who occupy marginalized social locations, experiences of mistreatment and violence extend beyond the familial and relational. Research is emerging on forms of mistreatment experienced by historically marginalized older adults that are often ignored, such as those related to forms of structural oppression including ageism, sexism, classism, and racism (Walsh et al., 2011). The recognition of structural and systemic forms of mistreatment, including the violation of human, legal, and medical rights; any deprivation of choices, decisions, status, finances, and respect; and any form of neglect, including social exclusion, isolation, and abandonment must be included as a fundamental aspect of elder mistreatment (World Health Organization, 2002, p. 10).

Finally, mistreatment and violence are experienced and understood differently across cultures. Using focus groups in a number of different countries (both in the Global North and the Global South) to understand how older adults understood and experienced mistreatment, researchers found that there were a number of differences in how older adults defined and experienced mistreatment and that beliefs about mistreatment were deeply embedded in a specific socio-cultural context (WHO/INPEA, 2002). Views about how older adults understand mistreatment is influenced by the norms, traditions, and beliefs that are central to their socio-cultural and geo-political context. This includes family roles and responsibilities, the role and status of Elders within the family and society, gender norms, and the roles and responsibilities of the state in the provision of care. For example, Doe, Han, and McCaslin (2009) posit that many Asian countries are slow to acknowledge the existence of Elder mistreatment because the tradition of filial piety (the respect and care for one's Elders) prevents them from doing so. The core values of collectivism, family harmony, filial piety, and gender role distinctions can shape whether individuals identify a specific act as abusive. In this case, a lack of respect and not caring for one's parents or Elders (for example by encouraging placement in long-term care) could be interpreted as "mistreatment".

A framework to explore and understand violence and mistreatment in older adults' lives

This section starts by defining violence and delineating the ways in which it is categorized (see textbox 10.2).

Textbox 10.2

Violence is the intentional use of force or power to dominate and control others. It can result in injury, death, psychological harm, maldevelopment, or deprivation. The WHO (2002) categorizes violence in the following ways:

Self-directed: done to oneself (suicide, self-harm).
Interpersonal: between individuals and includes family, intimate partner violence, and community (child abuse, youth violence, elder mistreatment).
Collective: groups against other groups or sets of individuals (war, genocide).

We have described some of the current problems with how elder mistreatment is conceptualized that do not necessarily fit into an AOP framework. To address this, Fraser and Seymour (2017) have drawn on a multi-dimensional framework articulated by Johann Galtung (1990) that addresses the different forms of violence that can impact individuals and communities – that goes beyond the individual experience. As well as defining **direct, structural, and cultural violence**, Galtung emphasized the **interaction** among the three and how they justify the existence of each other. According to Fraser and Seymour (2017), this framework allows for a shift away from "individually focused, behaviourally oriented conceptualizations of violence and abuse (symptoms)" (p. 22) to situating it within a broader socio-cultural context (causes). Table 10.1 provides a representation of this framework with applications to aging and older adults. **Direct violence** consists of specific actions and events that happen directly to individuals or groups. It is considered the most "visible" form of violence in that it is recognizable and prominent in cultural discourse. **Structural violence** centres around social injustice, a type of violence that explains how some groups are prevented from equal access to opportunity, resources, services, and power that are needed to fulfill human needs. **Cultural violence** represents the socio-cultural values and practices that justify and legitimize direct and structural violence (Galtung, 1990, p. 291).

Figure 10.2 provides an example of what this framework looks like when applied to sexual violence against older women. In this example, you will see how the interaction of all three forms of violence enables, embeds, and perpetuates violence against the Other. Structural and cultural violence (ageism, sexism) provides a socio-cultural context for the existence and experience of sexual violence against older women (direct violence). Galtung (1990) notes there is "a causal flow from cultural via structural to direct violence" in that the culture "teaches, admonishes, eggs on, and dulls us into seeing exploitation and/or repression as normal and natural, or into not seeing them at all" (p. 295). This is how these types of violence remain hidden. While only direct violence may be "visible" or is "identified", in cases like this example, these acts of violence remain more hidden than they may be with younger

Table 10.1 Galtung's (1990) framework of violence

Types of Violence	Description	Examples as Applied to Older Adults
Direct Violence (visible)	*actions and events*	Under the umbrella term of elder abuse and neglect: • Physical • Psychological • Sexual • Financial • Neglect Can also include: • Disease and chronic illness prevalence • Intimate-partner violence across the lifespan • Institutional mistreatment in communal care settings • Civil conflict and war (veterans, survivors)
Structural Violence (invisible)	*systems and pro- cesses*	• Enforced retirement • The Indian Act • Health care access for LGBTTsIQ older adults • High malnutrition rates for older adults • Poverty of older women • Immigration policies that exclude older adults in reunification
Cultural Violence (invisible)	*ongoing and enduring*	• Biomedical discourses on aging • Neoliberalism • Familism • Colonization • Assuming Normalcy (sanism, heterosexism, ableism)

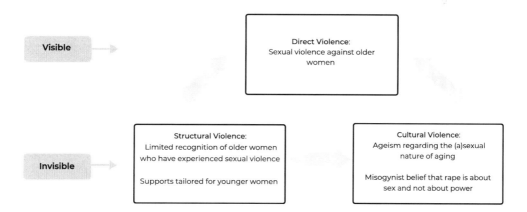

Figure 10.2 Types of sexual violence

women, primarily because of the intersectional nature of ageism and sexism and its relationship to sexual violence and older women (Bows, 2018).

Direct violence and older adults

Social workers and other professionals and organizations working to intervene with mistreatment and violence are more apt to recognize and relate to direct violence, because of its relative "visibility". Yet within the context of aging, the invisibility of even direct violence is problematic. Recent Canadian research on the prevalence of elder mistreatment noted that 8.2% of older adults aged 55 years and over who were surveyed reported experiencing some form of mistreatment, the most common being psychological (2.7%) and financial (2.6%) (NICE, 2015). A meta-analysis of global prevalence found that 15.7% of people age 60 years and over reported that they have been subjected to some sort of abuse or mistreatment, The pooled prevalence rates were highest for psychological (11.6%) and financial (6.8%) abuse (Yon, Mikton, Gassoumis, & Wilbur, 2017). These numbers do not sum to 15.7% as respondents could report more than one form of abuse. Moreover, these statistics do not represent the true extent or breadth of the issue. Under-reporting and under-recognition occur because these experiences are hidden and untreated but also because some experiences are less well examined or valued than others. Some happen to individuals by other individuals, but others happen because systems and structures themselves enact and perpetuate mistreatment and violence on older individuals.

There are a number of reasons older adults under-report, do not disclose, or do not identify what is happening to them as mistreatment or violence. As you read through the list below, consider how some of these may be situated in the *personal* (shame, fear); in the *relational* (fear of retribution, loss of relationship); and the *structural* (oppression, discrimination, exclusion).

This list is a summary of the findings of the literature on this topic, including the voices of older adults themselves:

- Ageism (not being heard, feeling powerless, feeling a lack of personhood and citizenship);
- Isolation;
- Stigma of being seen as a "victim";
- Loss of relationship;
- A lack of appropriate (cultural, linguistic, and age-specific) supports and services to report to;
- Shame, denial, and discomfort about the topic;
- A fear of retribution that may deter them from identifying incidents as "abusive";
- Language and terminology that do not represent people's experiences;
- Cultural norms and values about the treatment of older adults;
- Acceptance of mistreatment and violence across the life span that older adults may not attribute to being "old";
- Experiences of oppression that render marginalized groups invisible and ignored, so they do not disclose or are fearful of triggering past traumas.

Health and social care professionals (including social workers) are also not particularly adept at identifying when mistreatment or violence are present. Cohen (2011) notes that the rates of mistreatment and violence identified by professionals and care providers are low – even lower than the rates that are actually reported. The literature in this area posits a number of reasons professionals "miss" or ignore these signs. These include:

- Lack of awareness, education, or formal training;
- Lack of access to screening tools;
- Lack of understanding of what the "signs" of mistreatment are;
- Understanding the definition as being limited to the individual and/or relational;
- Lack of identification of structural or systemic abuses;
- Not seeing it as part of their scope of practice;
- Personal unease with the sensitivity and content of the problem;
- Time constraints in professional interventions;
- Respecting privacy for older adults;
- Skepticism that mistreatment is happening;
- Lack of knowledge about different cultural values and norms related to the treatment of older adults.

While older adults themselves often do not or cannot disclose mistreatment and violence, we should also address the fact that as practitioners (experts), we are often "disconnected" from older adults' lived experiences when they do not fit into neat definitional boxes constructed about social problems such as mistreatment.

Structural and cultural violence

As noted earlier, it is difficult to explore any of these forms of violence (relational, structural, and cultural) separately from one another because there is an interaction between them. While structural violence is enacted by the social, political, and economic policies and practices that impede or prevent well-being, they are justified and supported by cultural violence. A structural and cultural violence lens is very rarely applied to the experiences of aging, but it can be useful when exploring and understanding the relationship of mistreatment and violence to older adults who occupy marginalized positions (see, for example, Figure 10.1).

Trans and gender non-conforming older adults, for example, experience high rates of physical and sexual violence (direct violence) (Cook-Daniels & munson, 2010). In turn, they experience high rates of trauma exposure, repeat victimization, barriers to victim supports, and poor mental and physical health outcomes (Brotman, Ferrer, Sussman, Ryan, & Richard, 2015; Finkenauer, Sherratt, Marlow, & Brodey, 2012). The structural violence perpetrated against older trans and gender non-conforming adults is further facilitated and perpetuated by the intersection of transphobia and ageism experienced inside the LGBTTsIQ community and in homophobia, ageism, and transphobia within the broader society.

The experiences of Indigenous Elders with respect to elder mistreatment and violence also illustrates the impacts of structural violence across the life course. Violence, oppression, and discrimination are fundamental features of colonization (both historic and current). Indigenous Elders' current vulnerability with respect to mistreatment and violence is invariably linked to their lived experience of the products of colonization, such as residential schools, the sixties scoop, and restrictions placed on cultural practices and institutions by the state. This includes the destruction of the family structure and the loss of roles experienced by

Elders within it; poor socio-economic status, especially in rural and remote settings; and exposure to intergenerational violence in the home. The definition of violence and mistreatment that impacts Elders must be expanded to "reflect the complexities of colonial power relations and the intersecting and inter-related forms of violence experienced by Indigenous people" (Dumont-Smith, 2002, p. 11), in order to support the recognition of the impacts of historical oppression and violence upon current everyday experiences (Gray, LaBore, & Carter, 2018).

The risks for mistreatment and violence

Research shows that there are identifiable "risk" factors linked to the potential mistreatment and violence in older adults' lives. In its current conceptualization, this is often located in the *vulnerability* of older adults and their exposures to "risk" (Garnham & Bryant, 2017). Individual risk factors for mistreatment are linked to cognitive and physical impairments (biological) caused as a result of aging. Biological risk factors related to physical illness or disability should not be understood as something inherent to being older, rather as something that is socially determined and constructed (Canadian Centre for Elder Law, 2011b; Enguidanos, Deliema, Aguilar, Lambrinos, & Wilber, 2014). A diagnosis of dementia is not inherently a challenge; rather, the social construction of dementia (and people being diagnosed with dementia) creates the conditions for increased vulnerability to mistreatment (Jackson, 2016).

The risk of mistreatment and violence in older age has also been linked to experiences across the life course, such as child abuse, intergenerational family violence and abuse, intimate partner violence, trauma, micro-aggressions,[1] and discrimination (Walsh, Ploeg, Lohfeld, Horne, MacMillan, & Lai, 2007). The National Survey on the Mistreatment of Older Canadians (NICE, 2015) used a life course framework to understand mistreatment and found that predictors of mistreatment for older adults significantly correlated to "abuse" at earlier stages of their lives (p. iv). There needs to be a move from a practice that focusses exclusively on the examination of individual attributes and vulnerabilities as the only risk factors – (being old, being a woman, being in a caregiving relationship, being cognitively or physically frail) – to include social and structural conditions and factors that create and maintain vulnerabilities and risk (age-based segregation and isolation, violence across the lifespan, poverty, racism, institutionalization, homophobia, transphobia, ageism).

To address these missing links, the World Health Organization (2015) and Pillemer, Burnes, Riffen, and Lachs (2016) have identified the importance of looking beyond the individual and relational to include community, socio-cultural, and structural risk factors. These factors include social isolation, ageism, sexism, racism, other forms of oppression and discrimination, the cumulative impacts of trauma and violence across the life course, and the impacts of dependence within care relationships (Brandl, 2016; Hamby, Smith, Mitchell, & Turner, 2016; NICE, 2015). Table 10.2 charts risk factors, integrating some of the ideas addressed above. An understanding of these broad categories will assist you in your work with older adults.

Interventions

Interventions in social work are reflexive (*Why do I do this? What have I learned?*) or technical (*What do I do? What are the goals?*) in nature. The reflexive nature of

Table 10.2 Risk factors

Individual	Relational	Community	Socio-Cultural	Structural
• Cognitive and physical health • Age • Gender • Racial or ethno-cultural group membership and other identity positions • History of trauma • Socio-economic status • Disability	• Caregiver stress • Reciprocal violence in care relationships • Pre-existing relationship dynamics and dysfunction • Family roles • Living arrangements • Dependence	• Social isolation • Geographic location (urban centre vs. rural and/or remote town) • Lack of appropriate community supports • Loss of support networks	• Erosion of intergenerational family bonds (i.e., through collective traumas like colonization and genocide) • Socio-economic factors • Ageist stereotypes about older adults (i.e., frail, dependent) • Social disorder • Changing family structures (i.e., as a result of migration or employment patterns) • Systems of inheritance • Lack of systems that support aging or care	• Immigration • Social policy • Oppression (i.e., ageism racism, sexism, sanism, transphobia, ableism) • Legislation and protections • Human rights

interventions requires social workers to consider and reflect upon how our interventions impact older adults, including balancing their rights with their safety, and how interventions may reinforce and replicate disempowering, oppressive, and intrusive practices. Beaulieu and Leclerc (2006) note that when working with older adults on experiences of mistreatment, social workers should clarify their own positions by engaging in ethical and critical self-reflection. Central to this is an examination of beliefs and values as they relate to autonomy, risk, and decision-making and balancing this with the obligation to intervene. *Do we assume older adults have the capacity and right to make decisions even if we do not endorse them? How do we define safety?*

One challenge faced by social workers is that when we hear terms such as "abuse and neglect", "violence", or "mistreatment" applied to a case, we can become reactive and immediately want to "protect". Because we are working with adults, we need to recognize that the need to "protect" must be balanced with the right to self-determination and the right to live with (some) risk. This balance can be challenging in the context of practice, due to competing interests and emergent ethical dilemmas specific to each unique situation (Donovan & Regehr, 2010). Harbison (1999) calls this practicing "relative inaction", an approach that runs counter to the ethos of practitioners and organizations who have been charged with intervening in cases of elder mistreatment.

The technical nature of interventions in this area of practice (see Table 10.3) can also be challenging for social workers, especially for those who want prescribed guidance on "*what they should do*". There is very limited guidance in the tools that practitioners can use to identify and address mistreatment and violence. The interventions and solutions that do exist tend to focus specifically on the individual and neglect the structural and cultural causes that create and maintain mistreatment and violence (Harbison et al., 2012). Institutionalized intervention approaches (e.g., in the legal system or through specific legislation) can result in disempowerment by drawing on ageist assumptions about older adults' abilities, behaviours, and capacities (they need protection) and by assuming that these problems are best addressed and "fixed" by professionals given their "technical expertise" (Harbison, 1999). Interventions with older adults at the individual, legal, and organizational level are connected to the subordinate status they have in our society (as dependent, vulnerable, and frail) and is a "consequence of the ageism that is cultivated in late-modern society that is riddled with risk and anxiety" (Brozowski & Hall, 2010, p. 1954).

These three models represent the current options for practice. The choice of one particular model over another is related to decision-making capacity, jurisdiction, setting (institutions or community), and the severity of the mistreatment (i.e., whether it is a criminal act). In the case of decision-making capacity, when working with older adults who are assessed as not being capable of making decisions, social workers may require more support and guidance from the jurisdictional legal systems that are in place to address this (such as health care consent, guardianship, or decision-making legislation; see **Moral, legal, and ethical issues**). Institutional settings such as hospitals and nursing homes have specific policies and procedures for reporting and intervention attached to licensing that social workers are required to follow. There is less guidance for older adults residing independently in the community, when there is reluctance to engage with and accept interventions and ambiguity and ethical dilemmas abound.

The decision to engage and accept services voluntarily will vary by the type of mistreatment being experienced and associated factors such as gender, ethnicity, and socioeconomic status, past (and current) experiences of oppression, and the relative position

Table 10.3 Models of intervention

Model	Focus	Pros	Cons
Legal and Legislative	Criminal law (federal)Adult Protection and Guardianship legislation (provincial) Example: Criminal Code of Canada Physical Abuse: Sections 265 and 268 for assault and aggravated assault. Nova Scotia: Adult Capacity and Decision-making Act (2017) https://novascotia.ca/just/pto/adult-capacity-decision.asp	Provides concrete protections Reporting and interventions can be built in	Can infantilize Not always specific to older adults Can violate independence and decision-making abilities Inconsistent across provincial jurisdiction[2]
Education and Advocacy	Educating and supporting older adults as to their rights Advocacy at different systems and levels Example: Advocacy Centre for the Elderly www.advocacycentreelderly.org/	Older adults treated as capable actors in their own lives Education based Least intrusive and restrictive Rights based model	Acting on this information may be challenging Accessibility Does not address hesitancy to disclose and engage
Integrated Community Services	Multi-disciplinary and holistic Coordinated community approach Example: BC Association of Community Response Networks www.advocacycentreelderly.org/ Elder Abuse Response Team Kirby Centre (Edmonton, Alberta) www.kerbycentre.com/general/supportservices/elder-abuse-resource-line/	Addresses issue holistically (i.e., social services, health, legal) through multi-disciplinary teams Takes context into account	Can be time consuming and costly Funding issues dependent on systems of care delivery

of power held in relation to the individual, institution, system, or structure responsible for the mistreatment. Regarding financial abuse, for example, women, despite having fewer economic or structural advantages, tend to access supports more than men, who may feel more shame and stigma due to "historically socialized gender expectations to provide" (Burnes, Rizzo, Gorroochurn, Pollack, & Lachs, 2016, p. 1050). Marginalized older adults may have a historical mistrust of institutions and structures represented in the intervention process (health care, legal, and social services) and may show resistance to accessing services. They may be excluded from the process of identifying the mistreatment they are experiencing, and they may not be offered any services or supports. For example, LGBTTsIQ older adults' fear of exposure to abuse and mistreatment in the context of care has prompted many to avoid necessary medical intervention or impelled them to hide their sexual and gender identities in order to protect themselves when seeking treatment and formal care support (Brotman, Ryan, & Cormier, 2003).

Social workers therefore need to be aware that older adults may not voluntarily engage, or when they do, they may be resistant to specific approaches, especially those that are perceived as disempowering, discriminatory, and paternalistic (Canadian Centre for Elder Law, 2011a). Anti-oppressive approaches to working with older adults require responses that de-centre individual problems and situate them in a wider social-cultural and political context (Garnham & Bryant, 2017). These include identifying and addressing the intersection of different forms of oppression that could explain risks to exposure, how people react to mistreatment in particular ways, and/or why they may be reluctant or resistant to accessing support.

As well as understanding their legal and ethical responsibilities, and the services and resources available in their practice jurisdictions, AOG social workers need to critically reflect on how they can work with older adults in ways that:

- acknowledge the embedded nature of violence and mistreatment in their lives (individually, structurally, and culturally);
- take into account and include diverse lived experiences and perspectives, especially including those older adults on the margins; and
- avoid replicating disempowering practices and dynamics of interventions.

This can be done in the following ways:

1. Acknowledge the embedded nature of violence and mistreatment in the lives of older adults.

The presence of mistreatment and violence in older adults' lives can be challenging to detect and explore. Patterns of trauma, violence, and mistreatment are often well established in older adults' lives, making immediate change unimaginable for them (Brandl, 2016). Certain forms of mistreatment and violence may be visible; others (structural and cultural) are not and/or are sanctioned and perpetuated by the very structures and systems older adults inhabit and where social workers practice. Structural and cultural forms of violence and mistreatment, like colonization, racism, transphobia/cisgenderism, and ageism are often ignored or not taken into account through assessment and intervention and so go unaddressed. As a form of assessment and intervention, counter-storytelling can provide an alternative to professional narratives that are framed around dominant discourses of aging, mistreatment, and violence – such as older adults as being vulnerable, at-risk, incapable, and in need of our protection. This should not be undertaken in a way that minimizes the seriousness of the outcomes of these actions and events in older adults' lives, but rather in ways that make explicit "what is not told or known" about these experiences.

2. Take into account and include diverse lived experiences and perspectives, especially for those older adults on the margins.

Working with people who are potentially being mistreated or exposed to violence, especially those who do not identify the actions or events as "problematic", requires the social worker to "start where the person is at". This allows for recognition of the diversity and complexity of mistreatment and violence; how older adults attach meaning to their experiences, including narratives of resilience and resistance; and situating these experiences within a specific socio-cultural context. Burnes (2017) notes the importance of considering how problems are "individually-constructed realities" because this will determine how the problem is understood, what a successful outcome would be, and the path required to get there. This infers that a one-size-fits-all approach to intervention does not work (Jackson, 2016) and that social workers must be flexible in the way they approach each case.

3.   Avoid replicating disempowering practices.

Social workers must start from the position that a person is capable of making a decision unless proven otherwise. Older adults must be able to determine the course of action they wish to take, even if these decisions may appear to compromise their safety. This can be particularly challenging when others (such as family and care teams) request/force protective interventions. As social workers, we are often asked to intervene when older adults are resistant to expert or outside assessments and evaluations. We are asked to "react" to situations that would benefit more from a proactive, empowerment-based stance, for example, through the development of supportive long-term relationships where the social worker watches for opportunities to help facilitate and navigate change with the older adult.

The application of a harm reduction approach[3] has been identified as useful in this context (Burnes, 2017). Harm reduction is based on the assumption that the actions and events older adults experience may never be fully resolved or eradicated when we cede choice and control to the older adult. It allows the social worker to be flexible with their approach to intervention and to be least intrusive, restrictive, and paternalistic (Burnes, 2017). It also recognizes that people in abusive and violent situations have to live with the consequences of any intervention, including retribution (from the perpetrator), the loss of relationships, a reduction in the availability of material supports, and increased isolation. Social workers can work with older adults to put safeguards into place that address the potential for harm while allowing for choice and control. For example, in the case of potential financial mistreatment, ensuring that finances are being co-managed by money management services (either non-profit or for-profit), automatic bill payments through banks, and alerts for activity on accounts that seem out of the ordinary can reduce opportunities for their (re)occurrence.

Conclusion

Throughout this chapter, we have critically explored the hidden and contested nature of the mistreatment of older adults, as well as the social work practitioners charged with identifying and intervening in situations in which older adults may be exposed to or experience mistreatment or violence. We have given attention to types of violence and mistreatment, risk factors, and interventions that better integrate AOP principles of voice and self-determination.

Exercise

Read the following two case studies and reply to the series of questions:

Case 1: Is Mr. Chen Safe at Home?

Mr. Chen is a 78-year-old man of Chinese descent. He emigrated from Hong Kong 23 years ago with his wife to join their only child and his family who were already living in a medium-sized town in Southwestern Ontario. There is a very small Chinese community there. Mr. Chen speaks Mandarin and some English.

Mr. Chen comes to the hospital with a fractured arm after a fall at home. As the social worker, you are asked to meet with Mr. Chen because there is concern about his safety at home. His daughter-in-law says she believes that his arm was broken after Mrs. Chen pushed him and he fell.

When you meet with Mr. Chen, he is tearful but insists that everything is fine at home. Sometimes his wife gets frustrated with him because he has become more forgetful and weaker with age. He states that she has always been "angry" but that he has learned to "deal with it". He realizes he is a burden. He is also very embarrassed that his daughter-in-law thinks there is a "problem".

On your second visit to arrange some community supports for his return home, you find Mrs. Chen there. She becomes agitated with the suggestion that someone else assist Mr. Chen with his personal care. She does not want anyone in the house; she is already thinking that he needs to go to a nursing home and that she can move in with their son.

Case 2: Ingrid Isn't Lonely Anymore?

Ingrid is an 87-year-old woman living in her own home in a small rural town in PEI. You become involved with her as a community-based social worker because her daughter Susan is concerned about her being lonely and socially isolated. She is in relatively good health, but she is very anxious and feels fearful about going out to participate in any type of social activities.

She tells you that she is ashamed of being illiterate. She never learned how to read and write in school and always felt "stupid". She also tells you that she brought up six children by herself after her husband died, in rural PEI where she had no running water or electricity.

Susan calls you in a panic to state that her estranged brother George has moved into Ingrid's house and that she is very concerned. He has been isolating Ingrid from the rest of the family and has told Susan that he will now be taking care of Ingrid's finances because he thinks Susan has been "ripping her off". Susan tells you that George has a history of substance use. She is fearful for her mom's safety.

When you call Ingrid – she tells you she is happy that George is with her – because now she is not so lonely.

In each case, think about the following:

- Do you think that the older adult is being mistreated or experiencing violence? Why or why not?
- What types of mistreatment or violence do you think are present? (Refer to Table 10.1 and Figure 10.1)
- What are some important risk factors to take into account for both cases? (Refer to Table 10.2)
- What do you think some challenges would be to identifying mistreatment and/or violence in these cases?
- How would you intervene in these cases? What would be most challenging?
- Identify the different stakeholders involved in each case.
- What skills would you draw on when communicating with the numerous stakeholders involved?
- How does your organizational and regional context (where you work) potentially impact your choice of possible interventions?

Takeaways

- Elder mistreatment and violence are multi-dimensional in nature; they encompass a diverse and complex range of situations, issues, and experiences and require approaches to intervention that take these into account.
- Risks and outcomes for elder mistreatment and violence need to move beyond the individual and relational, to take into account the socio-cultural and structural.
- Older adults' experiences of mistreatment and violence are often different than expert-based definitions.
- Interventions are often not well articulated, which leaves social workers with inadequate information and tools to facilitate the inclusion of AOP.

Additional resources

- International Network for the Prevention of Elder Abuse: www.inpea.net/
- Violence Prevention Alliance: Global Campaign for Violence Prevention (WHO): www.who.int/violenceprevention/en/
- Elder Abuse in Aboriginal Communities Videos (Bear Paw Legal Education):
    - https://youtu.be/5AZjMe970w8
    - www.youtube.com/watch?v=rMFpS7-m3y8

Notes

1 See textbox 9.3 for definition of micro-aggressions.
2 For an overview of Canadian provincial legislation, please see Tables 5.2 and 5.3 in **Moral, legal, and ethical issues** and/or Canadian Centre for Elder Law (2011b) The Counterpoint Discussion Paper.
3 For a more complete discussion on harm reduction, please see **Mental health, mental wellness, and substance mis/use.**

References

Beaulieu, M., & Leclerc, N. (2006). Ethical and pyscho-social issues raised by the practice in cases of mistreatment of older adults. *Journal of Gerontological Social Work*, *46*(3–4), 161–186. doi:10.1300/J083v46n03_10.

Bows, H. (2018). Practitioner's views on the impacts, challenges and barriers, in supporting older survivors of sexual violence. *Violence against Women*, *24*(9), 1070–1090. doi:10.1177/1077801217732348.

Brandl, B. (2016). Working with older survivors of abuse: A framework for advocates. *National Clearing House on Abuse in Later Life*. Retrieved from www.acesdv.org/wp-content/uploads/2014/06/Working-with-Older-Survivors-of-Abuse.pdf.

Brotman, S., Ferrer, I., Sussman, T., Ryan, B., & Richard, B. (2015). Access and equity in the design and delivery of health and social care to LGBTQ older adults: A Canadian perspective. In N. A. Orel & C. A. Fruhauf (Eds.), *The lives of LGBT older adults: Understanding challenges and resilience* (pp. 111–140). Washington, DC: American Psychological Association. doi:10.1037/14436-006

Brotman, S., Ryan, B., & Cormier, R. (2003). The health and social service needs of gay and lesbian elders and their families in Canada. *The Gerontologist*, *43*(2), 192–202. doi:10.1093/geront/43.2.192.

Brozowski, K., & Hall, D. (2010). Aging and risk: Physical and sexual abuse of elders in Canada. *Journal of Interpersonal Violence*, *25*, 1183–1199. doi:10.1177/0886260509340546.

Burnes, D. (2017). Community elder mistreatment intervention with capable older adults: Toward a conceptual practice model. *The Gerontologist*, *57*(3), 409–416. doi:10.1177/0733464815581486.

Burnes, D., Rizzo, V. M., Gorroochurn, P., Pollack, M. H., & Lachs, M. S. (2016). Understanding service utilization in cases of elder abuse to inform best practices. *Journal of Applied Gerontology*, *35*(10), 1036–1057. doi:10.1177/0733464814563609.

Canadian Centre for Elder Law. (2011a). *A practical guide to elder abuse and neglect law in Canada*. Retrieved from www.bcli.org/sites/default/files/Practical_Guide_English_Rev_JULY_2011.pdf.

Canadian Centre for Elder Law. (2011b). *The counterpoint project discussion paper: Moving from scrutiny to strategy: An analysis of key Canadian elder abuse and neglect cases*. Retrieved from www.bcli.org/sites/default/files/Counterpoint_Project_discussion_paper.pdf.

Cohen, M. (2011). Screening tools for the identification of elder abuse. *Journal of Clinical Nursing*, *18*(6), 261–270.

Cook-Daniels, L., & munson, M. (2010). Sexual violence, elder abuse and the sexuality of transgender adults age 50+: Results of three surveys. *Journal of GLBT Family Studies*, *6*(2), 142–177. doi:10.1080/15504281003705238.

Doe, S. S., Han, H. K., & McCaslin, R. (2009). Cultural and ethical issues in Korea's recent elder abuse reporting system. *Journal of Elder Abuse & Neglect*, *21*(2), 170–185. doi:10.1080/08946560902780009.

Donovan, K., & Regehr, C. (2010). Elder abuse: Clinical, ethical and legal considerations in social work practice. *Clinical Social Work Journal*, *38*(2), 174–182. doi:10.1007/s10615-010-0269-2.

Dumont-Smith, C. (2002). *Aboriginal elder abuse in Canada*. Aboriginal Healing Foundation. Retrieved from www.ahf.ca/downloads/ahfresearchelderabuse_eng.pdf.

Enguidanos, S. M., Deliema, M., Aguilar, I., Lambrinos, J., & Wilber, K. H. (2014). Multicultural voices: Attitudes of older adults in the United States of America about elder mistreatment. *Ageing & Society*, *34*, 877–903. doi:10.1017/S0144686X12001389.

Finkenauer, S., Sherratt, J., Marlow, J., & Brodey, A. (2012). When injustice gets old: A systematic review of trans aging. *Journal of Gay and Lesbian Social Services*, *24*(4), 311–330. doi:10.1080/10538720.2012.722497.

Fraser, H., & Seymour, K. (2017). *Understanding violence and abuse: An anti-oppressive practice perspective*. Halifax, NS: Fernwood Publishing.

Galtung, J. (1990). Cultural violence. *Journal of Peace Research*, 27(3), 291–305. Retrieved from www.galtung-institut.de/wp-content/uploads/2015/12/Cultural-Violence-Galtung.pdf.

Garnham, B., & Bryant, L. (2017). Epistemological erasure: The subject of abuse in the problematization of elder abuse. *Journal of Aging Studies*, 41, 52–59. doi:10.1016/j.jaging.2017.04.001.

Gray, J. S., LaBore, K. B., & Carter, P. (2018). Protecting the sacred tree: Conceptualizing spiritual abuse against Native American elders. *Psychology of Religion and Spirituality*. Advance online publication. doi:10.1037/rel0000195.

Hamby, S., Smith, A., Mitchell, K., & Turner, H. (2016). Poly-victimization and resilience portfolios: Trends in violence research that can enhance the understanding and prevention of elder abuse. *Journal of Elder Abuse & Neglect*, 28(4–5), 217–234. doi:10.1080/08946566.2016.1232182.

Harbison, J. (1999). Models of intervention and 'elder abuse and neglect': A Canadian perspective on ageism, participation and empowerment. *Journal of Elder Abuse & Neglect*, 10(3–4), 1–17. doi:org/10.1300/J084v10n03_01.

Harbison, J., Coughlan, S., Beaulieu, M., Karabanow, J., Vanderplaat, M., Wildeman, S., & Wexler, E. (2012). Understanding 'elder abuse and neglect': A critique of assumptions underpinning responses to the mistreatment and neglect of older people. *Journal of Elder Abuse & Neglect*, 24, 88–103. doi:10.1080/08946566.2011.644086.

Jackson, S. L. (2016). The shifting conceptualization of elder abuse in the United States: From social services, to criminal justice and beyond. *International Psychogeriatrics*, 28(1–2), 1–8. doi:10.1017/S1041610215001271.

National Initiative for the Care of the Elderly (NICE). (2015). Into the light: National survey on the mistreatment of older Canadians. Retrieved from https://cnpea.ca/images/canada-report-june-7-2016-pre-study-lynnmcdonald.pdf.

Naughton, C., Drennan, J., Lyons, I., & Lafferty, A. (2013). The relationship between older people's awareness of the term elder abuse and the actual experiences of elder abuse. *Internal Psycho-Geriatrics*, 25(8), 1257–1266. doi:10.1017/S1041610213000513.

Pillemer, K., Burnes, D., Riffen, C., & Lachs, M. S. (2016). Elder abuse: Global situation, risk factors and prevention strategies. *The Gerontologist*, 56(S2), S194–S205. doi:10.1093/geront/gnw004.

Podnieks, E. (2008). Elder abuse: The Canadian experience. *Journal of Elder Abuse & Neglect*, 20(2), 126–150. doi:10.1080/08946560801974612.

Walsh, C. A., Olson, J. L., Ploeg, J., Lohfeld, L., & McMillan, H. L. (2011). Elder abuse and oppression: Voices of marginalized elders. *Journal of Elder Abuse & Neglect*, 23(1), 17–42. doi:10.1080/08946566.2011.534705.

Walsh, C. A., Ploeg, J., Lohfeld, L., Horne, J., MacMillan, H., & Lai, D. (2007). Violence across the lifespan: Interconnections among forms of abuse as described by marginalized Canadian elders and their care-givers. *British Journal of Social Work*, 37(3), 491–514. doi:10.1093/bjsw/bcm022.

World Health Organization. (2002). World report on violence and health summary. Retrieved from www.who.int/violence_injury_prevention/violence/world_report/en/summary_en.pdf.

World Health Organization. (2015). Addressing violence in aging: World report on violence and health. Retrieved from https://apps.who.int/iris/bitstream/handle/10665/42495/9241545615_eng.pdf?sequence=1.

World Health Organization/INPEA. (2002). Missing voices: Views of older person's on elder abuse. https://apps.who.int/iris/bitstream/handle/10665/67371/WHO_NMH_VIP_02.1.pdf.

Yon, Y., Mikton, C. R., Gassoumis, Z. D., & Wilbur, K. H. (2017). Elder abuse prevalence in community settings: A systematic review and meta-analysis. *The Lancet Global Health*, 5(2), 147–152. doi:10.1016/S2214-109X(17)30006-2.

Part 3

Revisioning gerontological social work

Chapter 11

Building inclusive communities

Questions to consider as you read this chapter

- How do you define "community" and "community social work"?
- What steps need to be taken to ensure that cities and neighbourhoods become "age-friendly"?
- How can social workers adopt a community-based approach in their practice?

Kimberly is a community organizer in a non-profit neighbourhood advocacy organization who is preparing for the annual "Fight Social Isolation" campaign. As part of the campaign, social workers visit different apartment complexes in the neighbourhood, knocking on doors to share news about local community events and services. This campaign is also meant to establish closer ties between community members and the organization and to check in on the growing and sizeable older population in the neighbourhood. It's winter-time in the Prairies, so part of this door knocking campaign is meant to check in on older people to make sure that their heat is on, especially during -40C weather. In one of her visits, Kimberly meets Ahnjong, an 81-year-old woman from South Korea. Ahnjong invites Kimberly to sit down, and they end up chatting for an hour. Kimberly soon learns that Ahnjong hasn't left her apartment for two weeks because of the weather. Her son, who sponsored her four years ago, was laid off and had to move to British Columbia to find work. As a result, Ahnjong was left behind in her apartment. Her son calls regularly but is unable to visit very often. Kimberly asks Ahnjong if she would be comfortable joining a community organization or social club so that she can have more contact with others. Ahnjong declines and explains that she is worried about slipping and falling outside given the frigid and temperamental weather. As they chat, Kimberly notices that Ahnjong's apartment is adorned with religious paintings and prayer books. Kimberly asks Ahnjong if she goes to the local church. Ahnjong replies that she doesn't because the nearest Korean-speaking church is more than 50 kilometres away and the local church is a different faith denomination than her own. Kimberly is familiar with the church and knows that a group of seniors run a volunteer-based friendly visiting program there. She hopes to complete a referral to the visiting program so that Ahnjong can increase her sense of belonging to the small-town community.

This chapter addresses how older people both define and create community in their later lives and the importance of community as people age. We explore how social workers within communities can better understand how community is defined by various stakeholders, including older adults themselves, in order to build a practice that facilitates social inclusion, civic participation, and belonging for older adults. We discuss what it means to build communities inclusive of older adults from equity-seeking groups, their families, and networks and how social workers can encourage agency (both resilience and resistance) in order to build community and advocacy initiatives.

The objectives of this chapter are to

- Introduce different definitions of "community" and "community social work";
- Explore the meaning of "age-friendly communities" in urban and rural settings;
- Identify community-based strategies such as lobbying, peer support, and advocacy;
- Reconsider what it means to belong and feel part of a community; and
- Situate experiences of aging within the larger structural forces that shape our definition of community.

Defining communities

The answers to questions such as "What is a community?" and "What is an inclusive community?" are likely "different for different people" (Pradeep & Karibeeran, 2017). For example, one can argue that a community refers to one's support networks. Another might say that community refers to one's local neighbourhood. Is a city a community? How about a rural setting? Do we consider nationhood to be our community? There are many complex relationships and issues to consider in defining community. Although this chapter will not exhaustively review the multiple ways in which community and community social work are understood in the literature (see Harris & White, 2013; Sherraden & Ninacs, 2014), we do believe it is important to call attention to the central concepts that have been used to define what is meant by "community". In general, definitions of community typically contain reference to both geographic space and social relationships. The term "spatial and relational" has been used by scholars in sociology to describe the central concepts inherent to all forms of community (Hamdi & Goethert, 1997). Spatial and relational are not binary or exclusive, however, since communities that are defined within local geographic boundaries are built through the development of relationships and social networks within borders. The same can be said for communities that are built through relationships, as relationships are typically developed through direct contact with others and imply spatial closeness or connectivity (Mason, 2000). For instance, this would be the case for both communities of interest or communities of people with shared identity who meet on a regular basis at the local café or YMCA.

In the context of increasing globalization and transnational migration and rise in the popular use of technologies, new forms of community that cross geographic and other spatial boundaries have emerged to contest the fundamental idea that community, even relational community, requires close geographic proximity. We only have to think of the proliferation of the Internet to understand how communities can be built virtually, leading to the popular use of the term "virtual community" (Maximova, 2011). As we will explore later in the chapter, both interest- and identity-based communities have used virtual and physical spaces to cross regions and borders transnationally in order to organize and build solidarity. While we may not typically think of older people as contributing to transnational or virtual communities, a central point to remember when defining relational communities in the context of aging is that older adults themselves actively engage in the creation of community. Older adults are not simply passive members of already existing communities. In the case of those who have been historically marginalized, the creation of informal communities to enhance safety and support has been fundamental to the development of a sense of belonging for themselves and younger members, in what would otherwise be a relatively hostile environment.

It is important to emphasize that the concepts of power and belonging are central to any definition of community (Anderson, 2006). One may impose a definition of community onto an individual or population, which is evident in the way in which geographic (such as a state or neighbourhood) and institutional (such as a school or residence) communities are constituted in policy. For example, think of our colonial history as a nation-state and of how Canadian geographic borders were forcefully and violently imposed over Indigenous nations and communities across Turtle Island.[1] This example brings to light the role of power in shaping who (1) defines geographic forms of community, (2) decides who belongs to it, and (3) imposes definitions on membership, rights, and entitlements to which community members are given access. On the other hand, we should not underestimate how powerful the creation of relational forms of community (including those which are interest and identity-based) can be to those who are otherwise subject to oppression within geographic and institutional borders. Relational communities can be considered forms of agency for individuals and groups of people, including older adults who belong to those relational communities because of shared values, experiences, and interests (real or virtual). We do not mean to romanticize these forms of relational community, however. It is important to remember that community is neither fixed nor free of conflict or disruption.

Communities can be challenging and challenged, both from within and from outside. Advocacy to shift what counts as community and who belongs within it can serve to enhance or limit a sense of belonging in a given time or context. People can belong to many communities simultaneously for many different reasons over the life course. Just as people can choose to belong to community, membership can also be imposed upon people. This makes the concept of community one that must always be understood as both time and context specific *as well as* fluid and contested.

Social workers have been involved in community work since the development of the profession (Sherraden & Ninacs, 2014). While the social work community organizing literature borrows somewhat from the sociological literature in order to define community in the context of practice, there are some points of distinction worth noting here. According to Shragge (2013), social workers practising at the community level have tended to focus most specifically on issue-based concepts of community (aligned with advocacy and social justice work) and support-based concepts of community (aligned with the development of services to enhance well-being and civic participation) within localized geographic boundaries, such as those at the neighbourhood level. Historically, there is a significant conceptual divide between social workers who engage in practice centred on community development/organization and/or policy (what we call indirect or meso–macro practice) and those who do direct (micro) practice with individuals, families, and groups. Although in recent years there has been increased recognition of the connections between community and individual/family practice, there continues to be somewhat of a disconnect between these fields. One has only to look to the ways in which social work is operationalized in both education and service delivery to identify distinctions in the ways in which social work is conceptualized and operationalized as either community practice-based or individual practice-based. Some social work scholars have aptly called our attention to the reality that, in fact, all social work is community-based because of our fundamental value of understanding individuals in context (Pradeep & Karibeeran, 2017). For example, social work is one of the few allied health professions that incorporates the "person in environment" approach to practice. This requires every social worker, even those who work exclusively with individuals in a therapeutic context, to understand and make use of the concept of community. Moreover, a sense of belonging within one's community is a fundamental aspect of well-being. Therefore, social workers must become more adept at both defining and including communities in their analyses of social problems and interventions.

This chapter is divided into three sections based upon the three distinct but related conceptual definitions of community described above, namely: (1) "community" created within localized geographic boundaries; (2) "community", which emerges through shared interest or concerns and leads to the development of initiatives such as advocacy or collective action; and (3) "community" that develops as a result of shared identity. In the first section, we take up the idea of spatially defined communities through the exploration of what "rural" community means and how it is defined, as well as through the examination of the global policy initiative "age-friendly communities" as a form of international policy. We examine how age-friendly communities have been operationalized across urban and rural contexts in Canada and some of the critiques that have emerged. In the second section, we explore issue-based relational communities through the lens of advocacy, social movements, and community organizing primarily led by older adults. We discuss how older people have engaged collectively in order to re-define what is meant by inclusive communities. Finally, in the third section, we explore some informal and fluid forms of community that emerge among older people due to shared identity in order to build or sustain relationships and enhance a sense of belonging, solidarity, and support. In this section, we highlight the importance of these alternative forms of community among historically marginalized older adults such as those from immigrant and trans communities. We argue that these informal communities have not been well recognized by sites and sectors of health and social care; and we suggest that identity-based relational communities among older adults from marginalized communities need to receive increased recognition in policy and practice. In the conclusion of this chapter, we further explore how social workers in direct practice can incorporate community practice more explicitly and strategically into their work on a daily basis.

Communities that begin in geographic space

A common way of talking about geographic communities is to situate them by size, as in the distinction "rural/urban". These perceptions of community might be useful in thinking about differences in aging across different geographic spaces, such as urban and rural spaces. To understand the complex task of defining what counts as a community, let us first consider the competing definitions of both "rural" and "rural community" (see textbox 11.1). Although commonly understood in relation to, and in opposition to, aging in urban spaces, there is no standard definition of rural aging. The Canadian government uses terms like rural and remote communities, although the definitions are applied somewhat inconsistently, and oftentimes they are clumped together. The *Oxford English Dictionary* (2019) defines "rural" as "connected with or like the country side". Phillipson and Scharf

(2005) argue that different explanations and conceptualizations of "rural aging" complicate any attempt to create a unifying definition of what counts as "rural". For instance, countryside has different connotations and connections to national identities and across nation-states. As such, Phillipson and Scharf (2005) suggest that we consider the social advantages and disadvantages that older adults in rural settings experience in relation to prevailing socio-political and economic structures in defining rural spaces.

Textbox 11.1

Rural is typically defined as connected with or like the countryside. In Canada, "rural" originally referred to the agricultural sector and evoked hard work, stoicism, and family ties. The definition of rural has changed over time to be less about occupation and shared values and more about population size, density, and proximity to urban centres. The idea of rural values or a rural way of life, often connected to the land and its inhabitants, is still real for many people aging in place in rural contexts as well as in-migrants (those who move/retire to the countryside).

To offer a clearer definition of rural community, the Federal/Provincial/Territorial (F/P/T) Committee of Officials created the Age-Friendly Rural and Remote Communities Guide in 2006. In this policy guide, rural and remote aging are defined together as geographic areas that are located outside towns and cities (see textbox 11.2). While the document offers helpful guidelines regarding the challenges of aging in rural versus urban settings, it is important to make distinctions between rural and remote aging. The statistical designation of a remote and isolated community refers to a settlement that is a long distance from, and/or that lacks transportation links typically found in populated spaces.

Textbox 11.2

Remote and isolated communities refer to settlements of between one and 1,000 people that are long distances from urban centres and/or that lack transportation links typically found in more densely populated spaces. One key difference between remote and isolated communities is that remote areas have year-round access, while isolated communities do not.

An urban centre is typically understood to be a concentration of a high-density population. Until 2011, Statistics Canada used the term urban to distinguish populations that had at least 1,000 people and a density of 400+ people per square kilometre (see textbox 11.3). Following 2011, Statistics Canada (2011) adopted the language of "population centre" in recognition of the continuum that exists when considering density to define a geographic community. Small population centres are classified as populations between 1,000 and 29,000 people; medium population centres are defined as communities between 30,000 and 99,999 people. Finally, large urban population centres are classified are those that are considered to contain 100,000 people and more.

Walmsley and Kading (2018) provide further nuances to the definition of urban centres by suggesting that "small cities", which are those with a population between 10,000 to 100,000 people, straddle the lines between large urban centres and rural towns, as they are cities yet are bound by rural history and traditions. Examples of small Canadian cities include Kamloops, BC; Miramichi, NB; and Peterborough, ON. Still, a definition focussed exclusively on population size and density reveals nothing about the nature of community other than its geographic boundaries. Instead, and particularly when attempting to understand concepts like "rural aging", we must draw upon how diverse older adults living within these boundaries actually experience their rural community, and the challenges and opportunities they face on a daily basis with respect to the development of a sense of belonging through participation, access to care support, and inclusion.

Age-friendly communities

Menec, Means, Keating, Parkhurst, and Eales (2011) suggest that we consider community within a geographic context along a continuum to account for the different needs and key issues across localities. One way that different countries have looked at key issues is through the World Health Organization's (WHO) *Global Age-Friendly Cities Project*, which draws upon the idea that community includes not only a recognition of geographic space, but also the ways in which communities facilitate social and structural relationships in support of aging members (WHO, 2018) (see textbox 11.4). The project gathered different stakeholders within a given city (such as older people and care providers) to discuss domains of community life that are or can become "age-friendly". These domains include (1) outdoor spaces and buildings, (2) transportation, (3) housing, (4) social participation, (5) respect and social inclusion, (6) civic participation and employment, (7) communication and information, and (8) community support and health services.

We focus on this policy initiative because the concept of age-friendly communities has gained prominence in recent years with the development of a global strategy that aligns and designs policies, services, and structures to help older people "age actively". While aging actively can mean different things to different people (as was highlighted in **Theorizing later life and social work praxis**), generally speaking, policies and programs that promote active aging speak to the physical and health barriers that older people face and identify initiatives that can address environmental adaptations to infrastructures and services to improve accessibility and civic participation amongst older adults. Proponents of age-friendly communities suggest that older people have a wide range of skills and abilities and their decisions and lifestyles are to be valued and respected. This being said, what does an age-friendly community actually look like? Some examples include ensuring that sidewalks are well maintained, buildings are adapted for accessibility (by having automatic door openers and elevators, for example) so that older people can actively participate in community activities. Being an "Age-Friendly Community" also means having affordable housing, safe and accessible neighbourhoods, transportation systems that cater to the needs of older adults, and community support services ensuring that older people can be socially active and take part in voluntary, political, and employment positions. The WHO (2018) recently modified the framework from that implemented in 2007 to include the following commitments: (1) fostering older people's autonomy, (2) enabling older people's engagement, and (3) promoting multisectoral action. The revised Age-Friendly Communities framework was adopted for the years 2016 to 2020.

It is important to note that the idea of "Age-Friendly Cities" has historical roots in Canada. In 1999, the principles of Age-Friendly Cities were agreed upon and later adopted by federal and provincial ministers. To date, the Government of Canada has considered inclusive communities through an initiative called "Age-Friendly Communities" (See www.canada.ca/en/public-health/services/health-promotion/aging-seniors/friendly-communities.html) and the Canadian intergovernmental secretariat – Federal Provincial, Territorial (F/P/T) – Seniors Forum adopted the "Aging and Place" document as a central strategy of inclusion. Four Canadian cities initially took part in the project including Saanich (BC), Portage la Prairie (MB), Sherbrooke (QC), and Halifax (NS). Later the F/P/T Age-Friendly Rural and Remote Communities initiative adopted the Global-Age-Friendly Cities framework for smaller and rural communities with populations under 5,000 people. The 10 communities included in this part of the initiative included Alert Bay (BC), Lumby (BC), High Prairie (AB), Turtleford (SK), Gimli (MB), Bonnechere (ON), Port Hope Simpson (NL), Clarenville (NL), Alberton (PEI), and Guysborough (NS).

Given the popularity of the framework, a number of social gerontologists have begun to assess and evaluate its effectiveness. Menec et al. (2011) examined Age-Friendly Communities from an ecological perspective, which considers the interrelationships between the environment and the person living within it. These scholars suggest that a basic benefit of age-friendly communities is that they promote social connectivity between older people and the environments in which they live (Menec et al., 2011). Personal characteristics (which the authors identify as age, socioeconomic status, cultural background, attitudes, preferences, health, and functional status) and environmental conditions change over time, and their relationship to social connectivity is dynamic. As such, there are certain "leverage points" (within the person or the environment) that are particularly key in determining the social connectivity of people and their environments (Menec et al.,

2011). Menec et al. (2011) define leverage points as key issues that play a disproportionally influential role in effecting change (e.g., when we ban smoking in public spaces in the interest of health promotion instead of persuading individuals to stop smoking).

Critiques of age-friendly communities

While the Age-Friendly Communities framework has resulted in important policy and programmatic initiatives to address challenges with aging in urban, rural, and remote communities, a number of critiques have been introduced by scholars and community members. Plouffe, Kalache, and Voelcker (2016) note methodological limitations in the ways in which a city is marked an "Age-Friendly Community". In particular, these authors note that the WHO adopts an arbitrary assessment tool (i.e., a checklist)[2] to determine whether a city meets and engages with the Age-Friendly model framework. Plouffe et al. (2016) argue that such assessment methods do not offer a comprehensive way of evaluating whether recommendations adopted by the WHO are being implemented in a meaningful way.

Another critique of the Age-Friendly Communities' framework is the way in which it unintentionally segregates older people in relation to the dominant society. In particular, Walsh, Scharf, and Keating (2016) note that nearly half of the existing literature on Age-Friendly Communities fails to integrate the concept of "social exclusion" in assessments of these communities. Generally speaking, social exclusion refers to the act of excluding people from full access to rights, resources, and opportunities as a result of their belonging to a particular group (such as being classified as an older person) (see Grenier and Guberman, 2009). To date, Age-Friendly Communities programs have not comprehensively examined how cumulative disadvantages play out across the life course of older residents of the participating communities. Moreover, few studies have examined the implications of migration and migratory pathways within aging age-friendly communities (Mirza, Liu, & Klinger, 2018).

The lack of attention to the experience of homelessness (see textbox 11.5), particularly in the context of aging, is another critique of the Age-Friendly Communities framework. According to Grenier, Sussman, Barken, Bourgois-Guerin, and Rothwell (2016a), homeless older people represent a diverse population whose experiences are under-reported due to a narrow focus on youth homelessness in research, policy, and practice. Existing research on aging and homelessness refers to the compounding impact of poverty, inequality, and rising housing costs on older adults. Homelessness among older adults is not necessarily a fixed state of either being housed or being "without a home" or "living on the streets" but can fluctuate when older people move from housed to homeless at various points in their life course or later in life. Among the challenges that older homeless people face are mental and physical health concerns as well as access to specialized medical care that may or may not be available in shelters (Grenier, Barken, Sussman, Rothwell & Bourgeois-Guerin, 2016b). Despite urgent calls to action by homelessness activists, advocates and researchers, the current Age-Friendly Community framework only peripherally engages with the problem of housing accessibility and homelessness. The lack of attention to the experiences of older people who are homeless within Age-Friendly initiatives raises questions about who is implicitly or explicitly excluded within Age-Friendly Communities; it speaks to dominant assumptions about what is considered an inclusive community.

> **Textbox 11.5**
>
> **Homelessness** describes the situation of an individual, family, or community without stable, safe, permanent, appropriate housing or the immediate prospect, means, and ability of acquiring it.

Issue-based relational communities: advocacy, social justice, equity, and inclusion

Alejandra is a 64-year-old woman born in Nicaragua who came to Quebec in her early 30s after working in Central America and the United States as a cleaner. She arrived under the Foreign Domestic Movement in 1985 to work as a domestic worker. She eventually left domestic work and was employed at a daycare. In her spare time, Alejandra does extensive volunteering at her local food bank. Despite living in Canada for decades, Alejandra finds that her job does not provide adequate compensation to cover daily necessities. In addition to her formal work (part time) and volunteer work, she also engages in under-the-table care work as do some of her South American women friends. The labour is somewhat piecemeal and is not enough for Alejandra, who is struggling to survive financially. She has tried to alleviate some of her costs by living with a roommate and has been on a waiting list for low-cost housing for over three years. Alejandra has also begun to reflect on her own aging experience as a result of meeting many older people who access the food bank where she volunteers. When she was younger, she never really noticed that most of the people accessing the food bank were older people, but now she has begun to question whether this will also be her future. One day at work, Alejandra speaks to an older woman from Bolivia, who discloses that she has been accessing the food bank for five years because her Old Age Security (OAS) is not enough to cover the high cost of food. The older woman also discloses that many of her friends are dealing with housing issues including landlords looking to increase rent applying pressure on their aging tenants to get them to move. Scared but motivated, Alejandra decides to meet with several people through the Food Bank network in the hopes of addressing this issue. She invites some of the older people that she has met at the food bank as well as the social worker who works there. As a first step, they decide that Alejandra should approach the local health and social care centre to ask what can be done. At the meeting she is frustrated that all the social service providers tell her is, "Just be patient. You're a year away from receiving your OAS, now is not the time to cause a fuss". Alejandra reports back to her support group, and they collectively decide to approach policy makers and politicians. They decide to attend the next town hall meeting, and in advance of it, they write a letter to their local member of parliament (MP) looking for solutions. While at the town hall, Alejandra and her support network are happy to see their MP, who has agreed to meet with Alejandra and this new group to discuss their issues. Alejandra is hopeful that her self-advocacy can begin to shed light on the precarious situation older people like herself are facing.

Advocacy initiatives with and by older people are important to consider in the context of community development and social work. Community organizing is a way to engage in social work practice and encompasses organizing, mobilizing, and educating people to build a sense of community (see textbox 11.6). Working with communities happens through grassroots organizing and aims to empower different forms of community, including those related to geographic region, those that are social and/or relational in nature (based on identity categories like age, class, or migration status) or those that are problem-focussed (e.g., issues of housing, transportation, healthcare). An example is the Age-Friendly Society of the South Cariboo, which hosts activities and information sessions for older adults living in 100 Mile House and other rural communities in the Interior of British Columbia.[3] Inspired by WHO's Age-Friendly Cities project that included two rural communities in BC, the Society was established in 2013 and now boasts over 100 members. A major issue for the members is transportation, as many live not only rurally, but also remotely, and quite a few live alone on farms or acreages. As there is no public transportation service, older adults must rely on family, friends, and neighbours to get to appointments in town. Thus, the Society proposed to the town council that the school bus be used to transport older adults while the children and youth are at school. This is an example of a creative – and intergenerational – solution that AOP social workers could support by advocating for its implementation and evaluation (to ensure sustainability).

Textbox 11.6

Community organizing is a way to engage in social work practice. Community organizing encompasses unifying, mobilizing, and educating people to build a sense of community.

Older adult activism through lobbying and the non-profit sector

Think about the last time you saw or heard about activism and advocacy related to older people. If you can't, then you're not alone. Most people do recognize older adults as having played a significant part in the historical development of Canada's universal programs such as health care and Old Age Security (OAS) in the 1950s and '60s. When the state attempts to reduce access to pensions, older adults become more visible in the public domain, including in the media. Yet other and more recent examples of advocacy and activism in relation to older people's issues is less common and reflects a general perception of dependence and invisibility in relation to the place of older people within Global North societies. Two more recent examples of older adult activism and lobbying are the Raging Grannies and the protests against increasing the age eligibility for OAS.

In Canada, the Raging Grannies is a group of older women that began in 1987 in Victoria, BC (Roy, 2006). The group was originally comprised of white, middle-class, educated women between the ages of 52 and 67 who initially protested against the presence of US Navy warships and uranium mining in the Victoria area. The group used different tactics such as singing satirical songs and dressing up in lab coats to protest and amplify their discontent with the provincial legislature's decision to allow nuclear-powered military vessels into Victoria's inner harbour. At the time, the group received considerable media attention for their protests. The Raging Grannies would eventually adapt their tactics to include parodies and stereotypical caricatures of older women as a means of challenging authority. The group has also been applauded for engaging in political messages that dispel dominant perceptions of older women through their active participation in social and environmentally conscientious events. In fact, there is a tribute to the Raging Grannies at the Canadian Museum of Human Rights in Winnipeg, in recognition of the role they have played in peace and social justice activism. To date, the Raging Grannies have spread nationally and into the United States and have expanded their membership to be more inclusive of diverse groups of older women.

Racialized communities have long and rich histories of activism, whether it be resisting racism and other interlocking forms of oppression or providing support to community members. Older adults have been central to advocacy and community development efforts that address social (in)justice, civic participation, social inclusion, and intergenerational transmission of knowledge about culture and history. Two such examples are The Council for Black Aging Community (CBAC) of Montreal and Action Dignity in Calgary, formerly the Ethnocultural Council of Calgary. CBAC is a charitable, non-profit organization in Montreal that works with Black Anglophone older adults. Founded in 1987, the CBAC addresses discrimination and invisibility in order to meet the growing needs of its older members. Action Dignity is a non-profit organization that addresses issues of diversity, human rights, racial inequities, and public participation (Action Dignity, 2013) and has developed innovative approaches that strengthen the role of ethnocultural communities in accessing and delivering services, domestic violence prevention, and neighbourhood engagement. In 2016, Action Dignity developed a Broker Strategy Program geared at older immigrant adults. Fifteen immigrant Elders received training and developed their capacity in (1) community outreach; (2) working on healthy relationships; and (3) developing basic mental health awareness. These 15 Elders went on to serve as community brokers who actively led focus group discussions with older adults and co-developed needs assessments with members of Calgary's ethno-cultural community based on their challenges with accessing services (e.g., interpretation services). The two examples presented above demonstrate how older adults actively participate in the building and development of inclusive communities.

Identity-based relational communities: creating inclusive communities through transnational and local informal networks

During my doctoral dissertation, I (Ilyan) worked as a community organizer for a grassroots organization that focussed on advocacy and education with the Filipino Canadian community in Montreal. At the time, I met Romero, an 82-year-old man from the Philippines who approached me with questions about his pension. Romero wanted to know whether there was a way to increase his monthly pension so that he could travel to the Philippines. Romero's children didn't want their father to return to the Philippines because they feared that he would quickly spend his pension on his extended family and close friends. Romero's children argued that it was more expensive to support Romero in the Philippines because of how quickly his allotment was spent there. However, Romero disclosed the need to leave for the homeland, noting feelings of loneliness and isolation in the suburban town in which he lived. Romero disclosed, "My children work and I'm alone with the grandchildren all day. I miss being around people. There's no daycare here because it's too expensive, and we're too far from everything". After hearing Romero's concerns, I began to think about meeting with the children to discuss the possibility of having Romero return to the Philippines on a part-time basis, knowing that OAS payments aren't reduced if older adults spend 6 months less a day in the homeland. I also reflected more deeply about Romero's definition of "community". Focussing only on community as existing within a specific neighbourhood/space made invisible how Romero conceptualized his community. Romero wanted to engage in transmigration because his community extended across national borders and included those with whom he felt a strong sense of belonging beyond his immediate family.

It is important to look at some of the ways in which older people themselves have defined and created a sense of inclusive community outside of the prescriptive programs and approaches put forth by policy makers and social service providers (see textbox 11.7). For example, we might want to consider what inclusive communities would look like, not only in the immediate vicinity, but also across Global North diasporas and in the Global South. This brings about important conversations about aging, space, and place. In this regard, paying attention to how older adults speak about community in the everyday is essential in order to enhance opportunities for the development of a sense of belonging among them as they age. The following section discusses inclusive communities among Canadian immigrant and transnational diasporas as an example of these issues.

Textbox 11.7

Inclusive communities are communities where the citizens and members feel safe, respected, and comfortable in being themselves and expressing all aspects of their identities. It is a place where each person shares a sense of belonging with the other members. It is home.

Relationships between people happen within and across numerous networks that transcend traditional borders and immediate family relationships. Since an important component of community is social and relational, and care networks and exchanges are closely connected to a sense of belonging, it is important to ask how a definition of inclusive communities can better account for transmigration/transnational caring relationships that extend beyond the immediate family (see textbox 11.8). Can aging communities be experienced transnationally? Ethnogerontological scholarship has begun to consider the identities, realities, and lived experiences of immigrant older adults in later life as active members of global families, who engage in caring exchanges across borders and communities (Baldassar, 2007; Warnes & Williams, 2006). These transnational communities and caregiving exchanges exist and occur despite immigration policy restrictions (further explored in **Policy and planning for an aging society**), demonstrating how older people participate in communities across space and time (intermittent time periods) (Phillipson & Ahmed, 2004; Sainsbury, 2006; Treas, 2008). The increasingly complex dynamics of immigration, which intersect with other life events such as labour force participation and retirement, often propel older immigrants, particularly those who are racialized, to take on an active role in caring for the family both locally and transnationally (Baldassar, 2007; Treas, 2008). These dynamics can often create communities that are not acknowledged by policy makers and service providers.

> **Textbox 11.8**
>
> **Transmigration** is the movement of people across natural and constructed borders and includes processes of leaving/fleeing one's home country and going to a foreign country for work or other opportunities, whether temporarily or permanently. This also includes continuous movement for older adults who cross borders for short or extended periods of time where they provide and receive care with transnational community members.

In an attempt to understand the complexities of care between older immigrants and their families, Sun (2014) suggests that older immigrants engage in a process of "reconfigured reciprocity" where care arrangements are constantly in a state of flux. Research with racialized and immigrant older people shows how older people engage in care exchanges where they are active participants in the provision of care (Ferrer, Brotman, & Grenier, 2017). In doing so, older people are participating and creating communities that cut across generations, borders, and time through three key contexts: the intergenerational, transnational, and chosen communal.

> *Let us return to Romero's story. Though people were friendly in his small suburban town, Romero missed speaking his language and seeing people in the village market. Romero wondered, "Is this my life now? What is life without community?" Romero wanted to tell his children that going to the Philippines for months at a time would allow him to be part of a community and to feel at home. While he understood his children's concerns over his spending, Romero spoke about how community, care, and support were intertwined.*

The financial support that older immigrants provide to transnational family and friends in the homeland represents a form of community that is not currently incorporated in the definition of community within the various sites and sectors of health and social care because it represents a form of community in which older people are both present and absent and so are not easily accounted for. However, the dynamics of care and community that exist within caring exchanges across national borders are nonetheless important forms of community. Older people speak about the importance of maintaining financial and emotional ties to their families and networks in the country of origin as an important means of maintaining a sense of belonging, even in cases where travel to the homeland is not possible for financial or health reasons. These considerations showcase how communities in the diaspora and homeland are actively created by older people and how older people can cross borders to participate in these different contexts. They also demonstrate the ways older people and their families situate and respond to austerity measures and "precarity" (see textbox 0.5 in the **Introduction**) with their accompanying scarcity of resources, both locally and transnationally, to ensure that caring needs are met across generations and borders. Informal networks within local jurisdictions in which older adults are active members can also be understood as an important form of community that serves to resist marginalization and exclusion. The following counter-story describes one such informal network:

Francesko and Chantale are partners and older members of the Haitian community in a major city in the province of Quebec. Francesko and Chantale are very active within a small group of older people and their church. Almost everyday their circle of eight to 10 older people meets at a local coffee shop to socialize and discuss current issues. Very few members of their tight-knit community speak French or English, but the support circle is adept at receiving information relating to discounts, pensions, news from their families, and other local community projects. The circle is fairly active in each other's lives and work to collectively address racism experienced by themselves, their children, grandchildren, and the community. Francesko and Chantale consider this circle to be their "second family". For instance, last month when Francesko had surgery, the close group of friends helped Chantale with housekeeping and other tasks to make it easier for Chantale and Francesko to deal with this major event.

Francesko and Chantale's story highlights how older people both create and rely upon chosen family, kinship ties, or informal networks to address both personal and structural issues. Older people with whom we have worked have often spoken about how members of their community become "like family", providing support that otherwise is not available or accessible. The establishment and reliance on these types of local community networks develops in response to difficulties accessing health and social care services and the realities of structural oppression. In response to gaps in available and accessible services and supports, many older people rely on their chosen support networks, comprised of fellow older people who share a common identity or ancestry in order to provide much-needed information on rights and entitlements and a sense of social belonging. As we saw at the beginning of the chapter with Kimberly and Ahnjong, local community organizations (such as food banks or socio-cultural groups) and public spaces (such as the mall or coffee shops) are important spaces in which informal networks organize. These reciprocal relationships reflect older people's need for support and contribute to continued agency in providing care within families and community. They also serve to prevent or decrease social isolation, which is of concern to gerontological social workers.

Finally, it is important to consider how community becomes the site for many reciprocal relationships that often go unnoticed with respect to older people as active members of community organizations and informal social groups (Ferrer et al., 2017; Pradeep & Karibeeran, 2017). Although traditionally viewed as a resource to offset social isolation among older people, these social support networks are considered more "like family" and often emerge in the context of a lack of accessibility of formal services and/or a lack of funding for local initiatives; they survive only because of the active participation of older adults themselves. For example, the LGBTTsIQ community is an example of a diverse and complex identity-based community made up of many communities. One can feel part of a local community and/or have a sense of belonging to a transnational community based on shared identity. In this regard, definition of community is, or can be, transnational because it invokes a social and relational definition, which exists across sites and borders (Pino, 2017).

Josephine is a 66-year-old trans person who considers them self to be part of the larger LGBTTsIQ community. Although Josephine has lived most of their life in a small town in New Brunswick, they enjoy travelling to St. John to be closer to their larger network of friends and acquaintances. Having had difficulties navigating space for themselves, Josephine keeps an eye out for younger members of the community to ensure that they find a place of belonging and support in a sometimes-challenging local environment. Josephine wants to make sure that young trans people and those that are aging are treated well and get access to the health and social care services they need. Josephine is sometimes called upon by the social worker from the local health agency, with whom they have developed a good relationship over the years, to speak to professionals and family members about trans realities and challenges in accessing care and support. They have even, a few times, opened their home to young folks from across the province who needed a place to stay after running away because of violence they experienced at home and in school. Josephine is happy to give back to the community in times of need. Recently, Josephine and a few friends they met while vacationing in Cuba started a trans aging social media website. They were surprised that, after only six months, the site had attracted over 200 members from around the world.

What can social workers do?

This chapter has offered a general overview of how policy makers, service providers, and older adults define communities and has presented examples of older adult activism and advocacy work. Building inclusive communities reflects geographic, social, emotional, and relational dynamics. As such, social workers can make important contributions to efforts intended to redress invisibility and correct access barriers among older adults in their daily work – particularly when it comes to advocating for more inclusive communities. Social workers must first recognize that older adults can be involved in advocacy and activism to address their needs and concerns. Advocacy and activism can take shape in different forms. For example, older adults can come together to discuss a specific issue and then generate ideas about communicating their message as we saw in Alejandra's case and with the Raging Grannies. Non-profit organizations (such as Action Dignity and the Age-Friendly Society of South Cariboo) can reach out to engage in capacity building with older people and develop programs that address older adults' realities and concerns.

As we have argued throughout this chapter, inclusive communities also include the informal and transnational networks to which older people belong. Despite health and financial concerns, older adults play a vital role in care exchanges across communities, contexts, boundaries, and sites. This fundamental aspect of what constitutes community is currently not well recognized within sites and sectors of health and social care. As social workers, we must deconstruct our current assumptions of what counts as "community". In this way, strategies and service delivery models can shift to both recognize and provide support to diverse older adults, their families, and informal networks. For example, in thinking about our tools for assessment and our intervention practices, intergenerational or chosen support relationships and transnational care exchanges are rarely considered or addressed. It is important to think about how to integrate support networks within and across communities and the ways in which older adults themselves define their communities of belonging into our daily practices. Social workers in different contexts, whether clinical, leadership, community development, group or individual practice, must adapt their work to be more inclusive of advocacy and pay attention to how broader definitions of community can link with both informal and transnational networks.

Exercises

- Think about one of the clients/cases in your practicum or place of work. Can you identify the different kinds of communities to which your client/case belongs? How are they situated locally/geographically? How about issue or identity-wise? Is your client/case a member of a transnational community, or might they want to be?
- Identify a community-based organization that does grassroots activism in your town or city. How can you, as a social worker, work within and/or with the organization in support of older adults?

Takeaways

- It is important to consider the ways in which communities are defined by policy makers, program planners, *and* older adults themselves.
- There are many definitions of community. However, most definitions include both spatial and relational components.
- Age-Friendly Cities is a World Health Organization initiative meant to build more inclusive communities. It has, however, been critiqued for unintentionally segregating older people and failing to take account of homelessness, for example.
- Transnational communities, both real and virtual, as well as informal identity-based kin networks must be more comprehensively integrated into assessment and intervention.

Notes

1 Turtle Island is what Indigenous people call/called the North American continent. As social workers, it is imperative that we recognize our colonial history and the role of social work in the nation-building project (see Baskin & Sinclair, 2015; Blackstock, 2006) and our complicity in ongoing practices of settler-colonialism (e.g., child apprehension/s).
2 The WHO (2015) checklist is a tool for a city's self-assessment and a map for charting progress. Among the items it measures are outdoor spaces and buildings, transportation, housing, social participation, respect for social inclusion, civic participation and employment, communication and information, and community and health services.
3 This story came from Researching Older Adult's Repositioning (ROAR), a research project conducted by Hulko, Mirza, and Seeley and funded by an Interior Health evidence-informed practice grant. We thank Noeman Mirza and Lori Seeley for allowing us to include it here.

References

Action Dignity. (2013). *Building bridges with ethnocultural communities: Training Resource, Information, Orientation Toolkit.* Calgary, AB: Ethnocultural Cultural Council of Calgary.

Anderson, B. (2006). *Imagined communities: Reflections on the origin and spread of nationalism.* New York: Verso.

Baldassar, L. (2007). Transnational families and aged care: The mobility of care and the migrancy of ageing. *Journal of Ethnic and Migration Studies, 33*(2), 275–297. doi:10.1080/13691830601154252.

Baskin, C., & Sinclair, D. (2015, October 05). *Social work and Indigenous peoples in Canada.* Encyclopedia of Social Work. Retrieved 14 Nov. 2019, from https://oxfordre.com/socialwork/view/10.1093/acrefore/9780199975839.001.0001/acrefore-9780199975839-e-953.

Blackstock, C. (2006). *Reconciliation in child welfare touchstones of hope for indigenous children, youth, and families.* Ottawa, ON: First Nations Child & Family Caring Society of Canada.

Ferrer, I., Brotman, S., & Grenier, A. (2017). The experiences of reciprocity among Filipino older adults in Canada: Intergenerational, transnational, and community considerations. *Journal of Gerontological Social Work*, 60(4), 313–327. doi:10.1080/01634372.2017.1327916.

Grenier, A., Barken, R., Sussman, T., Rothwell, D., & Bourgeois-Guérin, V. (2016b). Homelessness among older people: Assessing strategies and frameworks across Canada. *Canadian Review of Social Policy*, (74), 1–39. Retrieved from https://homelesshub.ca/sites/default/files/attach ments/39889-50157-2-PB.pdf.

Grenier, A., Sussman, T., Barken, R., Bourgeois-Guérin, V., & Rothwell, D. (2016a). 'Growing old' in shelters and 'on the street': Experiences of older homeless people. *Journal of Gerontological Social Work*, 59(6), 458–477. doi:10.1080/01634372.2016.1235067.

Grenier, A. M., & Guberman, N. (2009). Creating and sustaining disadvantage: The relevance of a social exclusion framework. *Health and Social Care in the Community*, 17(2), 116–124. doi:10.1111/j.1365-2524.2007.00804.x.

Hamdi, N., & Goethert, R. (1997). *Action planning for cities: A guide to community practice*. Chichester: John Wiley.

Harris, J., & White, V. (2013). *Community social work. A dictionary of social work and social care*. Retrieved from www.oxfordreference.com/view/10.1093/acref/9780199543052.001.0001/acref-9780199543052.

Mason, A. (2000). *Community, solidarity, and belonging: Levels of community and their normative significance*. Cambridge, UK: Cambridge University Press.

Maximova. (2011). Social aspects of internet communication: Virtual community and communication personality. *RUDN Journal of Sociology*, (1), 24–33. Retrieved from http://journals.rudn.ru/sociology/article/view/6291/5744.

Menec, V., Means, R., Keating, N., Parkhurst, G., & Eales, J. (2011). Conceptualizing age-friendly communities. *Canadian Journal on Aging/La Revue Canadienne Du Vieillissement*, 30(3), 479–493. doi:10.1017/S0714980811000237.

Mirza, R., Liu, A., & Klinger, C. (2018). Age-friendly initiatives and immigrant seniors: Addressing social isolation using technology. *Innovative Ageing*, 2(1), 168. doi:10.1093/geroni/igy023.605.

Oxford English Dictionary. (2019). *Cohort*. Retrieved from www-oed-com.ezproxy.lib.ucal gary.ca/view/Entry/168989.

Phillipson, C., & Ahmed, N. (2004). Transnational communities, migration and changing identities in later life: A new research agenda. In S. O. Daatland & S. Biggs (Eds.), *Ageing and diversity: Multiple pathways and cultural migrations* (pp. 157–174). Bristol, UK: Policy Press.

Phillipson, C., & Scharf, T. (2005). Rural and urban perspectives on growing old: Developing a new research agenda. *European Journal of Ageing*, 2(2), 67–75. doi:10.1007/s10433-005-0024-7.

Pino. (2017). Older Filipino gay men in Canada: Bridging queer theory and gerontology in Filipinx Canadian studies. In R. Diaz, M. Largo, & F. Pino (Eds.), *Diasporic intimacies: Queer Filipinos and Canadian imaginaries* (pp. 163–182). Evanston, IL: Northwestern University Press.

Plouffe L., Kalache A., & Voelcker I. (2016). A Critical review of the WHO age-friendly cities methodology and its implementation. In T. Moulaert & S. Garon (Eds.) *Age-friendly cities and communities in international comparison. International perspectives on aging* (pp. 19–36). Cham: Springer. doi: 10.1007/978-3-319-24031-2_2.

Pradeep, M., & Karibeeran, S. (2017). The 'community' in 'community social work'. *IOSR Journal of Humanities and Social Science*, 22, 58–64. doi:10.9790/0837-2209015864.

Roy, C. (2006). The irreverent raging grannies: Humour as protest. *Canadian Women Studies*, 25(3/4), 141–148. Retrieved from file:///Users/ilyanferrer/Downloads/5901-5777-1-PB%20(1).pdf.

Sainsbury, D. (2006). Immigrants' social rights in comparative perspective: Welfare regimes, forms in immigration and immigration policy regimes. *Journal of European Social Policy*, 16(3), 229–244. doi:10.1177/0958928706065594.

Sherraden, M., & Ninacs, W. (2014). *Community economic development and social work*. Abington, UK: Routledge.

Shragge, E. (2013). *Activism and social change: Lessons for community organizing*. North York, ON: University of Toronto Press.

Statistics Canada (2011). Definition of population. Retrieved from https://www12.statcan.gc.ca/census-recensement/2011/ref/dict/geo049a-eng.cfm.

Sun, K. C. (2014). Reconfigured reciprocity: How aging Taiwanese immigrants transform cultural logics of elder care. *Journal of Marriage and Family, 76*(4), 875–889. doi:10.1111/jomf.12119.

Treas, J. (2008). Transnational older adults and their families. *Family Relations, 57*(4), 468–478. doi:10.1111/j.1741-3729.2008.00515.x.

Walmsley, C., & Kading, T. (Eds.). (2018). *Small cities, big issues: Reconceiving community in a neoliberal era*. Edmonton: Athabasca University Press. doi: 10.1080/13691830600927617.

Walsh, K., Scharf, T., & Keating, N. (2016). Social exclusion of older persons: A scoping review and conceptual framework. *European Journal of Aging, 14*(1), 81–98. doi:10.1007/s10433-016-0398-8.

Warnes, A. M., & Williams, A. (2006). Older migrants in Europe: A new focus for migration studies. *Journal of Ethnic and Migration Studies, 32*(8), 1257–1281. doi:10.1080/13691830600927617.

World Health Organization (WHO). (2015). *Measuring the age-friendliness of cities: A guide to using core indicators*. Geneva: WHO. Retrieved from http://who.int/ageing/publications/Age_friendly_cities_checklist.pdf.

World Health Organization (WHO). (2018). *The global network for age-friendly cities and communities: Looking back over the last decade, looking forward to the next*. Geneva: WHO. Retrieved from http://who.int.

Chapter 12

Policy and planning for an aging society

Questions to consider as you read this chapter

- What are the social policies that impact older adults?
- What are the social policies that impact your current placement or place of work?
- How can social workers engage with social policy in ways that promote policy change?

> *In 2018, I (Ilyan) was invited to speak at a roundtable titled "Social and Economic Inclusion: Views on Canadian Seniors". Hosted by the federal government, the roundtable was meant to share views and insights on the challenges and opportunities related to improving the social and economic inclusion of older people in Canada. The Honorable Jean-Yves Duclos (Minister of Families, Children and Social Development) was in attendance to listen to different stakeholders from across the country.[1] The roundtable was attended by 22 academic and community organizations who work with various social service sectors and across provinces in Canada. There was also generative discussion about initiatives to enhance social and economic inclusion of older adults, including a national housing strategy, income security programs, grants and contributions to support communities, and a poverty reduction strategy (Employment and Social Development Canada, 2018). Despite the important conversations about aging and including older people more intentionally into Canadian policies and programs, only one organization represented ethnic minority communities and another four organizations spoke on behalf of First Nations, Inuit, and Métis communities. In fact, I was only one of five racialized people sitting at the Roundtable. I began to think about the following questions: Whose voices are predominately heard in policy development? How can policy makers be more inclusive of all the voices that should be part of policy discussions? How do we connect our social work practice, community organizing, and research to affect policy changes? What specific steps do we need to follow in order to enact social change?*

The story above is an example of how social workers can be involved in the development of and discussion about social policies. Some of us might find ourselves working with social policies and programs with local institutions and non-profit organizations, while others might be speaking to government officials as Ilyan did at the *Social and Economic Inclusion Roundtable* (Council of Canadians with Disabilities, 2018). Social workers might also work directly with social policy and programs in municipal, provincial, or federal contexts, while others could find themselves working in non-profit organizations advocating for better policies and/or programs. Take a look at Table 12.1, and see if you recognize these social workers who work in government and have had direct roles in developing and implementing policies.

Table 12.1 Social workers and social policy

Dr. Wanda Thomas Bernard is currently a member of the Canadian Senate. The Honourable Dr. Thomas Bernard is a social worker, educator, researcher, community activist, and advocate for social change. She is also a founding member of the Association of Black Social Workers and a full professor at Dalhousie University's School of Social Work.

Judith Seidman is a member of the Canadian Senate. She holds a BSW and MSW from McGill University's School of Social Work and is a PhD candidate in the Department of Epidemiology and Biostatistics at McGill University. The Honorable Seidman is an active member of the Standing Senate Committee on Social Affairs, Science and Technology and the Senate Committee on Human Rights.

Ginette Petipas Taylor is a member of the Liberal Party of Canada and a BSW graduate from the Université de Moncton. On August 28, 2017, the Honorable Petitpas Taylor was appointed Minister of Health, and on June 17, 2019, she announced the release of *Together We Aspire: Canada's first dementia strategy.*

Joe Ceci is an MSW graduate of the University of Calgary. From 2015 to 2018, he served as the New Democratic Party's (NDP's) Minister of Finance and president of the Treasury Board in the Alberta Cabinet.

Irfan Sabir earned social work and law degrees from the University of Calgary. From 2015 to 2018, he served as the NDP's Minister of Community and Social Services in the Alberta Cabinet.

Dave Barrett was the 26th premier of British Columbia from 1972 to 1975 and was responsible for implementing 369 bills and social policies over three years. He was an MSW graduate of St. Louis University and loved speaking to social work students about not only his time in government, but also his practice experience in corrections. Mr. Barrett lived with Alzheimer's disease until his death in 2018.

Brenda Shanahan is a BSW graduate from McGill University's School of Social Work. She was elected to the Legislative Assembly in 2015 under the Liberal Party. Her expertise centres on financial management and financial literacy. Ms. Shanahan served on the Special Joint Committee on Physician-Assisted Death.

As emerging AOP social workers and AOG practitioners, it is important to understand how social policies are developed and the ways in which they shape perceptions and expectations of aging. As we learned in **Age/ism: age as a category of difference**, social policies contribute to our perceptions and expectations of who is an older person and the types of benefits they (should) receive later in life. Take a moment to think about the kinds of policies that directly impact older people. How do these policies impact the social, economic, physical, and mental health of older people? How do these policies describe older people? Do they have age requirements? Who is included? Who is excluded? In this chapter, we examine different policies that affect the lives of Canadians and older people. We also discuss the ways in which social workers play a role in social policy development, revision, and implementation. In the second half of the chapter, we discuss how we might engage social policy through an equity, diversity and inclusion (EDI) lens. In particular, we see human rights, equity, social inclusion, and citizenship as integral social work values that should underpin aging policies, rather than an exclusive focus on prioritizing and meeting needs.

The objectives of this chapter are to

- Define social policy and explain how social policies are made at institutional and governmental levels;
- Identify and understand how policies impact experiences of aging;
- Appreciate the potential for effecting social change through policy (advocacy, analysis, and creation); and
- Become familiar with policy making principles aligned with AOP like equity, diversity and inclusion (EDI and a particular framework known as GBA+ (gender-based analysis+)that operationalizes intersectionality.

What is a social policy?

Joseph is a white cis-gendered male in his late 20s. He works at a geriatric rehabilitation centre, where for the last two years he has been responsible for discharge planning for outgoing clients. Most of Joseph's cases are transfer files from the hospital where clients had been admitted after a stroke or a fall. Joseph enjoys working with his interdisciplinary team of doctors, nurses, and other allied health professionals like himself (e.g., physiotherapist, occupational therapist, dietician). He has especially good relationships with his clients. Knowing the difficult journey that his clients face post-recovery and at the rehabilitation centre, Joseph takes pride in making sure that his clients have the necessary social supports to transition back to the community or to a long-term-care facility. Living with his mother, who is also aging and has a physical disability, makes his job as much personal as it is professional. As someone who is relatively new to the field, Joseph is also learning about the different social policies that impact older adults. For instance, Joseph realizes that he needs to be aware of the various social programs and policies that might benefit his clients when assisting them with discharge planning. On a number of occasions, he has received questions from clients' families who want to know whether they can receive additional resources or support from the government or community after their older family has been discharged from the rehab centre. While Joseph is familiar with basic benefits, he reflects on how he needs to know more about disability benefits such as the Canada Pension Plan (CPP) disability pension and the CPP post-retirement disability benefit.

What is your definition of a social policy? Do you think it is a term or concept that applies to government, to people, and/or to communities? Generally, a social policy is defined as the practice and organized system/form of administration in the conduct of public affairs (Oxford English Dictionary, 2019). Social policy is primarily concerned with how society meets human needs for security, education, work, health, and well-being (Rice & Prince, 2013). For instance, policies might be aimed at reducing inequalities in accessing services or establishing more support for equity-seeking groups based on needs or realities (Westhues & Wharf, 2012). As such, policies shape our daily lives, not only as social work practitioners, but also as citizens. They address local and global issues such as social, demographic, and economic challenges including poverty, immigration/migration, and globalization (Graham, Swift, & Delaney, 2012; Westhues, 2003; Westhues & Wharf, 2012). Social policies can also identify stakeholders (all those who have a stake in the issue the policy is meant to address) who can be considered responsible for providing services or support. These services and supports can include child and family support, schooling and education, housing and neighbourhood renewal, income maintenance and poverty reduction, unemployment support and training, pensions, and health and social care (McKenzie & Wharf, 2016; Westhues & Wharf, 2012). When we hear about social policy, we probably think about municipal, provincial, and federal programs or lawmakers. However, social policies also apply to private sector and non-profit organizations, community groups, and individuals (see textbox 12.1).

Textbox 12.1

Social policies are guidelines, principles, and legislation that are meant to improve the living conditions and quality of life of citizens.

One important question you might be asking is whether social policy is the same as social welfare. Graham et al. (2012) suggest that social policy is more concerned with the "big picture" of society and deals with issues related to social justice, equality, human rights and freedoms, (re)distribution of wealth, employment, health care, criminal justice, and mutual aid. Social policies are also concerned with identifying and implementing remedies (such as welfare programs) or solutions to a particular issue (Graham et al., 2012). Given the scope that social policies are meant to address, issues of power, control, and representation are important considerations in policy. Social welfare, on the other hand, refers to governmental support for the well-being of people and society (see textbox 12.2). A welfare state is a political system in which state mechanisms (enacted by government) assume some measure of responsibility for the health, education, and welfare of society (Graham et al., 2012). If social policies are the general "beliefs" and "principles" for how society is governed, including the rights and responsibilities of citizens, social welfare is the range of programs that governments offer to ensure that the basic needs of citizens are met (Graham et al., 2012).

Textbox 12.2

Social welfare is the range of programs that governments offer to ensure that the basic needs of citizens are met.

Through your social work history and policy courses, you are probably familiar with Canada's nation-building project and settler-colonial past (Blackstock, 2017). Before the welfare state, parents and families were considered the basic support system of society, and there were distinctions between the "deserving poor" and the "undeserving" poor. The deserving poor were considered the most vulnerable members of society through no fault of their own and therefore were provided compassion and support (Lightman & Lightman, 2017). The three groups covered by Elizabethan poor laws, for example, were children, persons with disabilities, and older adults (Graham et al., 2012). Until the onset of World War II, the capitalist economy was thought to be self-regulating, and the state had no specific role in intervening when there were periods of economic instability or unemployment. The Great Depression shifted how governments thought citizens could cope under an unregulated market economy and the role of the state and state interventions during times of financial crisis, unemployment, and poverty. The Canadian welfare state emerged following World War II and ushered in the notion of collective responsibility and expansive social policies/programs meant to better society. Armitage (2003) provides a list of seven types of programs or services that are quintessential features of the welfare state:

1. Cash programs such as Old Age Security, Canada Child Tax Benefit, Canada Pension Plan, and postsecondary student loans;
2. Fiscal measures, including tuition-fee deductions, child-care expense deductions, and RRSP exemptions;
3. Goods and services measures, such as hospital insurance, legal aid, and education;
4. Measures related to employment, including minimum-wage legislation and employment equity programs;
5. Occupational welfare measures, such as pension and insurance plans and sports and recreational facilities;
6. Family care and dependency programs such as home-care provisions; and
7. Voluntary/charitable programs, such as shelters, soup kitchens, and food banks.

The policies and programs listed above are aimed at "redistribution". The purpose of a redistributive policy is to promote equality (sameness) and to provide protective rights for at-risk groups in the workplace, at home, or in the community. Given the list above, a common question is whether policies are meant to be universal or for specific groups of people. The answer depends on the type of policy and the goal of the policy. Some policies are considered "universal" – that is, they apply to every citizen regardless of social or economic status, while others are considered selective transfers – where benefactors must demonstrate they meet specific eligibility criteria. The latter process is referred to as means-testing. Some redistributive policies provide compensation by way of tax credits (e.g., elder care), while other redistributive policies offer incentives (e.g., reduced rates for child care, work requirements to access social assistance benefits).

Adding more nuance to the purposes of social policy, Westhues and Kenny-Scherber (2012) argue that there are four policy types. **Strategic social policies** seek to improve the well-being of vulnerable groups either globally or locally (e.g., the United Nations Declaration on the Rights of the Child). A second type are **legislative or regulatory policies** that achieve a government's objectives through the use of regulation, laws, and other instruments to deliver social and economic outcomes that benefit the lives of citizens (OECD, 2018). An example of regulatory policies are safety and health regulations. **Program policies** are a third type of social policy and define program objectives, delivery structure, and implementation plans. The fourth and final type, **operational or administrative policies**, require decisions to implement specific protocols and procedures of the program.

If social policies are meant to address social inequalities and identify who is responsible for providing social services, then are they considered laws? Policies can lead to laws or they can arise from legislation, but policies and laws are two distinct social artefacts. While policies are meant to guide actions toward a desired outcome, laws are rules of conduct imposed by authorities and are a set of standards, procedures, and principles that all citizens must follow (see textbox 12.3). For instance, breaking the law could mean prosecution or some form of reprimand whereas choosing not to abide by a policy is seen as an individual choice. One might lose one's job for not following policy; however, one is unlikely to be imprisoned.

Textbox 12.3

Laws are the rules of conduct imposed by authorities and a set of standards, procedures, and principles that all citizens must follow.

When we address Canadian laws in the context of social work education and practice, we tend to pay particular attention to the **Canadian Constitution** and the **Canadian Charter of Rights and Freedoms**. This is because these documents speak specifically to the rights of individuals and groups in society, which is a central concern of social workers and a fundamental value of the profession. Introduced in 1982, the Charter determines a person's rights and freedoms, including the right to speak freely, believe in any religion or no religion, meet with or join any group (except a terrorist organization), live and work anywhere in Canada, and participate in peaceful political activities (Constitution Act, 1982). Because the Charter outlines the democratic rights and fundamental freedoms of citizens and oftentimes guides laws in Canada, it represents an important frame for understanding what is considered "equality" in a Canadian context. The Canadian Charter of Rights and Freedoms is a part of the Canadian Constitution and specifically addresses the rights and freedoms guaranteed within the Constitution. Section 15, which came into effect in 1985, establishes the "equality rights" of Canadian citizens (see textbox 12.4). Over time, Canadian courts have rendered hundreds of decisions based upon Section 15 of the Charter, including challenges to better include equity-seeking groups not previously identified within the Charter (see textbox 12.4). Human rights advocates (including social workers) have engaged the Charter as a powerful tool in the fight against discrimination in Canada.

Textbox 12.4

Human rights are entitlements all individuals should be able to access without fear of discrimination on the basis of race, sex, nationality, ethnicity, language, religion, or any other category of difference. According to the United Nations General Assembly (1948), specific human rights include life, liberty, freedom from slavery and torture, freedom of expression, the right to work, and education. **Section 15** of the **Canadian Charter of Rights and Freedoms** guarantees that every individual is considered equal before and under the law and has the right to equal protection and equal benefit of the law without discrimination (based on race, national or ethnic origin, colour, religion, sex, age, or mental or physical ability). Section 15 also protects equality on the basis of other characteristics that are not specifically indicated (e.g., sexual orientation, marital status, citizenship).

Section 15 of the Charter details the prohibited grounds for discrimination; thus, it is critical for AOP social workers to familiarize themselves with this section of the Charter. Provincial laws, policies, and programs related to human rights flow from Section 15 of the Charter. You may wonder why mandatory retirement was permissible when age is a prohibited ground for discrimination. This had to do with the definition of those who were of working age in employment legislation, which did not cover those over the age of 65.

State and institutional policies

After months of campaigning, a new provincial government is elected in Joseph's province. Within five weeks, the new government announces massive restructuring and cuts to health and social services. The new premier had campaigned on balancing the provincial budget and explicitly blamed rising costs on the inefficiencies of the care system. As a result, rehabilitation services, which previously had been aligned with hospital and clinical services, are now being integrated more into community health centres. Although Joseph had originally applauded the restructuring, he begins to wonder how these changes to the health and social care sector will affect his work. He becomes worried after chatting with colleagues who express fears of being laid off, especially the nurses who are the largest employee group. Joseph is reassured by the fact that he is one of only four full-time social workers.

As Westhues and Kenny-Scherber (2012) note, different levels of government and organizations are responsible for public policy. These authors introduce the concept of "scale" to understand the various levels of responsibility in the policy arena (Westhues & Kenny-Scherber, 2012). In Canada, the federal and provincial governments have different jurisdictions over social policies. For instance, while provinces are responsible for the "establishment, maintenance and management of hospitals, asylums [and] charities" (Constitution Act, 1982), the federal government is responsible for providing funds through the Canada Health and Social Transfer. Local municipalities are also responsible for policies, but at a much more limited scale as they focus on local matters including land and water use, infrastructure (e.g., roads and libraries), and municipal taxes (Westhues & Kenny-Scherber, 2012). It is important to note that broader social policies and agendas that are negotiated and set at the federal, provincial, municipal, and even international scales inform and enact social policies at the institutional/organizational level. Just as social policies take on many different forms, they can also be created in a number of different ways. One way of understanding the policy-making process is through the "policy cycle" (Lasswell, 1956), which outlines the phases of policy development.

- Phase 1: Agenda setting or problem definition helps policy makers decide problem areas to address;
- Phase 2: Policy formation is when stakeholders identify various needs and desires and engage in debates about budgetary issues, constraints, and existing programs;
- Phase 3: Policy legitimation is when the polices go through a legislative process and when they can be implemented (if adopted);
- Phase 4: Policy implementation is putting the policy into action;
- Phase 5: Policy evaluation includes assessments that determine whether the policy and its outcomes were effective; and

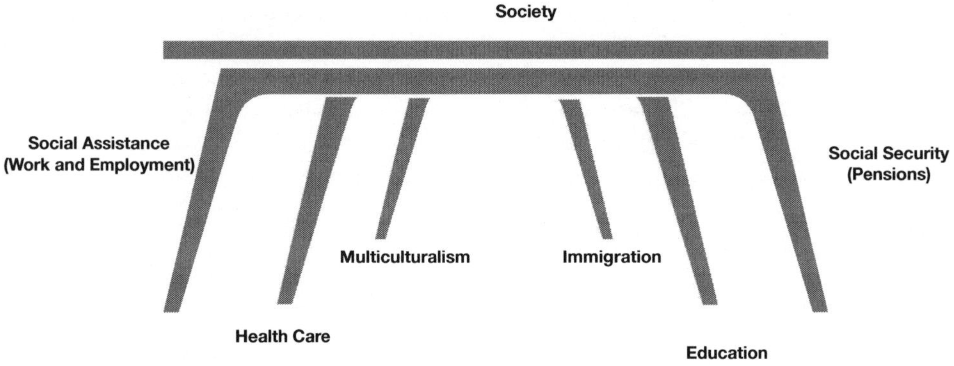

Figure 12.1 Social policy as a table metaphor

- Phase 6: Policy maintenance, succession, or termination is the phase where policies are consistently gauged for relevance and use. When new issues arise, the policy-making cycle begins again, helping governing bodies successfully address new and important challenges.

Main policy areas impacting Canadians

It is sometimes useful to think about social policy as a four legged-table that holds up the public or the overall well-being of society. The legs that hold up society are generally *health care, education, social assistance* (such as work and employment insurance), and *social security programs* (such as pensions). The table metaphor is a classic interpretation of how social policies tend to be organized for different members of society, in particular how they are made for people based on their specific needs. It is worth noting that a number of policies shape and structure how older people live their lives. Thus, when gerontologists think about social policies as a table, we envision more legs (see Figure 12.1).

Social policy and aging among Indigenous communities

As social workers, we are keenly aware of the policies that have impacted Indigenous communities in Canada. The Indian Act created in 1867 and enacted in 1876 effectively allows the federal government to control status, land, resources, wills, education, and band administration among First Nations communities (Inuit and Métis people are not governed by this law) (Baskin, 2018). Provisions within the Indian Act, such as the Residential Schools (which were active between 1879 and 1996), had devastating and intergenerational impacts on First Nations. For the most part, state policies have been used as mechanisms for surveillance and control of First Nations, as well as Métis and Inuit communities (Baskin, 2018; Blackstock, 2009). For instance, the White Paper of 1969 was a Canadian policy that sought to abolish legal documents such as treaties and attempted to assimilate Indigenous people and communities into the Canadian state. Despite this history and legacy of control, Indigenous people and communities have engaged in forms of resistance through grassroots advocacy and policy change. The Idle No More movement, which started as a series of teach-ins in Saskatchewan and later evolved into a mass protest movement against parliamentary bills seeking to control and undermine Indigenous sovereignty, is but one example.

The relationship between the Canadian government and Indigenous communities demonstrates the ways in which past and current policy can impact both individuals and a community (Baskin, 2018; Blackstock, 2009). For instance, Beatty and Berdahl (2011) noted that older adults from Indigenous communities (reserves, Northern areas, rural, urban) face a number of socio-economic and health concerns as a result of past (e.g., residential school) and current policies (e.g., homecare policies in urban centres). In particular, chronic health issues have meant that Indigenous older adults spend a disproportionate amount of time in healthcare systems in their communities and in urban centres. Issues and disjunctures between long-term-care and homecare programs and policies result in Indigenous Elders and their families expressing difficulties in navigating these health systems. For instance, did you know that some provincial transportation services for older adults and persons with disabilities such as handyDART or Wheel-Trans cannot pick up or drop off Elders who live "on reserve"? Jurisdictional issues such as these are everyday realities for Indigenous Elders and can be daily reminders that First Nations people are still "wards of the state".

Social policies directly impacting older adults

Several months have passed since the massive restructuring of health and social services. Joseph is thankful that neither he nor any of his colleagues were laid off. However, he does notice that there is a much more explicit protocol of how clients are expected to be discharged. One change that was implemented is the "First Available Bed policy". Hospitals and other tertiary care facilities (such as rehabilitation centres) have implemented a discharge policy where older patients must accept transfer to the first available bed in any long-term-care facility. If clients refuse the first available bed, the health authority assumes that a client's need is not urgent, and their names will be removed from the priority access list. The client has the option of applying to a private care facility. Joseph finds himself having difficulty adjusting to this policy. He finds there is much more onus on discharge and less consideration for how his older clients adapt while they are in the facility. Joseph believes that it is important to find a good fit for his clients, knowing the difficult transitions that clients face post-rehabilitation.

For most older Canadians, health and social care, caregiving, work and retirement, immigration, and housing are examples of the many policies and programs that can offer support. Returning to the social policy as a table metaphor, we see that for some older adults the social policy table has six legs, while for others the table can have as few as three legs (see Figure 12.1). Let us now take a look at a few social policies that affect the lives of older people in Canada: health care, social security, immigration, and housing.

Social policy and the Canada Health Act

One of the more well-known Canadian policies is "Medicare", our publicly funded, single-payer health care system. Adopted in 1984, *the Canada Health Act* specifies the conditions and criteria for which provinces and territories offer universal health insurance to constituents. Provinces and territories must conform to these criteria in order to receive federal transfer payments under the Canada Health Transfer. Understanding these jurisdictional relationships is important because it explains why health care is administered by provinces and territories (and therefore a provincial/territorial jurisdiction) yet funded by the federal government. As such, jurisdictional tensions oftentimes arise about who is considered eligible to receive services, who is to pay for complicated services and treatment, and who makes decision related to health care regulations. For example:

- While the federal government is responsible for providing health care benefits and income support to Canadian veterans, most veterans rely on provincial services for mental health issues;
- The federal government is responsible for providing care and support to Indigenous people living on reserves, but has been criticized for failing to provide equitable funding for child and family services on reserves. In 2016, the Canadian Human Rights Tribunal ruled that the federal government discriminates against First Nation children by failing to provide child welfare services that exist off of reserves (Blackstock, 2016); and
- Although we might assume that health care is universal to all Canadians, sponsored family members under the Parent and Grandparent Program (to be discussed later in this chapter) and refugee claimants do not receive the same health care benefits as citizens or landed status immigrants.[2]

While we have a universal health care system, no policies, existing national strategy, or seniors' framework addresses the health care needs of older adults. In 2015, the Canadian Medical Association (CMA) published a policy framework to guide a national seniors' strategy and influence health care transformation (Canadian Medical Association, 2015). The CMA stressed the need in particular for health promotion and illness prevention. As we learned in **Theorizing later life and social work praxis**, the notion of healthy aging is often used to promote the improvement of physical and health status. Guided by the World Health Organization (WHO), healthy aging is an approach to policies and programs that promote the mental health and social connections of older adults in order to improve physical health. The idea is that by increasing self-efficacy, self-esteem, coping skills and social supports, policies, and programs can empower individuals and communities and ward off chronic issues such as loneliness, isolation, and dependency. While a national seniors' strategy does not exist to date, Canada does have a federal strategy on dementia that was also championed by CMA (see **Dementia, personhood, and citizenship as practice).** The Alliance for a National Seniors Strategy, a network of healthcare organizations, proposed an evidence-based national seniors strategy based on four pillars: the first two pillars reflect the discourse of healthy and active aging: (1) independent, productive, and engaged citizens and (2) healthy and active lives (Sinha et al., 2016).

Social policy, work, and retirement

When people enter retirement, they are expected to financially support themselves and can do so in multiple ways. One mechanism is through the workplace. Depending on one's employer, a working person might have contributed to a workplace pension (wherein the employer also provides a contribution). Upon retirement, the retiree would receive back the contributions or they would receive specific benefits for the rest of their life. The difference between these two scenarios depends on whether the retiree had a *defined contribution* plan or a *defined benefit* plan. The former is subject to the vagaries of the marketplace; thus, it is less secure than the latter, which assures the retiree of benefits regardless of whether there is a recession. However, not everyone is able to save, and not everyone can find employment that allows for individual contributions. It is also important to recognize that not everyone has access to pensions. Pensions are very much gendered and classed.

The state does offer a pension scheme to ensure that Canadian citizens have access to funds in their later lives. Through government transfers (basic entitlements) and contributory schemes Canada's pension structure ensures a standard of living for older Canadians (Financial Consumer Agency of Canada, 2015). Think of the Canadian pension scheme as a pyramid, where at its base is Old Age Security (OAS). The OAS is a universal government transfer program whose purpose is to reduce poverty in later life (see Figure 12.2). When the OAS is insufficient, older adults can be eligible for the Guaranteed Income Supplement (GIS), which is a means-tested supplement (Service Canada, 2014). Another base of the pension pyramid is represented by the contributory programs such as the Canadian Pension Plan/Quebec Pension Plan (CPP/QPP), into which all Canadian workers formally contribute throughout their labour history in Canada (Ferrer, 2017). Finally, the top of the pension pyramid is represented by private pension programs (e.g., Registered Pension Plan and Registered Retirement Savings Plan (RRSP) and Mutual Funds). Private pensions come in the form of employer and/or individual contributions. Those who are self-employed, which includes both professionals such as accountants and lawyers as well as "working poor" people like seamstresses or those working predominantly within the secondary and peripheral labour market,[3] are responsible for saving for their own retirement should they need more than the OAS and GIS to survive, let alone thrive, in old age.

Feminist scholars have argued that the Canadian retirement pyramid reflects the gendered and stratified labour market in Canada (Marier & Skinner, 2008; Young, 2011).

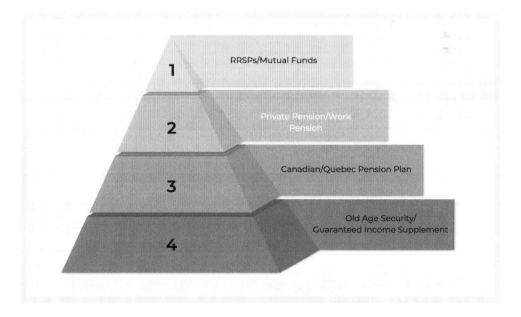

Figure 12.2 Retirement programs in Canada

According to Marier and Skinner (2008), older women disproportionately access the GIS, which, as of 2019, has a maximum benefit of approximately $14,000. These realities exist in large part because of the ways in which Canadian retirement policies are structured to benefit full-time and continuous work (Kodar, 2012; Young, 2011). Ferrer (2017) notes that the "persistence of low incomes is closely tied to the eligibility rules governing Canada's OAS and GIS programs, which are particularly restrictive to newcomers, and have a disproportionate impact for immigrant women who cannot access and benefit from pension programs in the same way as their Canadian-born counterparts" (p. 16). For instance, scholars have noted that Canadian immigrants tend to receive fewer public and private social benefits because of their time of arrival and consequent contributions to their pensions.

Social policy and immigration: Canada's growing and aging multicultural society

Immigration programs, and the consequent processes of migration, shape and structure the composition of the family unit and the ensuing availability of family members to provide care. As such, immigration is another important social policy area that requires attention and unpacking. Canada is lauded as a multicultural country that welcomes new cultures and supports a mosaic of communities.[4] To this point, Canada does have a multicultural policy meant to preserve the cultural freedom of all individuals and ethnic groups (see textbox 12.5). Yet scholars and activists have questioned whether such policies are welcoming (or perhaps hindering) the lives of racialized immigrants, particularly older ones. What impact does multiculturalism have on immigration specific to older people?

Textbox 12.5

Multiculturalism: Introduced in 1971, Canada's multiculturalism policy was implemented to preserve the cultural freedom of all individuals and ethnic groups within Canadian society. The government committed to supporting multiculturalism in four specific ways: (1) through assistance to cultural groups in their development and growth; (2) assistance to members of cultural groups to overcome barriers to full participation in society; (3) promotion of creative exchanges between cultural groups; and (4) assistance to immigrants in learning French or English.

Racialized older immigrants in Canada are largely comprised of two groups (Durst, 2010; Koehn, Spencer, & Hwang, 2010). The first group is composed of older adults who have aged-in-place after arriving under the Economic Class program during the mid-20th century. During this time, Canada's immigration programs were said to be liberalized after eliminating explicitly discriminatory admissions criteria and facilitating channels for reunification of family members (Durst, 2010; Koehn et al., 2010). While immigrants during this time period are said to have had longer opportunities for adaptation and integration, structural barriers and forms of exclusion (for instance, experiences of poverty and predominant work in the secondary and peripheral labour market) have meant that some immigrants who arrived earlier in life continue to experience economic inequities in later life (Galabuzi, 2006).

A second group of racialized older immigrants in Canada is comprised of new-comers who arrive under the Family Sponsorship category. An important provision of this sponsorship program is its "dependency clause" where sponsored older immi-grants are reliant on their sponsors (usually younger family members) for basic needs such as food, clothing, shelter, and dental and eye care for a period of 20^5 years. Stipulations of the Parent and Grandparent Program deny older immigrants from full access to health care services, and the basic income security programs for older adults discussed above (OAS and GIS). The imposition of a dependency clause, which restricts access to basic pension entitlements, creates structured dependencies on spon-sors who bear the economic cost and responsibility for necessary services and resources. In addition to a dependency clause, the federal government imposes an annual cap on the number of applications it processes and accepts (Ferrer, 2015). However, to allow older parents to join their children in Canada, the federal govern-ment allows temporary visits through the "Parent and Grandparent Supervisa[6]". While immigration and migration programs like the Parent and Grandparent Super-visa are meant to address application backlogs by providing an efficient and stream-lined method for family reunification, they in reality require considerable effort from adult children who must coordinate applications transnationally.[7] These age-specific immigration and migration programs call into question the survival of the interge-nerational family unit, the perpetuation of the cycle of poverty (including the femin-ization of poverty), and the imbalanced power dynamics given the structured dependency of older parents on their adult children.

Social policy and housing

In 2017, the Government of Canada adopted the first National Housing Strategy, which is a 10-year \$40-billion plan that will "give more Canadians a place to call home". The strategy aims to reduce chronic homelessness by 50%; it will result in 100,000 new and 300,000 repaired housing units. The new housing initiative is meant to build communities that are close to transit and public services and offers the Canada Housing Benefit, which is a rights-based approach to housing to ensure that "the National Housing Strategy prioritizes the most vulnerable Canadians including women and children fleeing family violence, Indigenous peoples, **seniors**, people with disabil-ities, those dealing with mental health and addiction issues, veterans and young adults" (National Housing Strategy, 2018). As we discussed in **Building inclusive commu-nities**, one critique of the housing policy is its lack of attention to homelessness *among older adults*. Among the issues that homeless older people face are health, housing, and social care needs that are distinct from those of their younger homeless counterparts. For instance, older homeless people are more likely to have mental and physical health concerns that might require specialized care (Grenier, Barken, & Mcgrath, 2016). Des-pite their emerging numbers, older homeless people are generally perceived as a sub-population whose issues are treated as chronic rather than structural. In response, social gerontologists and social work practitioners have called for attention/action on the unique housing issues facing older homeless people and the structural barriers contrib-uting to their experiences of marginalization.

Social policy in the context of neoliberalism and globalization

> *Joseph has noticed the impact that the First Available Bed policy is having on his team. What was once a collaborative interdisciplinary team is now struggling under the weight of growing caseloads and the push to discharge clients (i.e., "get them out the door"). In fact, Joseph has observed clients expressing concerns, frustration, and anger over being required to accept the first available bed because of how far the facility is from their families and familiar environment. Most clients eventually accept their placement because they cannot afford private long-term care. An example of this is Mr. Nguyen, a 90-year-old Vietnamese man who does not speak English or French. Joseph relies on an interpreter and the help of Mr. Nguyen's grandchildren to discuss his discharge plans. Mr. Nguyen is ready to be discharged but requires long-term care support and is therefore unable to return home. The first available bed is 40 km away from his grandchildren and does not have anyone on staff who speaks Vietnamese. Through an interpreter, Mr. Nguyen expresses his fear of going to a placement so far from his grandchildren and his inability to communicate his needs to staff. Concerned about how Mr. Nguyen will adapt to this facility, Joseph decides to advocate on Mr. Nguyen's behalf with his supervisor. In particular, Joseph hopes to discuss how the First Available Bed policy fails to account for language, culture, family circumstance, ability, class, and other categories of difference that determine one's social location.*
>
> *The meeting between Joseph and his supervisor does not go well. The manager of the rehab centre claims that they have far too many cases pending, and he doesn't want Mr. Nguyen to "bed-block" when he has been cleared for discharge. When Joseph tries to argue that there isn't a Vietnamese speaking staff member at the long-term care facility, his manager responds with, "I understand, but Mr. Nguyen doesn't need our services right now. He needs long-term care. Think about how much it costs for him to stay here while another person who needs rehab waits for Mr. Nguyen. At this point, it's about capacity and numbers, Joseph. I hope that we have resolved this issue because you're the only one raising this as an issue, and you're the only social worker who is falling behind on their caseloads".*

Now that we know some of the social policies that impact older Canadians, we return to the concept of neoliberalism discussed in **Sites and sectors of health and social care**. You will recall that neoliberalism is an ideology underpinning political and economic arrangements that promotes the free flow of capital (i.e., privatization) and a limited role for the state so that the private market can thrive (Harvey, 2007). Some scholars have argued that both neoliberalism and globalization have radically transformed growing interdependence between nations and that relationships between the economic and labour markets have transformed policies such as immigration into global capital.[8] In other words, state social policies are increasingly de-regulated in favour of privatized interventions. As we see in Joseph's counter-story, one of the ways that neoliberalism manifests itself in the workplace is through reduced resources, funding cuts, increased caseloads, and pressure for social workers to work faster and more efficiently. The First Available Bed policy (see endnote 3 in **Moral, legal, and ethical issues**) is an example of how efficiency and cost-savings are prioritized over the suitability of interventions or services.

The implications of neoliberalism and globalization for older people create dynamics where social programs are increasingly de-funded. Moreover, people are increasingly finding it difficult to access existing resources and services. Those accessing services find that they have to meet eligibility criteria to "prove" that they are in need. If we look at the policies that we have discussed in this chapter, we see that most social policies and services on aging are structured to narrowly address people's ongoing needs. There are very few universal programs.

Our vision of AOG and a human rights perspective on equity, inclusion, and citizenship

Disappointed with his meeting with his manager, Joseph speaks with the Nguyen family to inform them that there isn't much that he, as their social worker, can do. However, Joseph encourages the family to link with a non-profit organization that advocates for older people living in long-term care facilities. Given that the "First Available Bed" is a relatively new policy, Joseph believes that an advocacy organization would be better positioned to understand provincial laws and offer suggestions on how to better advocate for the family. Joseph also suggests that the family write to their local member of the legislative assembly (provincial) and member of parliament (federal) and media to shed light on this issue. The family agrees to these suggestions and asks Joseph to continue to offer his guidance. Although Joseph is invested in helping Mr. Nguyen, he is also wary of his supervisor's veiled threats about going against policy. He explains to the Nguyen family that while he personally believes the policy is unjust, he can't afford to risk losing his job.

Discouraged and frustrated with this case, Joseph begins to think about one of his BSW policy classes where he was asked to write a policy/issue brief. He then gets an idea to write a briefing note about the "First Available Bed" policy to identify problems and potential solutions. He hopes that this briefing note will be useful for his clients, colleagues, and other long-term care stakeholders.

Thus far, this chapter has discussed some of the social policies that shape and constrain the lives of older people in Canada. You might have noticed that most social policies were developed to address a *social need*. Rice and Prince (2013) attribute this to the colonial and gendered history of policies in Canada and note that most social policies were meant to offer income support in a limited, means tested fashion. In fact, you might have observed that most social policies we have discussed are tied to some form of economic outcome. How can social policy integrate intersectionality and related concepts like equity, diversity, and inclusion? As authors, we argue that social policies are integral to people's human rights, equity, social inclusion, and citizenship (see textbox 12.6 for definitions on social inclusion and citizenship). By adopting a rights-based approach to policies and programs, we can begin to assess people's experiences informed by a consistent set of values and principles based on their social location and lived experiences as well as the socio-cultural and geo-political contexts in which they live.

Textbox 12.6

Social Inclusion is the process of improving the terms of participation in society. Examples include enhancing the ability, opportunity, access and dignity of people and groups, particularly those who are disadvantaged on the basis of their identity/social location.

Citizenship encompasses legal status, rights, participation, and belonging, and as such evokes images of national identity, sovereignty, and state control. Citizenship is usually defined as a form of membership in a political and geographic community. When we think about social work practice and the social policies that impact our work, we must consider how human rights, social inclusion, and citizenship are implicated, as well as their relationships not only to one another but to our professional values and ethics. One important policy development in Canada is the introduction and integration of **gender-based analysis +** (GBA+) as a means of operationalizing principles of equity, diversity and inclusion (EDI) through an intersectional lens. EDI is currently the favoured discourse amongst policy professionals and decision makers, particularly in the post-secondary education (PSE) sector; however, it remains to be seen if these (potentially) powerful words will be translated into concrete and measurable actions to redress longstanding inequities, position diversity as a strength, and promote social inclusion and citizenship of those from equity-seeking groups. GBA+ goes beyond words as it is a framework with associated tools to support the analysis, development, and evaluation of policies from an intersectional perspective. In 2005, the Canadian government introduced the GBA approach to ensure that the development of policies, programs and legislation includes the consideration of differential impacts on diverse and equity-seeking groups. In 2015, the Status of Women was mandated to ensure that government policy, legislation, and regulations were sensitive to the impacts of social policy decisions on Canadian men and women. A GBA+ framework asserts that people's experiences are affected by intersecting parts of their identities, the contexts in which they find themselves, and their lived realities. As such, GBA+ expands on GBA to address categories of difference in addition to gender. Although the emergence of GBA+ represents an important and significant shift in Canadian policy (insofar as it is an attempt to mainstream intersectionality as part of policy analysis), by 2016 only 29 of approximately 110 federal organizations had committed to GBA+ (Hankivsky & Mussell, 2018). See textbox 12.7 for a definition of GBA+.

Textbox 12.7

GBA+ is a framework for undertaking a gender-based and intersectional analysis when developing and assessing policy, legislation, and government decision-making. The categories of difference on which it currently focusses are sex, gender, race, ethnicity, religion, age, disability, geography, culture, income, sexual orientation, and education.

As social workers, we engage in advocacy in ways that support people, ensuring voices are heard, and safeguarding rights. Throughout this book, we have argued that AOG is a reflexive process that includes identifying and working with people's stories of agency, resistance, and resilience. When we talk about agency, we are referring to actions or interventions that people are able to enact or engage in to produce a particular and desired effect. When we speak about resilience and resistance, we are calling for building capacity to overcome, recover from, and resist forms of oppression. In thinking about the AOG principles we discussed at the beginning of the book, how would you respond to the following questions?

- How do policies take into account identity, including questioning taken-for-granted privilege and the rationale for dominance in society?
- How do policies address social difference as an issue of power and equity rather than a matter of cultural and ethnic variation?
- How do policies examine the ways that individual and everyday oppressive acts are entrenched and (un)consciously supported by institutional structures?
- How do policies address social justice as both process and goal, which entails sharing power in interactions with patients, clients, and/or service users?
- Do policies value individuals as self-determining and interdependent actors who have a sense of their own agency as well as a sense of social responsibility?

Let's take a moment to think about Joseph's story and his decision to write a briefing (or issue) note. As social workers, it is important to think about how we make connections between policy and practice. A briefing note is an effective way of presenting findings and recommendations regarding an issue or policy to a non-specialized audience. The purpose of a briefing note is to convince your target audience of the urgency of the current problem and the need to adopt the preferred alternative or course of action. The key to a successful briefing note is tailoring your message to your particular audience. Briefing notes are effective ways for your readers to understand and likely make decisions about social policy. Let us take a moment to go through the steps of creating a briefing note.

Exercise[9]

Working with a colleague or classmate, prepare a briefing note of no more than two pages that describes and analyzes the "First Available Bed" policy discussed in Joseph's story.
   Guidelines:

Step 1: Identify context and importance of the problem

- Contextualize the social issue (in this case, the First Available Bed policy) and provide a rationale for why it may be a problem. You may want to include existing research that presents the social issue as a problem and the implications for specific communities/stakeholders. Be as succinct as possible (i.e., no more than two paragraphs).

Step 2: Present existing policy

- Write a few more paragraphs about the existing policies and programs to address your issue. This step is important because it allows your reader to get a sense of what is currently being done to address the social issue. This section of your briefing note should flow into the content that you develop in step 3.

Step 3: Critique existing policy

- Identify any shortcomings of the policy and possible improvements. What are the critiques of the existing policy/issue? How have researchers and community stakeholders addressed the issue? Again, this section should be no more than two paragraphs.

Step 4: Make policy/issue recommendations

•   This section provides a detailed explanation of the steps that need to be taken to address the issue. Bullet points may be helpful to the reader.

Step 5: Include appendices/recommended sources

•   Have a section on recommended sources to which your reader can refer for more information. Consider whether any of the detailed information that you have included in your briefing note could be made into an appendix (i.e., would it be helpful – but non-essential – for the person making the decision to have ready access to a specific document?)

Generally speaking, briefing notes summarize content in such a way that a professional but not overly academic audience can make a decision. The brief should be evidence-based, succinct, understandable, and accessible. Think about your audience and how they might receive your briefing note. At the end of the chapter, we provide a list of additional resources and samples from non-profit/advocacy organizations as well as other important resources from these groups on how to write and engage with social policy and social justice issues.

Takeaways

•   As emerging social workers and AOG practitioners, it is important to understand the ways in which policies shape perceptions and expectations of what aging should look like. Social policies also help build perceptions and expectations of who is considered an older person and the types of benefits they should receive in later life.
•   There are a number of policies that impact experiences of growing older, including (but not limited to) housing, immigration, health care, caregiving, work, and retirement.
•   Think about our AOG principles and how social policies can be argued to be rights (as opposed to simply responding to needs that are means-tested).
•   Briefing notes are effective ways to influence understandings of how social policies affect specific groups of people and structure their lived experiences, and to advocate for policies that support or promote the rights of older adults to social inclusion and citizenship.

Additional resources

•   Canadian Centre for Policy Alternatives: www.policyalternatives.ca/
•   CARP (Canadian Association of Retired Persons): www.carp.ca/
•   Federal/Provincial/Territorial Ministers Responsible for Seniors Forum: www.canada.ca/en/employment-socialdevelopment/corporate/seniors/forum.html
•   National Seniors Council: www.canada.ca/en/national-seniors-council.html
•   Vanier Institute of the Family: https://vanierinstitute.ca/
•   Canadian Center for Elder Law: www.bcli.org/elder-law-resources/tools-and-resources

Notes

1 The Council of Canadians with Disabilities provides an account of the Roundtable here: www.ccdonline.ca/en/publications/chairpersons-update/2018/se
2 The federal government does offer temporary coverage of health care benefits under the Interim Federal Health Program to refugee claimants and to people who are not eligible for provincial or territorial health insurance.
3 The secondary labour market is defined as high-turnover and low paying jobs within the service sector (Galabuzi, 2006).
4 Note that immigration is a federal jurisdiction with the exception of Quebec, where the province is responsible for its own immigration policy.
5 Previous iterations of the Parent and Grandparent Program (prior to the program's changes in 2014) imposed a 10-year dependency period.
6 The Parent and Grandparent Supervisa is a streamlined visa program that allows older parents to temporarily reunify with their families in Canada (Ferrer, 2015).
7 These costs include fees for applications, passports, medical/health checks, medical insurance, and other travel related costs.
8 According to Castles and Miller (2009), globalization is a phenomenon that has promoted the growth of cross-border flows of investment, trade, cultural products, and the proliferation of transnational networks.
9 The following exercise was adapted from the University of North Carolina at Chapel Hill's Guideline to writing a policy brief (https://writingcenter.unc.edu/policy-briefs/).

References

Armitage, A. (2003). *Social welfare in Canada*. Don Mills, ON: Oxford University Press.
Baskin, C. (2018). Sovereignty, colonization, and resistance: 150 years of social work with Indigenous peoples. *Canadian Social Work*, 20(1), 35–49.
Beatty, B. B., & Berdahl, L. (2011). Health care and Aboriginal seniors in urban Canada: Helping a neglected class. *The International Indigenous Policy Journal*, 2(1), 1–16. doi:10.18584/iipj.2011.2.1.10
Blackstock, C. (2009). The occasional evil of angels: Learning from the experiences of Aboriginal peoples and social work. *First Peoples Child & Family Review*, 4(1), 28–37. Retrieved from www.fncfcs.c
Blackstock, C. (2016). Toward the full and proper implementation of Jordan's Principle: An elusive goal to date. *Paediatrics & Child Health*, 21(5), 245–246. doi:10.1093/pch/21.5.245
Blackstock, C. (2017). The occasional evil of angels: Learning from the experiences of aboriginal peoples and social work. In S. Hick & J. Stokes (Eds.), *Social work in Canada* (pp. 54–63). Toronto, ON: Thompson Educational Publishing.
Canadian Medical Association. (2015). *A policy framework to guide a national senior's strategy for Canada*. Ottawa, ON: The Association. Retrieved from www.cma.ca/Assets/assets-library/document/en/about-us/gc2015/policyframework-to-guide-seniors_en.pdf.
Castles, S., & Miller, M. J. (2009). *The age of migration: International population movements in the modern world*. New York: Guilford Press.
Constitution Act. (1982). *Canadian charter of rights and freedoms*. Schedule B of the Canada Act, 1982. Ottawa, ON: Government of Canada.
Council of Canadians with Disabilities. (2018). *Roundtable on social and economic inclusion: Views of Canadian seniors*. Retrieved from www.ccdonline.ca/en/publications/chairpersons-update/2018/se
Durst, D. (2010). Elderly immigrants in Canada: Changing faces and greying temples. In D. Durst & M. MacLean (Eds.), *Diversity and aging among immigrant seniors in Canada: Changing faces and greying temples* (pp. 15–36). Calgary, AB: Detselig Enterprises Ltd.

Employment and Social Development Canada. (2018). *What we heard report on the roundtable on social and economic inclusion: Views of Canadian seniors.* Ottawa, ON: Author.

Ferrer, I. (2015). Examining the disjunctures between policy and care in Canada's parent and grandparent Supervisa. *International Journal of Migration, Health and Social Care, 11*(4), 253–267. doi:10.1108/IJMHSC-08-2014-0030

Ferrer, I. (2017). Aging Filipino domestic workers and the (in)adequacy of retirement provisions in Canada. *Canadian Journal on Aging, 36*(1), 15–29. doi:10.1017/S0714980816000684

Financial Consumer Agency of Canada. (2015). *Pensions and retirement.* Retrieved from www.canada.ca/en/services/finance/pensions.html.

Galabuzi, G. E. (2006). *Canada's economic apartheid: The social exclusion of racialized groups in the new century.* Toronto, ON: Canadian Scholars' Press.

Graham, J., Swift, K., & Delaney, R. (2012). *Canadian social policy: An introduction.* Toronto, ON: Pearson Canada.

Grenier, A., Barken, R., & McGrath, C. (2016). Homelessness and aging: The contradictory ordering of 'house' and 'home'. *Journal of Aging Studies, 39*, 73–80. doi:10.1016/j.jaging.2016.11.002

Hankivsky, O., & Mussell, L. (2018). Gender-based analysis plus in Canada: Problems and possibilities of integrating intersectionality. *Canadian Public Policy, 44*(4), 303–316. doi:10.3138/cpp.2017-058

Harvey, D. (2007). *A brief history of neoliberalism.* Oxford: Oxford University Press.

Kodar, F. (2012). Pensions and unpaid work: A reflection on four decades of feminist debate. *Canadian Journal of Women and the Law, 24*(1), 180–206. doi:10.1353/jwl.2012.0005

Koehn, S., Spencer, C., & Hwang, E. (2010). Promises, promises: Cultural and legal dimensions of sponsorship for immigrant seniors. In D. Durst & M. MacLean (Eds.), *Diversity and aging among immigrant seniors in Canada* (pp. 79–102). Calgary, AB: Detselig Enterprises.

Lasswell, H. D. (1956). *The decision process: Seven categories of functional analysis.* College Park, MD: University of Maryland Press.

Lightman, E., & Lightman, N. (2017). *Social policy in Canada.* Don Mills, ON: Oxford University Press.

Marier, P., & Skinner, S. (2008). The impact of gender and immigration on pension outcomes in Canada. *Canadian Public Policy, 34*(Supplement 1), S59–S78. doi:10.3138/cpp.34.Supplement.S59

McKenzie, B., & Wharf, B. (2016). *Connecting policy to practice in the human services.* Don Mills, ON: Oxford University Press.

National Housing Strategy. (2018). *Canada's national housing strategy.* Retrieved from www.placetocallhome.ca/pdfs/Canada-National-Housing-Strategy.pdf

Organisation for Economic Co-operation and Development. (2018). *Regulatory policy.* Retrieved from www.oecd.org/gov/regulatory-policy/

Oxford English Dictionary. (2019). *Policy.* Oxford University Press. Retrieved from www.oed.com/view/Entry/146842. Accessed 17 July 2019.

Rice, J. J., & Prince, M. J. (2013). *Changing politics of Canadian social policy.* Toronto, ON: University of Toronto Press.

Service Canada. (2014). *The old age security pension.* Ottawa, ON: Author.

Sinha, S.K., Griffin, B., Ringer, T., Reppas-Rindlisbacher, C., Stewart, E., Wong, I., Callan, S., & Anderson, G. (2016). *An evidence-informed national seniors strategy for Canada* (2nd ed.). Toronto: Alliance for a National Seniors Strategy. Retrieved from www.nationalseniorsstrategy.ca

United Nations General Assembly. (1948). *Universal declaration of human rights (217[III] A).* Paris.

Westhues, A. (2003). *Canadian social policy: Issues and perspectives.* Waterloo, ON: Wilfrid Laurier University Press.

Westhues, A., & Kenny-Scherber, C. (2012). The policy-making process. In A. Westhues & B. Wharf (Eds.), *Canadian social policy: Issues and perspectives* (pp. 23–42). Waterloo, ON: Wilfrid Laurier University Press.

Westhues, A., & Wharf, B. (2012). *Canadian social policy: Issues and perspectives*. Waterloo, ON: Wilfrid Laurier University Press.

Young, C. (2011). Pensions, privatization, and poverty: The gendered impact. *Canadian Journal of Women and the Law, 23*(2), 661–685. doi:10.3138/cjwl.23.2.661

Chapter 13

Everyday lives and realities

Questions to consider as you read

- How are older adults and their (chosen) families perceived by the various health and social care service providers with whom they come into contact?
- What are the parameters that shape social workers' understandings and interventions?
- What are the dominant and professional discourses that emerge in the stories presented?
- How might you rethink social work interventions in each story by using the intersectional life course approach?

This book has explored the realities of aging in Canada, moving from macro-level analyses of theories and perspectives driving discourses on aging to an exploration of the shape and nature of health and social care service delivery to older adults. We have called attention to some of the major longstanding and emerging topics in the field of social gerontology, including legal and ethical issues, mental wellness, risk, trauma, mistreatment and violence, caregiving, dementia and citizenship, and inclusive communities. Throughout the book, we have attempted to frame issues through the lens of those living these experiences on a daily basis. We hope that this has enhanced your understanding of the complex and diverse ways in which realities are structured, conceptualized, and positioned within the various sites and sectors with which older adults, their families, and communities interact. These are the spaces in which social workers work (as case managers, care coordinators, outreach workers, discharge planners, etc.), often within interdisciplinary teams, alongside other professional staff.

We believe that a more nuanced, particularized, and intersectional approach to our work can improve access, equity, and inclusion for older adults and their (chosen) families within health and social care services and better reflect our social work goals and values as change agents. In this last chapter, we want to bring home this message of the need to pay attention to intersectionality and interlocking oppressions in our work, in other words, to be anti-oppressive gerontologists, by telling a few stories about the everyday lives and realities of older adults, their families, and communities. These stories will centre on some "significant" issues that have come up in our own work and represent some of the major obstacles to the provision of care to older adults from marginalized communities.

The objectives of this chapter are to

- Present the stories of four older adults and the challenges they face in their inter-actions with various sites and sectors of health and social care as a starting point for questioning the way things operate and how they could be different;
- Introduce the intersectional life course approach and the life course lifeline as a tool of anti-oppressive analysis and intervention; and
- Engage students in counter-storytelling through a step-wise exercise.

We believe that stories of the everyday are the most powerful way to fully capture the impact of structural oppression on lived experience (Hulko, 2011). Unfortunately, there are few models to help support social workers in their efforts to fully understand how to query everyday lives and realities in a way that exposes the social structures that shape our understanding of social problems and, as a result, the ways these social problems are addressed within health and social care services. As such, social workers are left to rely mostly on their own individually developed "critical values" in order to make sense of the "presenting problems" of our older clients. This reality, coupled with pressures on our time and a lack of openness to a more nuanced, subjective, and holistic approach on the part of the sectors in which we work make it incredibly challenging to incorporate an analysis of "everyday lives and realities" into our intervention plans.

As described in **Age/ism: age as a category of difference**, applications of both intersectionality and life course perspectives can strengthen our understanding of the macro, meso and micro forces that shape experiences of aging among older people from equity-seeking groups (Brotman, Ferrer, & Koehn, 2019; Ferrer, Grenier, Brotman, & Koehn, 2017). Brotman et al. (2019) note that the intersectional life course approach "allows for the identification and consideration of the mutually reinforcing categories of (1) life events, timing, and structural forces; (2) local and globally linked lives; (3) identities and categories/processes of difference; and (4) domination, agency, [resilience], and resistance" (p. 4). Taking into account key events in people's lives, and the structural forces that shape these events enables researchers, policy makers and service providers to reflect and integrate how people both experience and make sense/meaning of these events (Brotman et al., 2019). For example, studies of neuro-diverse people's experiences of aging in Canada are greatly enhanced by considerations of disability, health and housing policies, and corresponding processes of transition, de-institutionalisation, social exclusion/inclusion, and discrimination. In parallel, the analysis of time situates people and systems historically, emphasizing the interconnection between contemporary realities and historic conditions (Daatland & Biggs, 2004). The intersectional life course's account of globally and locally linked lives presents aging as an intergenerational, collective, and relational experience that occurs across local and transnational regions (Brotman et al., 2019). Furthermore, the intersectional life course incorporates an understanding that people's identities are fluid, contextual, and shaped by both categories and processes of differentiation. Following the works of Brotman et al. (2019) and Ferrer et al. (2017), we argue that while systems of oppression can shape and often dominate people's lives, older people also demonstrate agency, in the forms of both resilience and resistance. Thus, "although systems of domination shape and structure experience, they can at the same time be countered and resisted" (Brotman et al., 2019, p. 5).

In this chapter, we draw from the methodology introduced to operationalize the intersectional life course in research (Brotman et al., 2019) and apply it as a practice framework. The methodology is partly based upon the life story narrative method (in conjunction with photovoice) and although designed as a tool for research, we believe it has the potential to be adapted for use in practice settings. Life story narrative (see textbox 13.1) can be a powerful tool for facilitating a rich, contextualized, and dynamic process of intervention that integrates structural critiques and social justice principles embedded within intersectionality and life course perspectives (Brotman et al., 2019). The insights to be gained from this practice tool have important real-world implications particularly with respect to enriching our understanding of the ways in which older adults are both vulnerable and resilient in their everyday interactions with the state (Dannefer & Settersten, 2010).

Textbox 13.1

Life story narrative is a research method that collects the life stories of people, focussing specifically on major life events and key meaningful moments as described by people, the meaning they attribute to these moments/events, and the ways in which they are shaped by social context, including socio-political and cultural themes within the broader society, institutions, and social history.

The life history approach is a narrative form of qualitative inquiry within the broader field of interpretive biography (Gardner, 2002) which has been recently adapted to the exploration of lived experiences in ways that remain true to the voices of affected populations (Denzin, Lincoln, & Tuhiwai Smith, 2008). The research lens of life story narrative pays particular attention to the contexts in which people are living or have lived and incorporates complexity and diversity into research design (Brotman et al., 2019). This can also be said of life story narrative as a practice tool. Life story narrative focusses on major life events and key meaningful moments, paying specific attention to both the ways in which these events are shaped by social context and how people understand and make meaning of them. A structural interpretation of life story narrative centres on interpreting how personal narrative and history are influenced by cultural themes within the broader society, institutions, and social history (Ferrer et al., 2017). Life histories are often gathered over an extended period using multiple interviews and can include other forms of intervention such as observation and visual methods (Denzin & Lincoln, 2008). Narrative tools of inquiry, such as the life history approach (Gardner, 2002), personal experience story (Drummond & Brotman, 2014; Grenier, 2007), lifeline (Brotman et al., 2019; Brotman & Kraniou, 1999), timeline (Ives, Denov and Sussman, 2015), and concepts of time, transition, and rupture (Grenier, 2012) can be used to inform practice and provide opportunities for the co-creation of contextualized understandings on the part of both social workers and their older adult clients. Life story narrative and lifeline tools of inquiry, used together, can amplify the voices of older people, enabling them to name and interpret their experiences of aging, key events over the life course, encounters of structural oppression and moments of resistance/resilience (Brotman & Kraniou, 1999; Brotman et al., 2019).

Lifeline Model

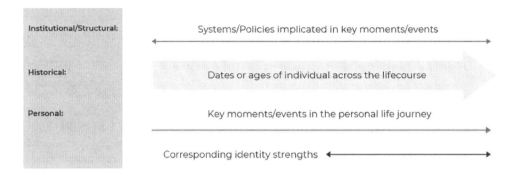

Figure 13.1 Lifeline model

Drawing from the life-history method, Brotman and Kraniou (1999) use a physical life-line (drawing) as a technique to engage in a conversation about significant events, memories, and relationships across the life course in order to yield rich stories about people's lives. Figure 13.1 highlights the components integral to the development of a lifeline.

For those older adults with cognitive or sensory impairments, the use of photo elicitation and third-party questioning is another research technique that can be adapted to practice, facilitating voice and inclusion and ensuring safety – cultural and physical (Hulko, 2014). The use of these various tools can deepen the potential for older adult clients to experience a sense of empowerment, both in terms of the capacity to reflect on their lived experiences and to articulate and describe their complex intergenerational, transnational, and community relationships that serve as supports and/or barriers (Cunsolo Willox, Harper, & Edge, 2013). They can also provide a mechanism for social workers to "rethink" their interventions and/or the policies that structure and shape these interventions and solicit feedback on older adults' experiences of health and social care.

Thinking holistically about people's lives across time and place, rather than simply focussing on "presenting problems", can open up avenues for consideration of intersecting identities and the challenges of multiple oppressions in concert with the strengths, resilience, and resistance strategies enacted by people and communities over the life course. Finally, social workers can use these life story narratives, either alone or with their clients, as the basis for the development of counter-stories: "re-writing" components of the narrative related to interactions with the state and their institutions as a means of visualizing change. That is, life stories can inspire counter-storytelling about the potential for alternative processes and practices, not as they were, but as they "should or could be". In other words, counter-stories can be applied to reconfigure encounters in the life story narrative for the purposes of re-imagining interventions, programs, and policies to better reflect transformative practice (see textbox 13.2). After assisting older adults to create counter-stories, AOP social workers can then use them for advocacy purposes (Hulko, Brotman, & Ferrer, 2017).

Textbox 13.2

Life story narrative as practice engages people in conversation about their life stories and the ways in which they make meaning of major life events. Life story narrative as a practice tool uses multiple methods for engaging in reflection about personal life history (including the use of a lifeline, drawing, journaling, and other art forms) in order to create space to share experiences that go beyond the immediate situation or problem. This enhances our capacity to foster a deep understanding of the connections between lived experience and the personal, historical, cultural, and structural contexts that shape this experience. It also facilitates a re-visioning of possible interventions that pay attention to life course factors that have contributed to current perspectives and realities.

Writing the life story narrative summary and drawing the lifeline

Below are questions to consider in the development of an analysis from the perspectives of both the older adult and the social worker. These questions are not hierarchical, but sit in conversation with one another in a fluid, iterative way. In developing a narrative summary and lifeline, it is common to move back and forth between these questions in order to create a holistic picture through which answers to these questions inform a story that pays attention to inter- and intra-personal, social, and structural dimensions.

Key questions in reflecting upon the situation of the older adult

- How does the person describe themself?
- How do identities, roles, and experiences interact?
- What are the key life events/relationships that have influenced them across time and place?
- What are the structural (social, institutional, relational) forces and processes that shape their experiences?

Key questions in developing a counter-story from the perspective of the social worker

- What is the current situation?
- Who are the significant players, and what are their roles?

- How do categories of difference (the social worker's own identity and social location) contribute to the challenges and opportunities for change faced by the social worker?
- What is the expected role of the social worker?
- What could the social worker have done differently?
- What would the story look like if all things were possible?

Four life story narratives

James's story

Born in 1947, James is a 72-year-old gay man who has lived with early onset Parkinson's disease since the age of 38 (see Figure 13.2). Since a young age, James has been interested in progressive ideas and wanted to be involved in changing the world for the better. James spent his adult life in Montreal being an activist in the anti-poverty movement and worked for many years as a community organizer in a local food bank. On weekends, he spent a lot of time riding his bike. James loved spending time alone riding his bike through all kinds of weather and reading for hours in local cafés. He was an avid reader and considered himself to be a bit of an armchair radical with an immense knowledge of history and philosophy. He loved to travel. James came out in his mid-40s. He had always known he was attracted to men but tried to suppress his feelings throughout his early teens and 20s due to shame and fear of hostility. Despite keeping his sexual identity from others, he experienced almost constant bullying in school because, as he explains, "I was too different, small and shy", and finally James decided to quit school in grade 10 and took off to travel. In his late 20s, James married Sheila, a woman he met while he worked at a local food bank. They had a son, Ben, in 1984. James tried his best to do what was expected of him, but he believes now that his need for independence and solitude was first rooted in his early life experiences of stigma.

When James was diagnosed with early-onset Parkinson's disease in 1985, things began to change. The stress of the diagnosis and rapidly fluctuating physical disability had a negative impact on his capacity to work, his ability to remain active, and the energy he could invest in others. For many years, James struggled with his disability and gradually began to isolate himself and to be isolated, giving up his beloved bike and his few social connections. His colleagues retreated, and he rarely had any visitors

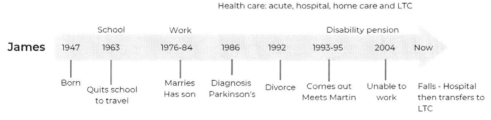

Figure 13.2 James' lifeline

or calls. Finally, he and his wife divorced in 1992. This prompted James to accept and declare his sexual orientation as a gay man. The progression of his degenerative illness made him feel as though he had little time left to "simply be who he was meant to be". This initially strained his relationship with his son, Ben, now living in Toronto, but they were able to reconcile in 2008. In the first few years after his divorce, while James still felt able, he explored his sexuality and met Martin in 1998 with whom he developed an intimate and long-lasting friendship. While they did not live together or identify as a couple, James says Martin is the closest friend he ever had.

After leaving his job in 2004 at the age of 57, James survived on a government disability pension that gave him a very modest income and lived under the poverty line in a low-cost disability-adapted social housing unit that he waited five years to get. He spent much of his time there, except for short walks in the neighbourhood when he was able. Gradually, James required more and more support to function and could go on fewer and fewer walks. Martin and Sheila (with whom James remained friends after the divorce) shared caregiving tasks, a reality that was not without its tensions. James was eligible for some homecare services. He received help with a shower once per week and someone to do light cleaning once every two weeks. As things got worse and after a significant fall in 2016, which put him in the hospital for over six weeks, his out-of-town family (two sisters who lived in the United States) agreed to provide financial support to enable him to have help three afternoons per week, and he was registered with Lifeline, a medical alert service. However, James was an independent man, and he perceived the Lifeline cord around his neck as an intrusion on his privacy. He also refused to use the walker he was given as he felt it obstructed his natural movement around his apartment and too visibly identified him in the neighbourhood. James was faced with much discrimination as a gay man and a person with a disability. People looked at him and his walker with pity and treated him with impatience on so many occasions that he did not want to take much more of that. So, the Lifeline cord often remained on the doorknob and the walker in the corner of his apartment despite the nagging of Sheila, Martin, and his homecare worker(s).

Things got progressively riskier for James, and last spring, after two months in hospital after a fall, he was deemed eligible for long-term/residential care. He was transferred to a nursing home in June. Although thankful for the increased attention and security he received in the nursing home and the good food, the adjustment to life in an institution for someone who prized his independence and autonomy to make decisions has been difficult. Although the staff found James to be kind and quiet as he rarely asked for anything, he was quickly identified as "resistant". He balked at the change in his medication regimen (they gave him his pills one hour later because of staff changeover) and did not like the fact that he could not lock his room door. He also continued to complain about being forced to use the walker and refused to join in on activities. Instead, James spent much of the day in his room listening to the CBC on the radio, another favourite activity throughout his life. Although he enjoyed watching sports on TV, the common room TV had no sports channel; it was "fixed" on a generic station that played what James called "empty-headed" programming. After three months, the requisite multidisciplinary meeting was to take place for James, the family, and the team to discuss James's transition and how things were going. James's ex-wife was asked by James's sisters to represent them at the meeting. The social worker, Amar, a racialized young cisgender man, had only met James once upon admission and had not reached out to either Sheila or Martin prior to this meeting. Although Amar would have preferred to talk with them in advance, he had little time as he was the only social worker in a setting with 150 residents, and he relied almost exclusively on the head floor nurse to identify "problematic residents or situations". Amar felt he had little power to change things and so kept his head down and his opinions to himself. Amar presented the team's perspective as a common front and began to list James's problems – that he refused to use his walker and that he was sitting in his room refusing to participate in activities. James was silent but visibly upset as they listed his faults and stated quietly that his walker didn't work properly. He shut down entirely when ideas for activities were repeatedly tossed around. He mentioned that the staff were refusing to let him out of the building on his own for fear of falls, which he resented. The physiotherapist conceded that the walker was a very old one, and she agreed to help find a better replacement and to assess him to see if he could go short distances without it.

Finally exasperated, Sheila spoke up. She told the staff about James's history as an activist and his joy of watching sports. She said, "If you could come up with other activities than Bingo – like something that has to do with what is going on in the real world – then maybe James might want to join in!" She blurted out that James was gay, much to the anger and frustration of James. The activities director looked at the papers in front of her, cleared her throat, and responded, "I see from your file that you are a Catholic. Would you like to attend church services?" James sat quietly and hung his head. The room went still, and the meeting ended with the physiotherapist reasserting that she would help James adjust to the walker. James agreed to join an exercise class twice per week, which in the end, he enjoyed. Martin recently purchased a television with all the sports channels, and James has been allowed to walk to the bathroom without the walker. He still is not allowed to go outside unescorted, and his interactions with the staff are limited to functional issues, but James sits quietly and enjoys what he can. Sheila visits monthly, and Ben drops in on his dad when he comes to town twice a year for a long weekend. Martin visits every two weeks and continues to identify himself as a friend. The staff say hello, but don't interact with him very much and never ask how he is. They say, "He is only a friend". James has demonstrated remarkable courage in the face of such identity negation. His attitude of taking things as they are has helped him to face incredible change and losses to his dignity and lack of recognition of his identity as other than a disabled body. James struggles on. Amar, the social worker, has not checked in or approached either Sheila or James since the meeting was deemed to end well, and the head nurse on the floor told him that "things remain quiet".

Peter's story

Born in 1951, Peter is a 68-year-old member of the Cree First Nation and lives in his home community north of Winnipeg (population of roughly 2,000 people) (see Figure 13.3). He is the youngest of five children in a big intergenerational network of family and community. His earliest childhood memories are of being treated like a toy by his older siblings, being swept up continually in the arms of his grandmother, and running

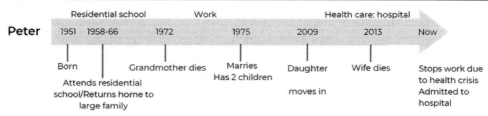

Figure 13.3 Peter's lifeline

into anyone's house when he felt cold or hungry. All of that changed when he and his siblings were sent to residential school about 400 kilometres from their home. Peter keeps his residential school experiences close to his chest; he is a quiet man who prefers to work with his hands than to talk at length on any topic. He went to residential school for the ages 7 to 15, eight years he says he would rather forget. When he arrived back home, his grandmother swept him up in her arms once again, despite the fact that he was already almost six feet tall, and "she never let go", according to Peter, until her death when he was 21. Peter married at 24 years old and settled into life as an ironworker, raising his daughters Pamela and Kay with his wife. Peter also enjoyed fishing whenever he had the chance.

Now an Elder in his community, Peter takes the responsibility for educating the younger generations about the history and cultural traditions of his people very seriously. He is well respected, and his home is a regular site of community gatherings. He serves as an Elder with the local Cree school that integrates culturally restorative practices. Peter visits the classroom regularly and teaches a woodcarving course. As a result of residential school, Peter and his siblings were separated for many years. Two have already died, and his middle sister lives in Vancouver. Only his older sister May (79 years old) lives nearby, and they remain close. Peter has lived with his daughter Pamela (40 years old) and her two boys (Nate, aged 12, and Brian, aged 14) for the past 10 years. His wife died from cancer in 2013. His daughter Kay married and moved to Yellowknife. The family often gathers to share meals, and Peter has taken his grandsons on many fishing trips. Pamela's ex-husband is not in the picture, and she has relied on her father for support over the years. Living with her father has enabled her to finish school and get a job as a teacher's aide. She is proud of her job and the time it gives her to be independent.

Recently, Peter had to travel a long distance to an urban centre in order to address the complications of his diabetes. An infection in his leg was not healing, and he was no longer able to walk on it. Peter still worked part-time in construction, but the problem with his leg required him to stop working. This made him frustrated and angry because he liked to keep busy and active and considered himself a strong man. He hid the problem from his family as long as possible because he did not want to go to the hospital in Winnipeg, but the pain had made it obvious to Pamela that something was wrong and she forced him to go check it out. Once there, he learned that he had a very bad infection and, in order to avoid amputation of his leg, he would need to be in the hospital for at least three weeks on intravenous antibiotics. His daughter made the trip with him in order to get the diagnosis and drove back and forth (1.5 hour trip) to ensure that he received appropriate care. For Peter, this was the first time he had been outside of his community for anything other than work in many years. The all-white institutional environment triggered early memories of living in residential school. He became agitated and restless, refusing to do what the doctors or nurses told him to do and trying to leave in the middle of the night. He fell and broke his arm trying to leave the hospital grounds one night, resulting in the hospital staff restraining him. When Pamela arrived the next day she found him incoherent and screaming that they were all trying to "cut him down" and demanding that his daughter take him home.

Pamela was stricken. She had never seen her father "lose it" like this and was concerned that he would not get the medical care he needed. She feared what would happen if she took him home and felt incapable of "doing a nurse's job". She tried speaking to the nurse at the desk about removing the restraints, but the nurse was adamant that the doctor requested this for her father's safety and that they needed him in restraints to protect him from himself. They told her that he was "trouble" for all of them, a "danger" to the staff because of his large size and angry demeanor, and without restraints they would have to medicate him further to keep him quiet. When Pamela raised her voice, an orderly was called and she was asked to leave until she calmed down. As she walked down the hallway, she heard one of the nurses exclaim, "We always have trouble with those people!"

Pamela ran to the social service department to see if she could speak to someone. The social worker, a white middle-aged woman who had worked at the hospital for over 15 years, opened the door and Pamela entered, crying. She didn't know what to do and was afraid to leave her father alone, but she had to get back to her home community in order to be home when her children arrived from school. They were already very upset by the absence of their grandfather and his ill health. Pamela crumbled in the chair, telling the social worker about how difficult it was to deal with the fact that her father did not tell her about his leg, how silent he was about any troubles, and how this silence had always made it very difficult for her, how she had to "pretend" everything was okay in front of others, even when it wasn't, so that her father could "keep face" in the community. She was desperate for him to get better and said that she could not manage on her own with the children, and while her job was very satisfying, it hardly brought in any money. She yelled that the hospital did not understand her father and was making things worse and that now he would die because of them.

The social worker immediately tried to calm Pamela down and told her that she would read through the file and discuss the situation with the head nurse on the floor and get back to her as soon as possible. The social worker had been very friendly with the head nurse since they started working together; she believed it was essential to keep on good terms with the floor nurses and doctors in order to provide the best possible outcomes for her clients. The next day, the social worker met with Pamela and immediately began to defend the actions of the hospital, explaining the safety issues, both for her father and the staff. Pamela read this immediately as patronizing and quickly changed her approach. She felt guilty for having spoken so openly without first assessing who sat in front of her. She demonstrated a veil of calm and said little else, simply asking when her father could be released. The social worker, although a bit confused, told Pamela that she would speak to the team to see if they could figure out a way to calm Peter down enough so that the restraints could be removed. Since compliance with the treatment was the only way to save his leg, the social worker reiterated that it was best for Peter to stay in hospital where he could be monitored. She offered to do a short-term counselling intervention with Pamela and her father to help them improve their communication. She explained to Pamela that as soon as the doctor deemed it safe for Peter to leave, they could discuss an appropriate plan for discharge. Until then, she recommended that Pamela and her father remain calm and accept the treatment plan, which is the "best care" the hospital can provide.[1]

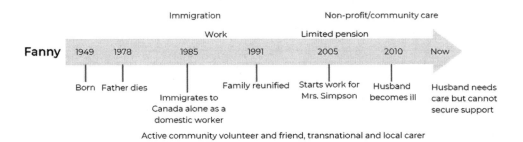

Figure 13.4 Fanny's lifeline

Fanny's story

Born in 1949, Fanny, now 70, moved from a small town in the Philippines to Sherbrooke in 1985 to work as a live-in domestic worker under the Foreign Domestic Movement (see Figure 13.4).[2] She was in her mid-30s and worked for a couple with three young children for over 13 years, after which she began working with two older women living with dementia. For the past 14 years, she has worked for Mrs. Simpson, now 92.

When she first moved to Sherbrooke, Fanny left her husband and two children (son, Jojo, age five, and daughter, Angel, age eight) behind in their home town in the Philippines with her mother and four other siblings. As the eldest in her family, Fanny was responsible for the care of her parents and three younger siblings. She was expected to look out for them and provide for their future. Her father died from a heart attack when Fanny was 29. This left the family in a very precarious financial situation, and finally, in 1985, Fanny made the hard decision to move to Canada to try to make more money to send home to her family and to support her younger siblings' education. She left her two children in the Philippines with her husband Paolo, and her mother was supporting him to raise the children.

It took Fanny a little over five years to earn her permanent residency and save up enough money to bring her husband and children to Canada in 1991 through the Family Reunification program. The time and distance caused a significant and long-lasting family disruption. Her now teenaged daughter acted out and was resentful towards Fanny. Her son became clingy and afraid – physically needing to be close to

Fanny – and had a hard time adjusting to his new school. Paolo had relinquished most of the childcare responsibilities in the Philippines to his mother-in-law because he worked long hours. However, in Sherbrooke, and without any French language skills, he had difficulty finding work and became the primary caregiver to the children, as Fanny was the one with a steady job. He accepted his duty but was depressed about his loss of capacity to provide for his family and struggled with this for the remainder of his life. Despite living in poverty and struggling to make ends meet, they scraped together everything they could to send money home to Fanny's family. Her mom, now aging in the Philippines, and Fanny's younger siblings back home, all needed financial support. The children both left home when they became adults.

The strain on Fanny's relationship with her daughter never really healed, and they now speak infrequently. Fanny feels that her daughter always seems angry and troubled. Her son, now 39, lives nearby and has children of his own. Her mother passed away in 2015, and Fanny still regrets not being with her. It causes her a lot of pain to think about it and motivates her to stay close and continue to provide support to her siblings struggling financially back home. She sends financial remittances every month and travels there every two years, but Fanny is getting increasingly tired and wishes that she could retire. A major issue is that there is no money to do so. Her husband, in and out of odd jobs since his arrival in Sherbrooke, has very little pension. He now has advanced arthritis in his hip and knees and struggles daily with pain and disability. Fanny will also have only a small pension, and so she plans to continue to work under the table for Mrs. Simpson for as long as she can. The work requires lifting, cleaning, and pushing a wheelchair, all of which is hard on Fanny's back and hands.

A local community-based non-profit homecare service comes to assess the situation to see whether Paolo and Fanny are eligible for homecare services, particularly to help Paolo with a shower once per week since his mobility has become severely compromised and he cannot get in and out of the bath easily. When the agency social worker discovers that Fanny is still working as a domestic worker, she says she does not understand why they need help at home. The social worker explains, "Fanny, you are fully capable of taking on this work for your husband, no? You do this every day!" When Fanny says that she cannot and that there is little money to pay for help from the agency, the social worker asks why this is the case. They are both 65 and should have adequate finances from their pensions. The social worker has no idea about the impact of immigration on access to pension entitlements or the realities of transnational care arrangements. The social worker asks why they are not asking for help from their son who lives close by. "Surely he can help Paolo take a shower!" Fanny explains that her son has financial and family troubles of his own and works long hours. They do not want to be a burden to him. When the social worker, on the way out the door, politely suggests that they should consider accessing the food bank and stop sending so much money back to the Philippines, Fanny closes the door and her heart against this cold, uncaring, ignorant woman and resigns herself to doing it all on her own.

Jeannie's story

Born in 1945 in East Vancouver, Jeannie, a 74-year-old cis-gender, white woman, has struggled all of her life with mental illness (see Figure 13.5). Diagnosed at 19 with

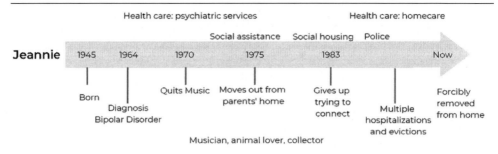

Figure 13.5 Jeannie's lifeline

bipolar disorder, Jeannie had no choice but to quit school. She was doing an under-graduate degree in music at the University of British Columbia, but she could not manage the stress and workload. She was hospitalized for a short period of time and had to take medication, but it made her feel tired and fuzzy, and she hated it. Jeannie felt that being on medication made her lose connection to her music, and she was not able to perform. She went off and on the medication for several years and struggled. Her mood swings and unpredictability were extremely challenging for her parents who constantly nagged her, she felt, to stay on the medication. Jeannie tried several times to go back to school, but she found it too difficult and spent a few years being aimless and fighting with her parents with whom she still lived. Her music and her animals (she loved cats) were her only solace. She gave all her love and caring to the creatures around her, taking in strays and nursing them back to health. Jeannie played guitar and was quite talented, having been in a band for several years, but there were a lot of drugs in the music industry and she felt she had to stay away or she would be in worse trouble. As a result, by the early 1980s Jeannie had lost most of her social contacts.

Finally, fed up with the number of animals in their home and the loud music Jean-nie played at all hours of the day and night, her parents gave her an ultimatum: stay on the medication or move out. Jeannie moved out when she was 30 years old and was determined never to speak to her parents again. This led to another mental health crisis and hospitalization. When she was released, Jeannie went on social assistance and moved into an apartment. She was supported by a community-based mental health social worker from the nearby tertiary mental health hospital. Over the years, she had many workers from the hospital; the names changed as professionals came and went. At the beginning, she tried several support programs and tried to connect with her workers but quickly got frustrated by the constant turnover and eventually gave up trying to make connections. Her real loves, her animals and guitar, sustained her throughout a lot of struggles and uncertainty. She collected all kinds of sheet music, albums, posters, t-shirts, and instruments when she could get them. She also collected items for her animals such as bowls, toys, stuffed animals, cat clothes, and figurines. Jeannie was proud that she was able to stay off the medication for long periods without a crisis.

Over time, and as she became more isolated, Jeannie began to see her animals, her music, and her collections as the only things she could count on. She had to move many times because of the number of cats she kept in her apartments. On a few occasions, Jeannie was evicted because of the smell and mess that emanated from her place. Her precarious housing situation meant that she was sometimes homeless and had to release her cats into the street. This would lead to a crisis, hospitalization, and then back into shelter. Now 74 years old, Jeannie is experiencing some disability and cognitive issues. Her hoarding and the fact that she currently has 12 cats is putting her again at risk of eviction. The social worker from the local healthcare centre is called by the landlord because of complaints from neighbours about the smell and noise. The social worker, a cis-gender, middle-class white woman arrives accompanied by a young, cis-gender first-generation (her parents emigrated from Eastern Europe) BSW student from the local university. The social worker sees the state of Jeannie's crowded dirty apartment and immediately wants to have Jeannie forcibly placed so that a clean-up can be undertaken. Jeannie flatly refuses and begins to scream at the social worker and student to leave. The social worker reacts strongly, turning to the student saying, "Crazy woman; if she touches me I am going to get bugs!" The student is visibly taken aback, but she tries her best to hide her reaction. The student has not disclosed to her supervisor that she also lives with mental illness for fear of experiencing stigma and discrimination. Based on her supervisor's reaction to Jeannie, she knows that hiding this information was the right thing to do. Still, the student feels a mix of despair and anger at witnessing the scene without being able to do anything to support Jeannie. The supervisor, who sees the mild shock on the student's face, tells her, "You're new to this country and don't yet understand how things work here, but don't worry, Jeannie won't hurt you". The police are called. Jeannie is put in restraints and into an ambulance. She is angry and frightened, and so is the student social worker.

Counter-storytelling: a stepwise exercise to enhance anti-oppressive practice

The four stories presented in this chapter offer opportunities for the reader to consider the themes emerging in this book through the lens of lived experience. While unique, each story reflects common processes and practices of marginalization and exclusion faced by diverse older adults, their families, and communities. Through the counter-story exercise, we provide the reader with an opportunity to reflect upon the unique and shared issues that emerge in the stories, practice AOG analysis, and create counter-stories of their own as a way of reimagining social work practice, institutional processes, policies, and structures. Counter-storytelling can be undertaken individually or in groups. We recommend working through each case one by one (James, Peter, Fanny, and Jeannie) and then stepping back to identify the common discourses, practices, and processes that shape current interventions across stories. Once the exercises and discussions/reflections have been concluded, you may choose to turn the page and note how our summary ideas compare with your own. We introduce the counter-story exercise as a stepwise procedure in the following paragraphs. Each step contains a series of questions to help you to focus your responses. The steps, although identified as separate components, can be undertaken in an iterative fashion. That is, you may want to go back and forth between steps to expand, or adapt, your previous responses.

Step One – The Personal-Historical: Before re-writing the endings of each of these life story narratives as counter-stories, try to re-imagine what the social work intervention might look like if anti-oppressive principles were practiced. It is important to understand the identity and social context of each older adult, paying attention to personal history, strengths, and challenges faced along the life course at multiple levels (micro, meso, macro), particularly those you interpret as having an impact upon the current situation. Try using the lifeline to identify key moments/events in the personal history of the older adult. In what ways has the older adult in each story faced structural disadvantage across the life course? What forms of agency (both resilience and resistance) are evident in their stories?

Step Two – The Structural: Identify the policies that shape each story. First, identify the policies implicated across the life course of the older adult. Try using the lifeline to "pull out" the policy areas related to key moments/events over the life course. Then turn to the policies that shape the particular site and sector in which the story takes place. Who is responsible for creating the policies you identified (government ministries, institutions, disciplinary bodies, etc.)? Refer back to **Policy and planning for an aging society** to support this analysis.

Step Three – The Institutional: What sites and sectors are implicated in the story? Refer back to **Sites and sectors of health and social care** to inform your analysis. Identify the institutional forces that shape the current priorities and practices of the sector and site in which events take place. What is the dominant discourse operating in the setting, and how does this potentially shape the parameters in which the social worker works? What facilitates and constrains the social worker's understanding and response? How are rights, entitlements, access, and equity operationalized?

Step Four – The Professional: What is the specific role of the social worker (and/or social work student) in the current context? How does this role compare with other professionals in the setting? What forms of power are granted and/or available to the social worker in this case? How might the social location of the social worker (and/or student) impact their understanding of, and intervention with, the older adults and (chosen) family members in the story? What about potential interventions and/or relationships with other professionals in the story? What challenges or barriers do they face in light of these categories of difference? Who must the social worker gain permission from in developing their plan? What are the professional discourses operationalized in this case? What approaches are used? Are these explicitly named or implicit? Refer back to **Theorizing later life and social work praxis** and **Sites and sectors of health and social care** to help frame your response to these questions.

Step Five – The Relational: Pay attention to the relationship between the social worker and the older adult and/or the (chosen) family introduced in each case. What does the relationship look like? What implicit and explicit forms of power are made evident in these encounters? Is trust building enacted in these stories and if so, how? How much time does the social worker have to undertake the work? What follow-up is put in place with respect to their intervention? How is the role of advocacy articulated?

Step Six – The Counter-story: Counter-storytelling is an opportunity to imagine what things would be like if anything was possible. In our book, counter-storytelling provides an opportunity to think about how social gerontology, and our work with older adults their families and communities, can be different and to imagine new forms of structure and power. It's important not only to dream big (in the sense of imagining the world transformed with unlimited funds at our disposal and with a greater voice in government decision-making) but also to think through possibilities that are different than what is currently available to us. It's important to remember that AOP is not only about thinking critically at the structural level, but also about embedding social justice and advocacy principles at the relational and professional level, in other words, in our everyday interventions. Although it's important to analyze historical and individual life course trajectories in order to more fully appreciate older adults' experiences and strengths, as well as the contexts that shape their current viewpoints and realities, we must also remember that we cannot change the past in our direct level interventions. So, our counter-stories must begin at the point of first contact. Begin your counter-story, in each case, at the point in which the social worker first appears on the scene. In your counter-story, think about how your intervention would change and what would remain the same. How would the social worker respond to the individual, to their colleagues? How might the social worker intervene at the client level, the departmental level, the institutional level, and the structural level? Should other sites and sectors be involved? If so, how? What kind of follow-up would you put in place? In making goals and objectives for your interventions, identify potential short-term and long-term priorities.

Linking the stories together [read this section after the counter-story exercise is completed]

For the purposes of analysis and reflection, the closing pages of this chapter provide a summary of some of the overlapping issues that surfaced in all four narratives across sites and sectors. In this summary, we highlight common constraints and processes of differentiation and oppression that we have identified in order to begin a conversation with the reader. This summary is in no way meant to be exhaustive. We also call attention to several forms of agency enacted by the marginalized older adult and their (chosen) families in the four narratives, which have largely gone unrecognized by the professionals involved.

Each life story narrative demonstrates unique configurations of intersecting forms of oppression including ageism, homophobia/heterosexism, colonialism, racism, sexism, classism, ableism, and sanism as they operate in the policies and practices of the health and social care sites and sectors in which these older adults find themselves: non-profit and community care (Fanny), homecare (Jeannie), health care (Peter), and long-term/residential care (James). While forms of oppression manifest differently in each case, there are evident common practices undertaken by professionals (including and most notably social workers) within these sectors that emerge from the particular roles and constraints governing interactions. The dominant and intersecting discourses of neoliberalism and bio-medicalization frame macro, meso, and micro structures and practices. For example, in Fanny's case, neoliberal discourse intersects with racism in the developing assumption of familism: that services do not need to be put in place for ethno-cultural minority older adults because it is assumed that their families will be available to provide care. The four narratives expose the shared processes of differentiation, most notably that of "othering", that currently operate as normative in health and social care delivery across sectors.

Several common threads link the stories together, some of which we describe here. In your reading of the stories, you may come up with other common threads, and we encourage you to write these down as part of this counter-storytelling exercise. Often-times, dominant discourses and the multiple and intersecting forms of oppression that operate at the structural level are difficult to identify. Entering into conversation between seemingly different stories and different contexts enables us to reconsider our perspectives and push the boundaries of our critical interpretation. We present here some of the ideas that have emerged in our discussions as co-authors for your consideration, evaluation, and critique.

First, the reader might note some of the relatively younger ages of the older adults in the stories we have presented. This was done purposely to reinforce the reality that lifelong marginalization often results in what has been called "early aging", a term that reflects the greater risk of morbidity among older adults facing stigma and discrimination across the life course, especially those living with complex chronic health conditions (see textbox 3.8). Another issue to consider is the ways in which older adults and their (chosen) families enact forms of agency in all four stories. Each story has within it different examples of resilience and resistance to micro, meso, and macro forms of exclusion and discrimination. Consider, for instance, how a "passive stance" (i.e., remaining quiet, demonstrating a passive demeanor or expression, asking for little) might be reinterpreted as resilience or resistance to authoritative "othering" and powerlessness. Resistance such as that expressed through anger and refusal should be reframed, not as non-compliance (which is the most common way that these acts are interpreted in health and social care) but as resistance to control and domination. Consider also the ways in which connections to people, animals, communities, spaces (i.e., neighbourhoods, home, organizations) and objects function as forms of resilience and resistance to structural and/or geographic exclusion.

Among professionals, we highlight the following realities as common in all four stories to varying degrees. In our analysis, we found that social workers and other professionals demonstrated

- a lack of knowledge of diverse realities and the consequences of marginalization on older people;
- processes of "othering" enacted explicitly or implicitly to create distance and assert power and control;
- fear of risk that functioned as a mechanism for stripping people of their rights and dignity;
- limited capacity for prolonged engagement, which exacerbated the already low levels of trust;
- identity erasure when problem-focussed interventions did not consider historic or current identity and experiences;
- well-meaning interactions that were underlined by negation of feelings and interpreted as patronizing and dismissive (i.e., repeatedly telling someone to calm down);
- the ways in which private-talk between professionals in public spaces takes place, revealing how prejudice is made manifest in the everyday, and particularly given the fact that these professionals assume that clients cannot hear or understand what is being said about them (dehumanization).

We also recognize how, even in cases where social workers or social work students noted that something was "amiss" in the organizational processes and structural conditions within sites and/or the attitudes of other professionals, they felt that they had little room or power to speak out or create change. Sustaining good working relationships with others within the site, a lack of time, and limited alliances within the setting were named as possible reasons for inaction. Concerns regarding potential risk of exposure to micro aggressions or other forms of exclusion were also factors in decisions to remain silent, especially in the case of the social work student in Jeannie's story.

We end this chapter by calling attention to the above-mentioned list of micro-aggressions (see textbox 9.3) specifically to assert that transforming micro- and meso-level practices does not always require increased funding or macro-level policy change, but simply a commitment to personal, professional, and organizational responsibility and the readiness or ability to take risks. Building alliances with others, both inside and outside our places of work, can help to enhance our capacity as social workers to make changes to discriminatory or disempowering organizational cultures and values.

Notes

1 Peter's story is adapted and expanded from the brief case study which first appeared in Grenier and Brotman (2010).
2 The Foreign Domestic Movement was a domestic caregiver program that offered permanent residence to caregivers after two years of live-in service (Ferrer, 2017).

References

Brotman, S., Ferrer, I., & Koehn, S. (2019). Situating the life story narratives of aging immigrants within a structural context: The intersectional lifecourse perspective as research praxis. *Qualitative Research*, 1–20. Pre-published October 14, 2019. doi:10.1177/1468794119880746

Brotman, S., & Kraniou, S. (1999). Ethnic and lesbian: Understanding identity through the life-history approach. *Afflia, 14*, 417–438. doi:10.1177/08861099922093734

Cunsolo Willox, A., Harper, S. L., & Edge, V. L. (2013). Storytelling in a digital age: Digital storytelling as an emerging narrative method for preserving and promoting Indigenous oral wisdom. *Qualitative Research, 13*(2), 127–147. doi:10.1177/1468794112446105

Daatland, S. O., & Biggs, S. (2004). *Ageing and diversity: Multiple pathways and cultural migrations.* Bristol: Policy Press.

Dannefer, D., & Settersten, R. A. (2010). The study of the life course: Implications for social gerontology. In C. Phillipson & D. Dannefer (Eds.), *The SAGE handbook of social gerontology* (pp. 3–20). London: SAGE Publications.

Denzin, N. K., & Lincoln, Y. S. (2008). *Collecting and interpreting qualitative materials* (3rd ed.). Thousand Oaks, CA: SAGE Publications.

Denzin, N. K., Lincoln, Y. S., & Tuhiwai Smith, L. (2008). *Handbook of critical and indigenous methodologies.* Los Angeles, CA: SAGE Publications.

Drummond, J., & Brotman, S. (2014). Intersecting and embodied identities: A queer woman's experience of disability and sexuality. *Sexuality and Disability, 32*(4), 533–549. doi:10.1007/311195-014-9382-4

Ferrer, I. (2017). Aging Filipino domestic workers and the (in)adequacy of retirement provisions in Canada. *Canadian Journal on Aging, 36*(1), 15–29. doi:10.1017/S0714980816000684

Ferrer, I., Grenier, A., Brotman, S., & Koehn, S. (2017). Understanding the experiences of racialized older people through an intersectional life course perspective. *Journal of Aging Studies, 41,* 10–17. doi:10.1016/j.jaging.2017.02.001

Gardner, K. (2002). *Age, narrative and migration: The life course and life histories of Bengali elders in London.* Oxford and New York: Berg.

Grenier, A. (2007). Constructions of frailty in the English language, care practice and the lived experience. *Ageing & Society, 27*(3), 425–445.

Grenier, A. (2012). *Transitions and the lifecourse: Challenging the constructions of 'growing old'.* Bristol: The Policy Press.

Grenier, A. & Brotman, S. (2010). Les multiples vieillissements et leurs representations. In M. Charpentier, N. Guberman, V. Billette, J. P. Lavoie, A. Grenier, & I. Olazabal (Eds.) *Vieillir au pluriel: Perspectives sociales* (pp. 23–34). Quebec: Presses de l'Université du Québec.

Hulko, W. (2011). Intersectionality in the context of later life experiences of dementia. In O. Hankivsky (Ed.), *Health inequities in Canada: Intersectional frameworks and practices* (pp. 198–217). Vancouver: UBC Press.

Hulko, W. (2014). Operationalizing intersectionality in feminist social work research: Reflections and techniques from research with equity-seeking groups. In S. Wahab, B. Anderson-Nathe, & C. Gringeri (Eds.), *Feminisms in social work research: Promise and possibilities for justice based knowledge* (pp. 68–89). New York: Routledge Press.

Hulko, W., Brotman, S., & Ferrer, I. (2017). Counter-storytelling: Anti-oppressive social work with older adults. In D. Baines (Ed.), *Doing anti-oppressive practice: Social justice work* (pp. 193–211). Toronto, ON: Fernwood Press.

Ives, N., Denov, M., & Sussman, T. (2015). Social work with aging populations. In N. Ives, M. Denov, & T. Sussman (Eds.) *Introduction to social work in Canada: Histories, contexts and practices* (pp. 327–343). Don Mills, ON: Oxford University Press.

Concluding thoughts

To conclude our book, we provide a brief summary of the main takeaway points and offer some final reflections. This represents our last opportunity to engage in a kind of virtual dialogue with you, the reader, by speaking to our experience of writing the book and challenging all of us to think about the issues raised in/by the stories we shared. We invite you to dialogue with those issues and stories by making use of your subjectivity, positionality, and critical reflexivity.

Revisioning gerontological social work through reflexive practice

Doing anti-oppressive gerontological social work requires us to be reflexive, as well as to think and act differently on a daily basis. Our eight principles of AOG identify the central concepts that we must be aware of in order to support this reflexive process. This idea of a *reflexive process* suggests that there is no fixed state of being at which point we become anti-oppressive practitioners. AOG as practice means learning to live in uncertainty and to question assumptions that are rooted in personal, cultural, and structural values, discourses, and ideologies. This involves learning how to be comfortable with discomfort and approaching our professional lives in this way. By doing so, we can remain open to the positions and opinions of others, particularly older adults, their (chosen) families, and communities with whom we work and also be humble about what we know and what we have yet to learn. Recognizing and paying attention to how power operates within and across individual, professional, organizational, and structural contexts is central to AOG. However, we cannot underestimate the reality that enacting AOG practice in sites and sectors of health and social care marked by neoliberalism and bio-medicalization will be challenging, if not significantly frustrating for social workers committed to AOP social work. Tensions are present no matter what sector we are working in, which was made evident in this book through our use of stories and cases.

One of our main take-home messages is that storytelling and counter-storytelling are powerful. This builds upon social work's commitment to learning through examining case studies, by re-visioning case presentations as an opportunity to engage in reframing and rethinking our own practices. The difficulty of moving from critical reflection to action, a common critique of AOP, is well known. Counter-storytelling can be a tool to redress this problem as it presents a way of re-imagining what we can **do** in our daily interventions. Re-imagining, not only the root causes of social problems, but also our daily social work interventions (such as those with clients, families, communities, colleagues, supervisors, organizations/institutions, and structures) can help us to push back against normative discourses and models of care. It's important to recognize that doing so puts us at risk because pushing back requires conflict and struggles over power in order to create opportunities for change. These power struggles are structural and professional, but they are also personal; they affect us and our relationships with others. The risks associated with pushing back are faced differently by each of us, depending on our individual social location: Where we stand or are positioned in relation to the margins and the centre of society based on various categories of difference, including age, gender (identity and expression), class, dis/ability, ethnicity, faith, sexual orientation, and race will necessarily affect our experiences and perspectives.

Shifting our lens

Anti-oppressive approaches to social work have not extended to working with older adults to a significant degree, although we can locate much in the critical gerontology literature to draw upon to build knowledge for AOG practice and apply important lessons from other areas of AOP social work to social gerontology. Key points to consider include avoiding homogenizing older adults, seeing older adults in the context of the life course (personal and structural), addressing the nature of ageism (on its own and in interaction with other forms of oppression), attending to the complexity of identity and specificity of social location, taking an intersectional approach, breaking down both binaries and barriers, and being willing to be a resister.

Teaching and learning are not technical processes per se; they require us to think critically and make the application to practice. Keeping the eight principles in mind provides a framework, rather than a set of technical steps, to do our work. This process takes time and requires identifying **what is in our power to do and what risks we are prepared to take** – *and* we must remember that small steps can lead to great change. No matter what barriers we may face in our work enacting AOG, this work will be challenging *and* satisfying. This is evidenced by a quote from a former student who presented in class a very profound idea on enacting advocacy in health care social work:

> I used to find it very frustrating to bring up my interest in developing a narrative approach in my work with patients to my colleagues who would simply tell me that I failed to understand my primary function which was to manage a speedy and appropriate discharge plan without getting into the patient's "whole life story". Over time I recognized that, as long as the paperwork was filled out correctly and in a timely manner, the way I engaged with my clients was pretty much in my own hands. So, I would remind myself on a daily basis that while the hospital owned the product, I owned the process, and that helped me better integrate AOP into my work. While it didn't necessarily lead to quick changes (to structural problems I encountered in my work), it gave me a window through which to share power with my clients, stay open to their points of view, and identify avenues for potential long-term organizational change.
>
> (Paulo Roberto Fumaneri, personal communication, March 20, 2017)

Staying the course (i.e., holding onto hope)

This reflection demonstrates that there are many possible **points of hopefulness** – moments of opportunity in which we can enact our AOG principles. Social work with older adults, their families, and communities is both a challenging and rewarding area of practice. In writing this book, we have drawn on our experiences from decades of work, including in the roles of case manager, community organizer, hospital social worker, policy advisor, service provider, activist, researcher, and educator intersecting all three sectors and across several sites. In recognition that our personal experiences inform our practice, we also integrate our roles and experiences as children, grandchildren, and caregivers to our analysis. In all that time, we have not lost the sense that working with older adults, their families, and communities is a privilege and a pleasure. The people and communities within which we have worked have fuelled our commitment to social change at all levels so that health and social care services are better able to advance access and equity principles and create opportunities to bridge the gap between the design and delivery of health and social care and the fundamental values of the social work profession. Living our social work values by raising the importance of social justice and equity at all times often means being the lone advocate or sole resister in the room. This requires strength and courage.

In order to do this work, it is important to build allies or accomplices who can validate and support our AOG practice interventions and join with us to create more inclusive communities and equitable social policies for older adults, their families, and communities. We know from our own work that social workers are often challenged in their work environments to develop best practice using AOP principles as a guiding framework. Therefore, we recommend identifying what power you hold or to which you have access and what you are willing to risk and then finding allies either inside or outside your organization to sustain you in this work. This can include colleagues from other disciplines who work in the field of aging as well as AOP social workers who specialize in other fields of practice such as immigrant services, child welfare, and community organizing, for example. As we were writing these concluding thoughts, one of our colleagues, who is the regional director of an Aboriginal health centre in Ontario and has a background in public health, stressed the importance of social work:

> I see social workers as being the sole resister in the room (i.e., the one who is willing to do more than say the right thing and to actually hold people accountable to do the right thing). This is even more important in clinical settings where social work can ensure that spiritual and emotional wellness are meaningfully considered along with the physical and cognitive dimensions of aging and health.
>
> (Danielle Wilson, personal communication, August 1, 2019)

The hope we still have ties directly to our experience with older adults as resilient and resistant to domination and oppression in their everyday lives across the life course. It is for this reason that we have written this text, a dream we have held individually and collectively for over a decade. We did not all know each other before sitting down to write this book, although each of us is connected with at least one other person in some scholarly and friendship capacity. In writing the book over the past two years, we have come to identify a shared vision as well as some tensions in the ways in which we articulate anti-oppressive gerontology and prioritize particular intersections of identity and interlocking oppressions in our work. The dynamic, and sometimes conflictual, space in which we have written is embodied in the current text. We hope that it has provided the reader room to communicate with the book, locate points of common understanding with their own perspectives and experiences, as well as points of tension through which they can engage in dialogue with their own practice, their colleagues either in school or at work, and the professional and counter discourses that are meaningful to them.

Acknowledging gaps and limitations

It is important to note that the intersecting identities and interlocking forms of oppression that we have chosen to foreground do not represent the full diversity present in social work practice and Canadian society. Further, although we tried to pay attention to the major themes and areas of practice in gerontological social work and included case studies and counter-stories reflecting a diverse cast of characters and issues, we are aware that there is room to include more topics such as neuro-diversity, homelessness, incarceration, and aging in other countries, as well as more examples related to rural and remote communities and trans and gender nonconforming people. We envision this book to be a jumping off point for the development of AOG knowledge and best practice: that is, social work with older adults that attends to the ways in which interlocking oppressions impact the lives of older adults, their families, and communities and values the diverse forms of meaning making, resilience, and resistance of older adults in a multitude of yet-to-be-articulated ways.

Table 14.1 Anti-oppression gerontology (AOG) principles version 2.0

1. Be critically **self-reflexive** and **humble**, understanding that you are part of the process and have your own biases and triggers.
2. Focus on the complex notion of **identity**, including questioning taken-for-granted **privilege** and the rationale for **dominance** in society and using **age** and **ageism** as starting points.
3. Explicitly name the issue of social **difference** as an issue of **power** and **equity** rather than a matter of cultural and ethnic variation.
4. Go beyond individual actions, prejudices, and ideas to examine the ways that individual and **everyday oppressive acts** are entrenched in and (un)consciously supported by **institutional structures**.
5. View **social justice** and **cultural safety** as both process and goal, which entails affirming **difference** and sharing **power** in interactions with patients, clients, and/or service users.
6. Value individuals as **self-determining and interdependent** actors who have a sense of their own **agency** and **social responsibility** and appreciate that **resilience and resistance** are important strategies of **agency** enacted by individuals and communities in response to oppressive forces.
7. Centre **voice** and **access** as foundational rights in the design and delivery of policy and services and make use of **GBA+** (gender-based analysis plus) in policy and planning to foreground **intersectionality** and related concepts like **equity, diversity** and **inclusion** (EDI).
8. Live your **values** and **ethics** by working towards a more **socially just** and **equitable** world.

An invitation to join our AOG community

Finally, we return to the eight principles from the introduction (see Table 14.1 above) that emphasize how gerontological social work practice can be re-visioned through an anti-oppressive lens and encourage students and practitioners to join with us and with older adults to put these into practice. We ask you to think about how the perspectives we have introduced in this book might inform your own social work practice and to challenge us by offering your critique of what you consider incorrect, incomplete, or missing from the book. By inviting you to be critical of our book and ourselves as authors, we are not asking you to simply *criticize*, but rather to be critically self-reflexive to help us nudge the field of gerontological social work forward in ways that better reflect our collective commitment to social justice and intersectionality and pursuit of a more equitable, caring, and socially just world.

Index